Handbook of Palliative Care

Second Edition

EDITED BY

CHRISTINA FAULL
MB BS, BMed Sci, MD, FRCP
Consultant in Palliative Medicine,
University Hospitals of Leicester and
LOROS – The Leicestershire and Rutland Hospice,
Groby Road, Leicester

YVONNE H. CARTER
OBE BSc MB BS MD FRCGP FMedSci
Dean,
Warwick Medical School,
The University of Warwick,
Coventry

LILIAN DANIELS
BNurs (Hons) RGN HV Onccert Cert. Ed
PhD Candidate. Formally Macmillan Research Lecturer,
Centre for Palliative Care and Oncology,
University of Central England, Birmingham

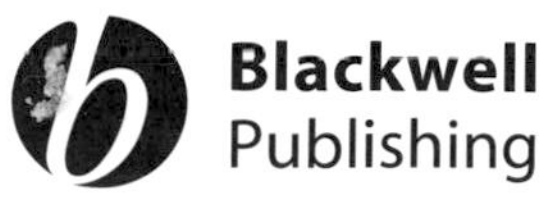

Blackwell Publishing, Inc., 350 Main Street, Malden, Massachusetts 02148-5020, USA
Blackwell Publishing Ltd, 9600 Garsington Road, Oxford OX4 2DQ, UK
Blackwell Publishing Asia Pty Ltd, 550 Swanston Street, Carlton, Victoria 3053, Australia

First published 2005

Library of Congress Cataloging-in-Publication Data
Handbook of palliative care / edited by Christina Faull, Yvonne Carter,
Lilian Daniels. – 2nd ed.
p.; cm.
Includes bibliographical references.
ISBN-13: 978-1-4051-2112-5
ISBN-10: 1-4051-2112-2
1. Palliative treatment—Handbooks, manuals, etc.
[DNLM: 1. palliative Care—Handbooks. WB 39 H23653 2005] I. Faull, Christina.
II. Carter, Yvonne, 1959– III. Daniels, Lilian.

R726.8.H355 2005
616′.029–dc22

2004026399

ISBN-13: 978-1-4051-2112-5
ISBN-10: 1-4051-2112-2
A catalogue record for this title is available from the British Library

Set in 10/13 Sabon by TechBooks, India
Printed and bound in India by Replika Press Pvt. Ltd.

Commissioning Editor: Maria Khan
Development Editor: Mirjana Misina
Production Controller: Kate Charman

For further information on Blackwell Publishing, visit our website:
http://www.blackwellpublishing.com

The publisher's policy is to use permanent paper from mills that operate a sustainable forestry policy, and which has been manufactured from pulp processed using acid-free and elementary chlorine-free practices. Furthermore, the publisher ensures that the text paper and cover board used have met acceptable environmental accreditation standards.

Contents

List of Contributors

RACHAEL BARTON *Consultant Clinical Oncologist, Department of Clinical Oncology, Princess Royal Hospital, Saltshouse Road, Hull, E. Yorks,* HU8 9HE

SARA BOOTH *Macmillan Consultant in Palliative Medicine, Director Palliative Care Service, Addenbrookes NHS Trust, Box 193, Hills Road, Cambridge* CB2 2QQ

MIKE BENNETT *Senior Clinical Lecturer in Palliative Medicine, St Gemma's Hospice, 329 Harrogate Road, Leeds,* LS17 6QD

ALISTAIR CHESSER *Consultant Nephrologist, Barts and The London NHS Trust, The Royal London Hospital Whitechapel, London,* E1 1BB

ANDREW CHILTON *Consultant Gastroenterologist and Hepatologist, Kettering General Hospital, Kettering, Northamptonshire* NN16 8UZ

CANDY M COOLEY *Palliative Care Development Manager for Worcestershire, South Worcestershire PCT, Shrub Hill, Worcester* WR4 9RW

FINELLA CRAIG *Palliative Care Consultant, Symptom Care Team, Great Ormond Street Children's Hospital, Great Ormond Street, London,* WC1N 3JH

LILIAN DANIELS *BNurs(Hons) RGN HV Onccert Cert. Ed, PhD Candidate. Formally Macmillan Research Lecturer, Centre for Palliative Care and Oncology, University of Central England, Birmingham,* B42 2SU

JACQUELINE EDWARDS *Research Fellow in Children's Cancer Nursing, 7th Floor, Old Building, Great Ormond Street Children's Hospital, Great Ormond Street, London,* WC1N 3JH

CHRISTINA FAULL *Consultant in Palliative Medicine, University Hospitals of Leicester and LOROS – The Leicestershire and Rutland Hospice, Groby Road, Leicester* LE3 9QE

KAREN FORBES *Consultant in Palliative Medicine, Department of Palliative Medicine, United Bristol Healthcare Trust, Bristol Haematology and Oncology Center, Horfield Road, Bristol,* BS2 8ED

ANN GOLDMAN *Consultant in Paediatric Palliative Care, Great Ormond Street Hospital for Children, London,* WC1N 3JH

DENISE HARDY *Harewood Farm, Whinfell, Kendal, Cumbria* LA8 9EL

FIONA HICKS *Consultant in Palliative Medicine, Leeds Teaching Hospitals Trust, St James Hospital, Beckett Street, Leeds* LS9 7TF

IRENE J HIGGINSON *Professor of Palliative Care and Policy, Department of Palliative Care and Policy Guy's, King's and St. Thomas' School of Medicine, King's College London, Weston Education Centre, Cutombe Road, London,* SE5 9RJ

CHRISTINE HIRSCH *Research Pharmacist, Compton Hospice, Compton Road West, Wolverhampton* WV3 9DH

GILLIAN HORNE *Macmillan Lead Cancer Nurse, Doncaster & Bassetlaw Hospitals NHS Foundation Trust, Armthorpe Road, Doncaster, South Yorkshire,* DN2 5LT

JEREMY JOHNSON *Medical Director, Shropshire and Mid Wales Hospice, Bicton Heath, Shrewsbury,* SY3 8HS

DANIEL KELLY *Senior Research Fellow in Cancer Nursing, St Bartholomew School of Nursing, City University, 24 Chiswell Street, London,* EC1Y 4TY

JONATHAN KOFFMAN *Lecturer in Palliative Care, Department of Palliative Care and Policy, Guy's, King's and St. Thomas' School of Medicine, King's College London, Weston Education Centre, Cutcombe Road, Denmark Hill, London* SE5 9RJ

BRIAN NYATANGA *Macmillan Senior Lecturer, University of Central England, Division of Oncology, Palliative Care and Macmillan Education Unit. Westbourne Campus, Birmingham.* B15 3TN

HAZEL PEARSE *Specialist Registrar in Palliative Medicine, Leeds Teaching Hospitals Trust, St James Hospital, Beckett Street, Leeds* LS9 7TF

NICKY RUDD *Consultant in Palliative Medicine, Leicestershire and Rutland Hospice and University Hospitals, Leicester, Osbourne Building, Leicester Royal Infirmary, Leicester* LE1 5WW

KEITH SIBSON *Specialist Registrar in Palliative Care, Symptom Care Team, Great Ormond Street Children's Hospital, Great Ormond Street, London,* WC1N 3JH

SURINDER SINGH *Department of Primary Care and Population Sciences, Royal Free and University College Medical School, Royal Free Campus, Rowland Hill Street, London* NW3 2PF

NEIL SMALL *School of Health Studies, University of Bradford, 25 Trinity Road, Bradford,* BD5 0BB

STEPHANIE TAYLOR *Department of General Practice and Primary Care, Barts and the London Medical School, Queen Mary, University of London, Mile End Road, London* E1 4NS

NICK THEOBALD *Thomas Macaulay Ward, Chelsea and Westminster Hospital, 369 Fulham Road, London,* SW10 9NH

ELIZABETH THOMPSON *Consultant Homeopathic Physician and Honorary Senior Lecturer Palliative Medicine, Bristol Homeopathic Hospital, Cotham Hill, Cotham,* BS6 6JU

ROSEMARY WADE *Consultant in Palliative Medicine, West Suffolk Hospital, Hardwick Lane, Bury St Edmunds, Suffolk* IP33 2QZ

MARY WALDING *Practise Development Nurse, Sir Michael Sobell House, 64 Weyland Road, Headington, Oxford,* OX6 8DN

DEREK WILLIS *Graduate Entry Moderator and Honorary Clinical Lecturer, Department of Primary Care, Birmingham Medical School, Partner Birmingham Medical Centre, 6 Bellevue, Edgbaston, Birmingham* B5 7LX

ANDREW WILCOCK *Macmillan Clinical Reader in Palliative Medicine and Medical Oncology, University of Nottingham, Hayward House Macmillan Specialist Palliative Care Unit, Nottingham City Hospital NHS Trust, Nottingham* NG5 1PB

JANE WORLDING *Consultant Clinical Oncologist, Walsgrave NITS Trust, Department of Radiotherapy & Oncology, 2 Clifford Bridge Road, Coventry* CV2 2DX

CATHERINE ZOLLMAN *General Practitioner and GP Educationalist, Bristol Vocational Training Scheme, Postgraduate Medical Centre, Frenchay Hospital, Frenchay Park Road, Bristol* BS16 1LE

Foreword

Since qualifying as a doctor, palliative care has pervaded my life. Be it as a junior hospital doctor, as a general practitioner working as part of a team of health care professionals, as a governor of a hospice or as an educator, I have been involved in palliative care. I have seen some of the best care possible but I have also been aware of the variation in the quality of care provided for patients. It was, therefore, a great pleasure to accept the invitation to write the foreword to this excellent book which should help health professionals improve the care that they provide for their patients.

Time was when lack of information and guidance were reasons for poor palliative care. Not now. This book brings readers up to date with recent developments and how to use them in palliative care.

Sadly and ashamedly many of us who work as health care professionals can recall patients whose expectations of a 'decent death' were thwarted by inadequate palliative care. However, reassuringly, we can also recall patients who did achieve a 'good death' with the help of effective palliative care services. One of the aims of this book is to address the unacceptable variation in practice.

The zeal of curative intent should be matched by the determination of a 'decent death'. Medicine has matured over recent years to realise that cure is not an option for all patients. Palliative care is acknowledged to be an important part of the work of most health care professionals but it has also come in from the twilight zone of medicine to become an identifiable and respected medical specialty in its own right.

Most patients wish to die at home. The majority of care that they receive in their last year of life is delivered by primary health care teams including general practitioners but many patients also spend a considerable amount of time in hospitals or hospices. It is important, therefore, that all health care professionals are competent in looking after dying patients. I believe that training programmes for all health care professionals must include palliative care in their curricula. In addition to teaching in aspects of palliative care, they need to be exposed to how care is provided for patients dying of cancer and other life-limiting conditions in a variety of settings. That includes doctors and nurses training for careers in hospital based specialties spending time learning in primary care. Health professionals once registered also have a responsibility to maintain their competence by keeping up to date with advances in palliative care. This book will help as part of their continuing personal and professional development programmes regardless of specialty or job description.

The book illuminates the importance of palliative care and deals systematically with the subject. It is well referenced which will help those who wish to search for the original evidence or just wish to read more about a subject access more information. I am sure that this book will help all those involved in caring for dying patients in their quest to provide the highest quality palliative care possible.

Professor Steve Field
Birmingham, UK
2004

Preface to the Second Edition

The first edition of this book was well received and to our great pleasure attained awards from our colleagues in both primary care and other specialities, winning the BMA *Book of the Year Award* in 1999. Most important to us was that it appeared to meet the needs of clinicians and successfully bridge the gap that sometimes occurs between a reference book and the patient in front of us. Our aim was to be as practical as possible and help enhance the quality of both everyday and unusual clinical practice. In this second edition we aim to respond similarly to recent developments in palliative medicine and the delivery of palliative care services and have incorporated both advances in symptom management and our growing knowledge of the palliative care needs of a diversity of patients and communities. The book continues to address in particular the increasing focus of care delivery in primary care and the multidisciplinary nature of palliative care.

Although palliative care for all patients has been promoted for some time, specialist expertise, knowledge and research has until recently largely focused on cancer. The growing understanding of disease trajectories and symptom burden in other advanced illnesses has allowed inclusion in this edition of chapters on palliative care in advanced heart, liver and renal disease, as well as updating and broadening chapters on care of patients with AIDS, and neurological diseases. Likewise, the chapters which focus on the management of specific symptoms address the needs of both cancer and non-cancer patients. We hope that such a resource will be especially helpful for primary care professionals who are required to care for patients with a variety of conditions requiring palliative care.

A key theme of this edition is the breadth and scope of palliative care provision, which is discussed specifically in a new chapter: 'Needs, rights and inclusion in palliative care'. The addition of this and chapters such as 'Palliative care for adolescents and young adults' demonstrates the objective of this handbook in highlighting diversity of need and tackling current inequalities within palliative care delivery.

Teamwork remains pivotal to palliative care and even more so as the patient group expands requiring incorporation in the team, professionals from specialities such as cardiology, renal, respiratory and neurological fields. There is an emphasis within this edition of the handbook on examining the strategies for better interdisciplinary team working, and in particular how the interface between primary and secondary care can be enhanced for more cohesive care of palliative patients.

Since the first edition we have seen a number of initiatives such as integrated care pathways, the Gold Standards Framework and the Palliative Care Outcome Scale, which reflect the current emphasis on the delivery of quality, evidence-based and equitable palliative care services. This year the National Institute of Clinical Excellence has issued guidance for improving supportive and palliative care for adults with cancer, which provide a framework for good practice. This handbook aims to provide a resource to professionals as they seek to implement the guidance and enhance the quality of palliative care provision in their practice area.

The second edition responds to evaluative comments on the first edition in strengthening its multidisciplinary focus and providing a broader professional approach through both the editorial team and contributors. The book therefore aims to respond to a wide audience of generic and specialist practitioners involved in the delivery of palliative care in the spectrum of clinical settings but with particular emphasis on the care of patients in the community by the primary care team. It aims, as before, to embrace practical issues as well as to provide an evidence-based and empirical approach.

Acknowledgments

This book has only been made possible by the hard work of many and we hope this edition does justice to the efforts of all the individuals who have given so much. We are aware of how much personal complexity some of the writing team have been dealing with and we should like to pay tribute to their commitment to this book and to ensuring high quality palliative care for all. We should also like to particularly acknowledge Richard Woof who contributed so much to the first edition and who's legacy brings much to this second edition.

Abbreviations List

Ach(m)	Acetylcholine muscarinic
AIDS	Acquired immune deficiency syndrome
ALS	Amyotrophic lateral sclerosis
CAMPAS	Cambridge palliative care audit schedule
CD	Controlled drug
CHF	Chronic heart failure
COPD	Chronic obstructive pulmonary disease
COX	Cyclo-oxygenase
CT	Chemotherapy
DMD	Duchenne muscular dystrophy
EORTC	European Organisation for Research and Treatment of Cancer
ERCP	Endoscopic retrograde cholangiopancreatography
ESRD	End-stage renal disease
GABA	Gammaamino-butyric acid
GP	General practitioner
GSF	Gold standards framework
HIV	Human imunodeficiency virus
5HT	5-Hydroxytryptophan
LANSS	Leeds assessment of neuropathic symptoms and signs
M3G	Morphine-3-glucuronide
M6G	Morphine-6-glucuronide
MLD	Manual lymphatic drainage
MND	Motor neurone disease
MNDA	Motor neurone disease association
MS	Multiple sclerosis
MST	Morphine sulphate continues tablet
NICE	National Institute for Clinical Excellence
NMDA	*N*-methyl-D-aspartate
NSAID	Non-steroidal anti-inflammatory drug
PCT	Primary care trust
PEG	Percutaneous endoscopic gastrostomy

POS	Palliative care outcome scale
PPI	Proton pump inhibitor
RT	Radiotherapy
SLD	Simple lymph drainage
SSRI	Selective serotonin reuptake inhibitor
STAS	Support team assessment schedule
TENS	Transcutaneous electrical nerve stimulation

Drug routes

i.m.	Intramuscular
i.v.	Intravenous
oral	Oral
p.r.	Per rectum
s.c.	Subcutaneous

Drug administration frequency

o.d.	Once daily
b.d.	Twice daily
t.d.s.	Three times daily
q.d.s.	Four times daily
stat	Straight away
prn	As required

Units

h	hour
l	litre
ml	millilitre
mm	millimeter
mg	milligram
μg	microgram

Addendum

The editors should like readers to be aware that since going to press the COX-2 inhibitor Rofecoxib has been withdrawn from the market because of adverse effects.

1: The Context and Principles of Palliative Care

CHRISTINA FAULL

Introduction

Palliative care is an important part of the work of most health care professionals, irrespective of their particular role. The care of people with advanced and terminal illness can be extremely rewarding [1], and this is enhanced by having confidence in core skills and knowledge of basic physical and non-physical symptom management. Palliative care is not an alternative to other care but is a complementary and vital part of total patient management.

> *I need my doctor to explain to me, to be cheerful, to share his experience and guide me, not only in the treatment but with my feelings as well. I need my doctor to discuss the possibility of death, and to find options that are unknown to me, because without him, I don't even know where to look for them. I would also like to feel free to talk to him about trying alternative treatments, without fear of his resentment or contempt, that would destroy my hope and enthusiasm, or spoil the relationship* [2].

The majority of care received by patients during the last year of life is delivered by general practitioners (GPs) and community teams. A systematic review of GP involvement in this care reported that [3]:

- GPs value this work and it is appreciated by patients.
- Palliative care is sometimes delivered less well in the community than in other settings.
- Some GPs are unhappy with their competence in this field.
- With specialist support GPs demonstrably provide effective care.
- The confidence of GPs and the understanding of the potential of team members increase through working with specialist teams.

Of course, many patients spend significant time in hospitals during their last year of life and it has been estimated that 10–15% of beds are occupied by patients with advanced disease. Despite the majority wishing to die at home, over 60% of these patients die in hospital.

There are a broad range of challenges in delivering high quality palliative and terminal care including professional competence and confidence, organisational factors and resources. Patients with advanced disease can present some of the most challenging ethical, physical, psychological and social issues and it is vital to have a grasp of the communication skills required to effectively explore these issues. It is also important to be able to identify when referrals to specialists and other services are needed.

This chapter outlines the development of palliative care, defines the principles that underpin effective care and presents an overview of the attainment and assessment of quality in palliative care. As Singer and Wolfson put it:

> *Twenty years ago, the challenge was to engage healthcare workers in the care of the dying. Ten years ago, the challenge was to engage healthcare organisations in quality improvement efforts on end of life care. Today, the challenge is to develop systematic and comprehensive information on the quality of end of life care at the population level* [4].

Without systematic information about patients' and their carers' experiences at the end of life, we will not know what we are achieving, whether we are improving and where we need to focus our efforts.

What are hospice and palliative care?

Much of our understanding and knowledge of the philosophy, science and art of palliative care has developed and grown through the work of the hospice movement. Dame Cicely Saunders worked with patients suffering from advanced cancer and undertook systematic narrative research to understand what patients were experiencing and needed. The bedrock of the hospice philosophy, in Western society at least, is that of patient-centred holistic care focusing on quality of life and extending support to significant family and carers (see Box 1.1).

> *What links the many professionals and volunteers who work in hospice or palliative care is an awareness of the many needs of a person and his/her family and carers as they grapple with all the demands and challenges introduced by the inexorable progress of a disease that has outstripped the possibilities of cure* [5].

Box 1.1 Etymology

The word 'hospice' originates from the Latin *hospes* meaning host; *hospitalis*, a further derivative, means friendly, a welcome to the stranger. The word *hospitium* perhaps begins to convey the vital philosophy of the hospice movement: it means the warm feeling between host and guest. Hence a hospice denotes a place where this feeling is experienced, a place of welcome and care for those in need.

The word 'palliative' derives from the Latin *pallium*, a cloak. Palliation means cloaking over, not addressing the underlying cause but ameliorating the effects.

Hospice has perhaps become thought of as solely a place of care. It is, however, much more than this and in essence is synonymous with palliative care. Both have a philosophy of care not dependent on a place or a building but on attitude, expertise and understanding. More recently the term *specialist palliative care* has been used to represent those professionals and services that concentrate on this area of health care as their main role and expertise, recognising that almost all health care professionals provide elements of palliative care for patients as part of their practice.

Palliative care has been defined for cancer patients as:

> *The active total care of patients whose disease is not responsive to curative treatment. Control of pain, of other symptoms and of psychological, social and spiritual problems is paramount. The goal of palliative care is achievement of the best quality of life for patients and their families. Many aspects of palliative care are also applicable earlier in the course of the illness, in conjunction with anticancer treatment* [6].

This definition is being refined in the light of both the recognition that patients with a broad range of terminal diseases benefit from palliative care and the need to define Supportive Care, a new direction of government strategy in cancer care (see below) [7].

The goals of palliative care are:

- the best possible quality of life for patients and their families;
- symptom control;
- adjustment to the many 'losses' of advanced and terminal illness;
- completion of unfinished 'business';
- a dignified death, with minimum distress, in the patient's place of choice;
- prevention of problems in bereavement.

To this end palliative care is a partnership between the patient, carers and a wide range of professionals. It affirms life and regards dying as a normal process, neither hastening nor postponing death. It integrates the psychological, physical, social, cultural and spiritual aspects of a patient's care, acknowledging and respecting the uniqueness of each individual.

> *You matter because you are you, and you matter until the last moment of your life. We will do all that we can to help you not only to die peacefully, but to live until you die* [8].

Specialist palliative care

Specialist palliative care came into focus with the founding of St Christopher's hospice in London in 1967 by Dame Cicely Saunders. It was here that an approach which formed the basis for the role of specialist services was developed:

- high quality care for patients and their relatives, especially those with complex needs;
- a range of services to help provide optimum care whether the patient was at home, in hospital or required specialist in-patient care;
- education, advice and support to other professionals;
- evidence-based practice;
- research and evaluation.

The subsequent, mostly unplanned, growth of specialist palliative care services has led to a wide variety of models of service provision, distribution and funding across the country, with some areas, and therefore patients, being better served than others. The Government in the UK has recently focused policy on ending the post code lottery and other inequalities in access to and quality of care.

Issues in palliative care worldwide

Fifty-six million people die across the world each year, 80% of deaths occurring in developing countries. The world population is estimated to increase by 50% in the next 50 years, almost all of this increase in population will be in the developing world. In addition, there will be a huge shift in age of the population with two- to threefold increase in population of over 60 years in the developed and developing world, respectively. The Barcelona declaration on palliative care in 1996 [9], like the World Health Organization in 1990 [6], called for palliative care to be included as part of every governmental health policy. Every individual has the right to pain relief. Inexpensive, effective methods exist to relieve pain and other symptoms. Cost need not be an impediment. It is estimated that globally a hundred million people would currently benefit from the availability of palliative care. We are a long, long way from achieving this. Tens of millions of people die in unrelieved suffering [10].

The challenges for palliative care in developing countries

A multiplicity of challenges faces the development of palliative care globally, but the issues are more pronounced in the developing world for several reasons—principally, poverty, the ageing population, the increase in smoking and the increase in cancer and AIDS-related deaths. Cancer caused 10% of deaths in 1985 and this figure is estimated to rise to 15% by 2015 [11, 12]. By the year 2015 it is estimated that two-thirds of all new cancer cases will occur in the developing world [12]. The problems are compounded by late presentation of cancer and the limited treatment resources available for cancer. The developing world has only 5% of the world's total resources for cancer control, although it must cope with almost two-thirds of the world's new cancer patients. Tobacco smoking causes death. Globally the annual number of tobacco-related deaths is expected to rise from three million to ten million by the year 2025 [13]. Much more than half of this increase will occur in the developing world, three million in China alone. The developing world is currently suffering from an epidemic of lung cancer making this cancer the most common worldwide. By 2015 about one million deaths in China will be from lung cancer.

There is also an AIDS epidemic. In the first edition of this book it was projected that the *cumulative* total of adults with HIV positivity would be 30–40 million. Now these numbers have vastly exceeded the previous projections. In 2002 there were 42 million people living with HIV/AIDS and during that year three million people died. Of those living with HIV/AIDS, 98% are in the developing world. The sociological effect of AIDS deaths in the developing world, especially sub-Saharan Africa where the adult prevalence rate is 8.8% and in some countries up to 35%, is catastrophic. It affects those most likely to be breadwinners for the extended three-generation family, and leaves many children orphaned. For example in Zimbabwe, life expectancy is expected to go down from 61 to 33 years by 2010 [10]. By then 25 million children will have been orphaned through AIDS.

Availability of opioids

Under the international treaty, *Single Convention on Narcotic Drugs* [14], governments are responsible to ensure that opioids are available for pain management. The 1996 report from the International Narcotics Control Board (INCB) showed that opioids are still not widely available for medical needs [15]. Eighty percent of the global morphine is used in ten industrialised countries.

The main impediments to opioid availability are: government concern about addiction; insufficient training of health care professionals; and restrictive laws over the manufacture, distribution, prescription and dispensing of opioids. There is also considerable reluctance on the part of the health care profession concerning their use, due to concerns about legal sanctions. This is made worse by the burden of regulatory requirements, the often insufficient import or manufacture of opioids and the potential for diversion of opioids for non-legitimate use.

International observatory on end of life care

This unique new initiative is an invaluable resource for anyone wishing to learn more about global issues in palliative care. The website http://www.eolc-observatory.net provides research-based information about hospice and palliative care provision internationally, presenting public health and policy data, as well as cultural, historical and ethnographic perspectives.

Unmet need and continued suffering in the developed world

The hospice movement and palliative care have come a long way in the past 30 years. There is a considerable body of knowledge and expertise, and services have grown enormously in number and character. There is, however, still a major unmet need. The majority of people are not living and dying with the comfort and the dignity that it is possible to achieve for most patients. Identified areas for improvement include:

- management of pain in advanced cancer [16–20];
- management of other symptoms [16, 20, 21];
- information and support for patients and carers;
- attention to comfort and basic care for those dying in hospitals [22];
- the needs of patients dying from non-malignant illness [23–28];
- the needs of patients out of working hours [29–31].

The major challenge for those who seek to improve the care for patients with advanced disease is to ensure that all health care professionals consider palliative care an important part of their role, and have adequate skills, knowledge and specialist support to undertake it effectively. This is of crucial importance in the 70% of the week that are 'out-of-hours' when patients are especially vulnerable to the deficits in health care systems.

Tackling inequalities and improving access in the UK

This key theme within the National Health Service (NHS) has very specific challenges for the delivery of palliative care. There are defined groups of patients who have poor outcomes, who underutilise specialist palliative care services, who have insufficient access to services and for whom service models should develop to meet their needs in an appropriate way.

Patients with non-malignant illness

Studies discussed in more detail in later chapters of this book indicate that these patients are considerably disadvantaged compared to those with cancer. Initiatives that are enabling this to be tackled include:

- National Service frameworks: those for heart disease [25] and older people [26] include sections on palliative care provision.
- New Opportunities Fund health grants programme.
- Disease specific charities such as the British Heart Foundation.

The National Council for Hospices and Specialist Palliative Care Services has begun to focus the national debate and help specialist services to consider how to develop new models of service, quality assurance, commissioning and fund-raising [27, 28]. As yet there is little literature on implementation of these strategies.

Ethnic diversity

Health professionals the world over recognise the fundamental human right to die with dignity. However, the notion of what constitutes a 'good death' may vary considerably between and within cultures. Whilst it has been shown that there are often greater similarities than differences between cultures when living and dealing with cancer [32], we know that it is more difficult for people from ethnically diverse communities to access or obtain information, support and services that will meet their needs. Issues of communication, cultural diversity, appropriateness of information, organisational and staff attitudes and discrimination are contributing factors across the spectrum of health and illness contexts, and having cancer is no exception to this experience [32–36]. For example, services such as counselling and psychological interventions in appropriate languages may not be available [32]. There may be difficulties in accessing self-help and support groups, Asian or African Caribbean wig types or prostheses and holistic pain control [37].

Compounding this disadvantage and poor quality of life is that people from diverse ethnic communities are more likely to be poor and have financial and housing difficulties [32]. In addition, evidence, although limited by inadequacy of ethnicity monitoring, suggests that people with cancer from diverse ethnic communities have poorer survival than others [38]. In these conditions, it is not surprising that people from ethnically diverse communities with cancer consistently wish for [39]:

- more information about cancer, cancer treatments and cancer care services;
- improved open communication and awareness about their condition;
- reduced feelings of stigma, isolation and fear;
- greater control and choice in their care;
- more effective care.

Migrant communities in Britain have proportionately higher death rates from diseases not related to cancer, compounding their disadvantage in accessing palliative care. Gatrad and colleagues [40] suggest that realising high quality palliative care for all will need fundamental changes on at least three fronts: tackling institutional discrimination in the provision of palliative care, progress in incorporating transcultural medicine into medical and nursing curriculums and a greater willingness on the part of health care providers to embrace complexity and in so doing develop a richer appreciation of the challenges facing people from minority communities in achieving a good end.

Enabling people to be at home

The National Cancer Plan 2000 [41] has required formalised Networks to provide support to the commissioning process and drive and coordinate improvement in service quality. High quality care at home for people with advanced disease is a key focus of the plan and of the guidance from the National Institute for Clinical Excellence (NICE) on Supportive and Palliative Care (Box 1.2) [42].

Box 1.2 Recommendations of the NICE guidance for Supportive and Palliative Care 2004, which are key for primary care [42]

12: Mechanisms need to be implemented within each locality to ensure medical and nursing services are available for patients with advanced cancer on a 24–hours, seven days a week basis, and that equipment can be provided without delay. Those providing generalist medical and nursing services should have access to specialist advice at all times.

13: Primary care teams should institute mechanisms to ensure that the needs of patients with advanced cancer are assessed, and that the information is communicated within the team and with other professionals as appropriate. The *Gold Standards Framework* provides one mechanism for achieving this.

14: In all locations, the particular needs of patients who are dying from cancer should be identified and addressed. The *Liverpool Care Pathway for the Dying Patient* provides one mechanism for achieving this.

THE GOLD STANDARDS FRAMEWORK

Thomas [43] has developed seven standards (Box 1.3) to help primary care teams improve their delivery of palliative care. Clear benefits have been demonstrated: more patients dying in the place of their choice,

Box 1.3 The seven 'C's': Gold standards for palliative care in primary care

Communication: Practice register; regular team meetings for information sharing, planning and reflection/audit; patient information; patient held records

Co-ordination: nominated coordinator maintains register, organises meetings, audit, education symptom sheets and other resources

Control of symptoms: Holistic, patient centred assessment and management

Continuity out-of-hours: effective transfer of information to and from out-of-hours services. Access to drugs and equipment

Continued on p. 10

Box 1.3 *Continued*

Continued learning: Audit/reflection/critical incident analysis. Use of PLT

Carer support: Practical, financial, emotional and bereavement support

Care in the dying phase: Protocol driven care addressing physical, emotional and spiritual needs. Care needs around and after death acted upon

fewer crises, better communication and co-working and increased staff morale [44]. Communication with and the quality of out-of-hours primary care services is of critical importance in achieving the goals of care.

HOSPICE-AT-HOME SERVICES

Hospice-at-home services are developing nationwide but vary in their name, composition, availability and referral criteria. In general, they are rapidly responding teams of nurses who support the district and Marie Curie nursing services to provide additional support for patients who are dying. Research into their benefits has had severe methodological impediments and there is no absolute clarity as to whether they do increase the home death rate or improve patient and/or carer experience [45, 46]. On balance it seems that they can do both these things.

The principles of palliative care

Knowing how to approach patients with advanced illness is the first step in achieving effective care.

- Consider the patient and their family/carers as the unit of care whilst respecting patient autonomy and confidentiality; acknowledge and encourage participation;
- Perform a systematic assessment: physical, psychological, social and spiritual;
- Communicate findings to the patient, providing information and support at all stages;
- Relieve the patient's symptoms promptly: "*There is only today*";

- Plan proactively and thoroughly for future problems;
- Use a team approach: listen to suggestions and views; involve resources for extra support at an early stage.

What do patients and their carers need?

The uniqueness of each individual's situation must be acknowledged and the manner of care adapted accordingly. The essence of what patients and their carers may need is outlined in Box 1.4.

Box 1.4 The rights and needs of patients and their carers

Patients have a right to confidentiality, pain control and other symptom management and, wherever possible, to choose the setting of death and the degree of carer involvement. They also have a right to deny the illness.

Information
The patient has a need for sensitive, clear explanations of:
- the diagnosis and its implications
- the likely effects of treatments on activities of daily living and well-being
- the type and extent of support that may be required and how it may be addressed
- expected symptoms and what may be done about them

Quality of life
The patient has a need for life that is as normal, congenial, independent and as dignified as possible

An individual's quality of life will depend on minimising the gap between their expectations and aspirations and their actual experiences. This may be achieved by:
- respect, as a person as well as a patient, from properly trained staff who see themselves as partners in living
- effective relief from pain and other distressing symptoms
- an appropriate and satisfying diet
- comfort and consolation, especially from those who share the patient's values and beliefs and/or belong to the same cultural community
- companionship from family and friends, and from members of the care team
- continuity of care from both the primary care team and other services

Continued on p. 12

Box 1.4 ***Continued***

- consistent and effective response to changes in physical and psychosocial discomfort
- information about support and self-help and other groups and services

Support for carers
The patient's family or other carers have a need for support at times of crises in the illness and in their bereavement. These needs include:
- practical support with financial, legal, housing or welfare problems
- information about the illness (with the patient's consent) and the available support
- respite from the stress of caring
- involvement of carers in the moment of death and in other aspects of care
- bereavement support
- special support where the patient's death may directly affect young children, or where the patient is a child or adolescent

It should be clear from this that communication skills (see Chapter 6) play a fundamental role in achieving good palliative care and quality of life for the patient.

> *Almost invariably, the act of communication is an important part of the therapy; occasionally it is the only constituent. It usually requires greater thought and planning than a drug prescription, and unfortunately it is commonly administered in subtherapeutic doses* [47].

Achieving good symptom management

Twycross, amongst others, has done much to ensure an evidence-based, scientific rigour in palliative care [48]. The management of any problem should be approached by:
- anticipation;
- evaluation and assessment;
- explanation and information;
- individualised treatment;
- re-evaluation and supervision;
- attention to detail;
- continuity of care.

ANTICIPATION

Many physical and non-physical problems can often be anticipated and in some instances prevented. Failure to anticipate problems and to set up appropriate management strategies (e.g. who should they call?) is a common source of dissatisfaction for patients [49]. Understanding the natural history of the disease with specific reference to an individual patient, awareness of the patient's psychosocial circumstances and identification of 'risk factors' allows planning of care by the team. For example, in a 45-year-old woman, recently found to have spinal metastases from her breast cancer, potential issues that could be anticipated are:

- Pain—may need NSAID, opioids and radiotherapy.
- Spinal cord compression—examine neurology if unsteady or 'numb'.
- Young children—may need help, practically and in telling the children.
- Work—may need financial and benefit advice.
- Hypercalcaemia—check blood if nauseated or confused.

EVALUATION AND ASSESSMENT

An understanding of the pathophysiology and likely cause(s) of any particular problem is vital in selecting and directing appropriate investigations and treatment. Deciding what treatment to use is based on consideration of the evidence of the mechanism of the symptom and of the treatment's efficacy and safety in the situation. This is illustrated by the following specific examples:

- Sedation for an agitated patient with urinary retention is not as helpful as catheterisation.
- Antiemetics for the nausea of hypercalcaemia are important but so too is lowering the serum calcium (if appropriate).
- A patient who is fearful of dying may be helped by discussing and addressing specific fears rather than taking benzodiazepines.
- Pain in a vertebral metastasis may be helped by analgesics, radiotherapy, orthopaedic surgery, TENS and acupuncture. A decision as to which to prescribe is made only by careful assessment.

Co-morbidity is common and should always be considered. For example, it is easy (and unfortunately common) to assume that pain in a patient with cancer is caused by the cancer. In one series almost a quarter of pains in patients with cancer were unrelated to the cancer or the cancer treatment [50].

The multidimensional nature of symptoms, such as pain, means that the use of drugs may be only one part of treatment. A holistic assessment is vital in enabling the most effective management plan.

EXPLANATION AND INFORMATION

Management of a problem should always begin with explanation of the findings and diagnostic conclusions. This usually reduces the patient's anxieties even if it confirms their worst suspicions—a monster in the light is usually better faced than a monster unseen in the shadows. Further information may be useful to some patients. A clear explanation of the suggested treatments and follow-up plan is important for the patient to gain a sense of control and security. Allow plenty of space for questions and check that what you meant to convey has been understood (see Chapter 6).

Mr H, with advanced liver disease, was very anxious in outpatients. He told me he had developed a tender lump on his chest. On examination this turned out to be gynaecomastia, most probably, I thought, due to the spironolactone. With the relief of this explanation he chose to continue the drug rather than have recurrence of his ascites.

Mrs S looked worried and was angry. We discussed the scan results she had had six months earlier, before her chemotherapy and surgery. "So what does that mean?" she asked. "I'm afraid that means the cancer cannot be cured" I said. She dissolved in tears and said "Thank you doctor. I have been thinking this but no one would tell me."

INDIVIDUALISED TREATMENT

The individual physical, social and psychological circumstances of the patient and their views and wishes should be considered in planning care. For example, lymphoedema compression bandages may be unused unless there is someone available to help the patient to fit them daily.

Treatment options need to be shared with the patient and their perspective on choices be explored. For example, Mr K developed arterial occlusion in his leg. Because of his other symptoms he was thought to have recurrent bladder cancer but this was not confirmed by scans. He needed to consider whether to have an amputation. It appeared most likely that he would die from his disease within the next weeks to months. He decided that he would only have the amputation if he had six months or more to live and declined the operation.

RE-EVALUATION AND SUPERVISION: BE PROACTIVE

The symptoms of frail patients with advanced disease can change frequently. New problems can occur and established ones worsen. Interventions may be complex (many patients take more than 20 tablets a day) and close supervision is vital to ensure optimum efficacy and tailoring to the patient.

ATTENTION TO DETAIL

The quality of palliative care is in the detail of care. For example, it is vital to ensure that the patient not only has a prescription for the correct drug but also that they can obtain it from the pharmacy, have adequate supplies to cover a weekend, and understand how to adjust it if the problem worsens.

CONTINUITY OF CARE

No professional can be available for 24 hours and seven days a week, but patients may need support at all hours of the day. Transfer of information within teams and to those that may be called upon to provide care (e.g. out-of-hours services) is one way of ensuring continuity of care. Patient held records, clear plans in nursing care records at the patient's house, team handover/message books and formalised information for out-of-hours services [51] are all ways to achieve this.

Limits of symptom control

There is always something more that can be done to help a patient but it is not always possible to completely relieve symptoms. Specialist advice should usually have been sought for help in the management of intractable symptoms. This extra support is in itself an important way of helping the patient.

In such situations an acceptable solution must be found to provide adequate relief of distress for the patient. For management of a physical symptom and sometimes of psychological distress this may be a compromise between the presence of the symptom and sedation from medications. It is hard for a team to accept suboptimum relief of symptoms and discussions with the patient and the family may be very difficult. It is important for the team to remember the great value of their continuing involvement to the patients and their carers; to acknowledge how difficult the situation is and not to abandon the patient because it is painful and distressing for the professionals.

Slowly, I learn about the importance of powerlessness.
I experience it in my own life and I live with it in my work.
The secret is not to be afraid of it—not to run away.
The dying know we are not God.
All they ask is that we do not desert them [52].

Attaining quality in palliative care

In the UK the quality of palliative and end-of-life care is an area of increasing focus. A special issue of the *British Medical Journal* in 2003 focused thought on what constitutes a good end of life [53]. New guidance from NICE interprets the evidence base for achieving high quality palliative and supportive cancer care (see the key recommendations for primary care in Box 1.2) and will now direct commissioning [42]. The government initiatives outlined in *Building on the Best* [54] will also aim to improve choice, quality and equality in end of life care, especially for those patients who do not have cancer.

At a national level assessment of some aspects of the quality of palliative and end-of-life care has been made through the national cancer patient survey [55], the Commission for Health Improvement [56] and the survey of specialist palliative care services [57]. Most Primary Care Trusts (PCTs) have undertaken a self-assessment of some aspects of their palliative care (mostly structural aspects, e.g. is there access to a syringe driver?) in the cancer baseline questionnaire. Systematically compiled information of structural, process or outcome measures is, however, not available at national or local levels and a primary care team or Trust will need to implement its own systems of quality assurance and audit.

Quality assurance

The general medical services contract focuses on the quality of the care provided by practice teams. The Gold Standards Framework (GSF) for palliative care described above [43,44] is one possible method for assuring high quality palliative care and achieves 23 points in the quality and outcomes framework. The practical use of frameworks such as the GSF is discussed further in Chapter 2. The use of a care pathway is another method of quality assurance and two such pathways have been developed for care in the last days of life [58,59]. This is discussed further in Chapter 21. Standards for palliative care have also been developed for community hospitals and nursing homes.

Clinical governance systems are a key component of quality assurance and examples relating to palliative care within this framework are shown in Box 1.5. In the future PCTs may develop novel enhanced level services in palliative care, driving up the quality in areas of poor performance.

Box 1.5 Examples of palliative care quality assurance within a clinical governance framework for a Primary Care Team and Primary Care Trust

Component of clinical governance	Example
A: Primary Care Team level	
Consultation and patient involvement	Are patients asked about their preferred place of death?
Clinical risk management	Is there a policy for the use of syringe drivers including rapid access to parenteral drugs?
Clinical audit	Are all patients taking morphine also prescribed appropriate laxatives?
Use of information about patient's experiences	How does the team reflect about those patients who die in hospital?
Staffing and staff management	Are there palliative care link nurses with performance reviewed job description?
Education, training and continuing professional development	Does the team use up-to-date symptom management guidance?
B: Primary Care Trust level	
Organisational and clinical leadership	Are there designated managers, doctors and nurses with lead responsibilities for palliative care?
Direction and planning	Is there a clear PCT strategy to address identified gaps in services?

Continued on p. 18

Box 1.5 *Continued*

Performance review	Does the PCT utilise its home death data and activity reports from specialist palliative care services to inform commissioning?
Patient and public partnership	How do cancer support groups work with the PCT?

Audit of quality

The Healthcare Commission will be a key auditor of the quality of primary care in the UK. Amongst other evidence they may explore will be evidence of audit of outcomes of care. Quality assurance frameworks such as the GSF and Dying Care Pathway are relatively easily audited with respect to goals of care. For example, a standard could be set by a PCT or practice that the place of choice for death should be known for at least 80% of patients and a death at home should be achieved for at least 80% of those desiring this. A variety of measures of outcomes in palliative care have been developed, with a breadth of validation work [60,61]. Only two, however, have good applicability to primary care: the Palliative Care Outcome Scale (POS) [62] and the Cambridge Palliative Audit Schedule: CAMPAS-R [63].

References

1 Redinbaugh EM, Sullivan AM, Block SD et al. Doctors' emotional reactions to recent death of a patient: cross sectional study of hospital doctors. *BMJ* 2003; 327: 185.
2 Kfir N, Slevin M. *Challenging Cancer: From Chaos to Control.* London: Tavistock/Routledge, 1991.
3 Mitchell GK. How well do general practitioners deliver palliative care? A systematic review. *Palliat Med* 2002; 16: 457–464.
4 Singer PA, Wolfson M The best places to die. *BMJ* 2003; 327: 173–174.
5 Saunders C. Foreword. In: Doyle D, Hanks GWC, Macdonald N, eds. *Oxford Textbook of Palliative Medicine.* Oxford: Oxford University Press, 1993: v–viii.
6 *Cancer Pain Relief and Palliative Care.* Technical Report Series: 804. Geneva: World Health Organization, 1990.
7 Tebbit P. *Definitions of Supportive and Palliative Care: A Consultation Paper* London: National Council for Hospice and Specialist Palliative Care Services, 2002.

8 Saunders C. Care of the dying—the problem of euthanasia. *Nursing Times* 1976; 72: 1049–1052.
9 The Barcelona Declaration on Palliative Care. *Prog Palliat Care* 1996; 4: 113.
10 Sternswärd J, Clark D. Palliative medicine—a global perspective. In: Doyle D, Hanks G, Cherny N, Calman K, eds. *Oxford Textbook of Palliative Medicine.* 3rd edition. Oxford: Oxford University Press, 2003.
11 Lopez AD. Causes of death: an assessment of global patterns of mortality around 1985. *World Health Stat Quart* 1990; 43: 91–104.
12 Bulato RA, Stephens PW. Estimates and projections of mortality by cause: a global overview 1970–2015. In: Jamison DT, Mosley HW, eds. *The World Bank Health Sector Priorities Review.* Washington DC: World Bank, 1991.
13 World Health Organization. Tobacco-attributable mortality: global estimates and projections. In: *Tobacco Alert.* Geneva: World health Organisation, 1991.
14 United Nations. *Single Convention on Narcotic Drugs, 1961.* United Nations sales No. E62.XI.1, New York: UN 1962.
15 International Narcotics Control Board. *Availability of Opiates for Medical Needs.* New York: United Nations, 1996.
16 Kutner JS, Kassner CT, Nowels DE. Symptom burden at the end of life: hospice providers' perceptions. *J Pain Symptom Manage* 2001; 21: 473–480.
17 Rogers MS, Todd CJ. The 'right kind' of pain: talking about symptoms in outpatient oncology consultations. *Palliat Med.* 2000; 14: 299–307.
18 Larue F, Collequ SM, Brasser L, Cleeland CS. Multicentre study of cancer pain and its treatment in France. *BMJ* 1995; 310: 1034–1037.
19 Cleeland CS, Gonin R, Hatfield AK et al. Pain and its treatment in outpatients with metastatic cancer. *N Engl J Med* 1994; 330: 592–596.
20 Addington-Hall J, McCarthy M. Dying from cancer: results of a national population-based investigation. *Palliat Med* 1995; 9: 295–305.
21 Valdimarsdottir U, Helgason AR, Furst CJ, Adolfsson J, Steineck G. The unrecognised cost of cancer patients' unrelieved symptoms: a nationwide follow-up of their surviving partners. *Br J Cancer.* 2002; 86: 1540–1545.
22 Mills M, Davies HTO, Macrae WA. Care of dying patients in hospital. *BMJ* 1994; 309: 583–586.
23 Jones RVH. *A Parkinson's Disease Study in Devon and Cornwall.* London: Parkinson's Disease Society, 1993.
24 Addington-Hall JM, Lay M, Altmann D, McCarthy M. Symptom control, communication with health professionals and hospital care of stroke patients in the last year of life, as reported by surviving family, friends and carers. *Stroke* 1995; 26: 2242–2248.
25 Department of Health. *National Service Framework for Coronary Heart Disease.* London: Department of Health, 2000. *www.doh.gov.uk/pdfs/chdnsf.pdf*
26 Department of Health. *National Service Framework for Older People.* London: Department of Health, 2001. *www.doh.gov.uk/nsf/olderpeople/pdfs/nsfolderpeople.pdf*
27 Tebbit P. *Palliative Care for Adults with Non-malignant Diseases: Developing a National Policy.* London: National Council for Hospices and Specialist Palliative Care Services, 2003.

28 Addington-Hall J. *Reaching Out: Specialist Palliative Care for Adults with Non-Malignant Diseases* Occasional, Paper 14. London: National Council for Hospices and Specialist Palliative Care Services, 1998.
29 Munday D, Dale J, Barnett M. Out-of-hours palliative care in the UK: perspectives from general practice and specialist services. *J R Soc Med.* 2002; 95: 28–30.
30 Shipman C, Addington-Hall J, Barclay S et al. Providing palliative care in primary care: how satisfied are GPs and district nurses with current out-of-hours arrangements? *Br J Gen Pract.* 2000; 50: 477–478.
31 Thomas K. *Out of Hours Palliative Care in the Community* London: Macmillan Cancer Relief, 2000.
32 Chattoo S, Ahmad W, Haworth M, Lennard R. *South Asian and White Patients with Advanced Cancer: Patients' and Families' Experiences of the Illness and Perceived Needs for Care. Final Report to Cancer Research UK.* Centre for Research in Primary Care, University of Leeds, January 2002.
33 Hill D, Penso D. *Opening Doors: Improving Access to Hospice and Specialist Palliative Care Services by Members of Black and Ethnic Minority Communities.* London: National Council for Hospices and Specialist Palliative Care Services, 1995.
34 Firth S. *Wider Horizons: Care of the Dying in a Multicultural Society.* London: The National Council for Hospice and Specialist Palliative Care Services, 2001.
35 Karim K, Bailey M, Tunna KH. Non-white ethnicity and the provision of specialist palliative care services: factors affecting doctors' referral patterns. *Palliat Med* 2000; 14: 471–478.
36 Gunarantum Y. Ethnicity and palliative care. In: Culley L and Dyson S, eds. *Ethnicity and Nursing Practice.* Basingstoke: Palgrave, 2001.
37 Faull C. Cancer and palliative care In: Kai J, ed. *Ethnicity, Health and Primary Care.* Oxford: Oxford University Press, 2003.
38 Selby P. Cancer clinical outcomes for minority ethnic groups. *Br J Cancer* 1996; 74: S54–S60.
39 Johnson MRD, Bains J, Chauan J, et al. *Improving Palliative Care for Minority Ethnic Communities in Birmingham.* A report for the Birmingham Specialist and Community NHS Trust and Macmillan Trust, 2001.
40 Gatrad AR, Brown E, Notta H, Sheikh A. Palliative care needs of minorities *BMJ* 2003; 327: 176–177.
41 Department of Health. *The NHS Cancer Plan: A Plan for Iinvestment, a Plan for Reform.* London: Department of Health, 2000.
42 National Institute for Clinical Excellence. *Guidance on Cancer Services: Improving Supportive and Palliative Care for Adults with Cancer.* London: National Institute for Clinical Excellence, 2004.
43 Thomas K. *Caring for the Dying at Home: Companions on a Journey.* Oxford: Radcliffe Medical Press, 2003.
44 Thomas, K. The Gold Standards Framework in community palliative care. *Eur J Palliat Care* 2003; 10(3): 113–115.
45 Grande GE, Todd CJ, Barclay SIG, Farquhar MC. Does hospital at home for palliative care facilitate death at home? Randomised controlled trial. *BMJ* 1999; 319: 1472–1475.
46 Grady A, Travers E. Hospice at Home 2: evaluating a crisis intervention service. *Int J Palliat Nurs* 2003; 9: 326–335.

47 Buckman R. Communication in palliative care: a practical guide. In: Doyle D, Hanks GWC, Macdonald N, eds. *Oxford Textbook of Palliative Medicine*. Oxford: Oxford University Press, 1993: 47–61.
48 Twycross R, Wilcock A. *Symptom Management in Advanced Cancer*, 3rd edition. Oxford: Radcliffe Medical Press, 2001.
49 Blyth A. An audit of terminal care in general practice. *BMJ* 1987; 294: 871–874.
50 Twycross RG, Fairfield S. Pain in far advanced cancer. *Pain* 1982; 14: 303–310.
51 King N, Thomas K, Bell D. An out-of-hours protocol for community palliative care: practitioners' perspectives. *Int J Palliat Nurs.* 2003; 9: 277–282.
52 Cassidy S. *Sharing the Darkness; the Spirituality of Caring*. London: Darton, Longman and Todd, 1988.
53 What is a Good Death? *BMJ* 2003; 327: 173–237.
54 Department of Health. *Building on the Best: Choice, Responsiveness and Equity in the NHS* London: Department of Health, 2003.
55 Department of Health. *National Surveys of NHS Patients: Cancer National Overview 1999–2000*. London: Department of Health, 2002.
56 Commission for Health Improvement. *National Service Framework Assessment 1: NHS Cancer Care in England and Wales*. London: Commission for Health Improvement, 2001.
57 National Council for Hospice and Specialist Palliative Care Services. *The Palliative Care Survey 1999*. London: National Council for Hospice and Specialist Palliative Care Services, 2000.
58 Ellershaw J, Ward C. Care of the dying patients; the last hours or days of life. *BMJ* 2003; 326: 30–34.
59 Fowell A, Finlay I, Johnstone R, Minto L. An integrated care pathway for the last two days of life: Wales-wide benchmarking in palliative care. *Palliat Nurs* 2002; 8: 566–573.
60 Hearn J, Higginson IJ. Outcome measures in palliative care for advanced cancer patients. *J Pub Health Med* 1997; 19: 193–199.
61 Clinical effectiveness working group. *The Which Tool Guide*? Southampton: Association for Palliative Medicine, 2002.
62 Hearn J, Higginson IJ. Development and validation of a core outcome measure for palliative care: the palliative care outcome scale. Palliative Care Core Audit Project Advisory Group. *Qual Health Care.* 1999; 8: 219–227.
63 Ewing G, Todd C, Rogers M, Barclay S, McCabe J, Martin A. Validation of a symptom measure suitable for use among palliative care patients in the community: CAMPAS-R. *J Pain Symptom Manage.* 2004; 27: 287–299.

2: Teamworking for Effective Palliative Care

LILIAN DANIELS

Introduction

Palliative care has a multi-disciplinary responsibility. A variety of health and social care professionals are involved in the delivery of palliative care services. These span a spectrum of care settings, from hospital through to hospice, community and nursing and residential homes. The success of palliative care delivery is reliant on the extent to which all professionals and care settings work together to provide seamless care for each individual patient. The basis of seamless care is effective teamworking.

Multi-disciplinary teamworking is not without its problems and palliative care is no exception to this. Indeed, the highly emotive circumstances of the patient and family can emphasise and expose the pressures and tensions in teamworking. This chapter will explore these challenges and set out some strategies for effective teamworking in the provision of palliative care. This will be achieved through:

- examination of teamworking and its problems,
- discussion of team-working in palliative care,
- outlining the roles and responsibilities of professionals involved in the delivery of palliative care,
- presentation of current guidelines for palliative care teamworking,
- strategies for the implementation of teamworking in palliative care in day-to-day practice.

This chapter focuses on primary care teamworking and the interface with professionals and teams in other care settings. The principles of teamworking and inter-team communication, however, are applicable to all those involved in palliative care delivery.

Palliative care: everyone's responsibility

The defining of 'palliative care approach' recognised that all health professionals, in all care settings, should incorporate the principles of palliative care in their practice [1,2]. The broadening of the scope of hospice and specialist palliative care to encompass many life-limiting conditions other than cancer requires the appropriate involvement of a broad range of professionals in the end-of-life care of many patients.

The provision of palliative care, therefore, is a multi-disciplinary and multi-agency responsibility. It embraces a host of professionals from general and specialist fields and involves integrating the work of professionals from hospital, community, hospice and other care settings such as residential and nursing homes. Increasingly, this will include professionals working in fields such as cardiology, neurology and respiratory medicine. The coordination of such a potentially large number of professionals in the provision of cohesive palliative care is a considerable challenge.

The majority of any patient's time is spent at home and most people wish to die at home. Hence the primary care setting should be the focus of care. The General Practitioner (GP) may be the first point of contact for the patient and the primary care team will be the consistent providers of care throughout the patient's journey. It is relevant, therefore, to start the examination of teamworking for palliative care in this setting.

Teamwork in primary care

The primary care team has been given a considerable remit in recent years with the emphasis on a primary care-led national health service [3]. The Department of Health (DoH) White Paper, 'Primary Care Delivering the Future', outlined the responsibility of primary care services in reflecting local health and social needs. It also stipulated that services should be coordinated with professionals aware of each other's contributions and with no gaps in service provision [3].

More recently, the National Health Service Plan [4] further emphasised the shifting of power to primary care services. The implementation strategies have identified primary care staff as being in a unique position to integrate health and social care services locally [5]. Primary care trusts (PCTs) have been delegated an increased responsibility and role for developing links, networks and patient pathways for seamless care [6].

The primary care team has been considered to have a central role in palliative and cancer care for some time [7,8]. However, the growing emphasis on primary-care-led services has been further reflected in the field of cancer and palliative care. This is demonstrated by the production of guidelines for care in the community for people who are terminally ill [9], and the promotion of strategies for the purchasing and delivery of primary-care-based palliative care [10].

Most recently the NHS Cancer Plan [11] has emphasised the role of primary care and teamworking within its recommendations. The development of cancer networks as a service model recognises the importance of multi-agency and multi-disciplinary teamworking. The plan [11] also recommends that PCTs appoint lead cancer clinicians who would take responsibility for leading cancer and palliative care service provision and integrate with the local cancer network. This model has also formed the framework for the National Institute of Clinical Excellence (NICE) guidelines *Improving Supportive and Palliative Care for Adults with Cancer* [12].

Multi-disciplinary teamworking is recognised as one of the key elements of successful primary care [13,14]. Teamworking is considered advantageous for a number of reasons. Ovretveit states "the point of a team is to bring together the different skills which a patient or client needs, and to combine them in a way which is not possible outside the team" [15]. The literature demonstrates that teamworking:

- enables a more coordinated service with earlier intervention and prompter referrals [16];
- promotes continuity of care [17];
- avoids crisis intervention [18];
- provides support and prevents burnout amongst professionals [19].

Problems in primary care teamworking

The literature highlights a number of issues regarding the delivery of primary care and teamworking in the community. A lack of continuity of care, poor coordination of services and the blurring of responsibilities are among the problems attributed to primary care teams [20]. Studies demonstrate that reasons for poor teamwork include: misunderstanding the roles of others [21], lack of regular meetings to define objectives and clarify roles, and differences in status and power [22]. The differences in decision-making and potential conflicts inherent within teams can often result from the differences in professional training, socialisation and culture [15].

Nationwide and local studies have highlighted a number of inadequacies in community-based palliative care of which poor teamworking was frequently identified [23–28]. Examples of poor multiprofessional working included:

- delays in communicating changes in a patient's condition or care between secondary and primary services;
- duplication of effort;
- patients 'falling through the net' [29].

The NHS Cancer Plan acknowledged that support for patients living at home with advanced cancer was sometimes poorly coordinated, with a particular lack of services available over 24 hours [11]. Following a review of empirical studies, Thomas concluded that lack of teamwork and poor communication and coordination were amongst the most common reasons for palliative home care failing to support patients adequately [30]. The review also recognised the need for generalists and specialists to work more effectively together.

In order to achieve the continuity of care between care settings and services, it is essential that each team functions effectively. In particular, the primary care team must work cohesively and in collaboration with other providers of care. The following sections will explore the construction and functioning of teams in the delivery of palliative care.

Who does what: professional roles in the delivery of palliative care

The key element of palliative care is that the patients and their families or carers are the focus of care and at the centre of teamworking [31]. Each individual and their family live within a community. Therefore, it is the GP and primary care team who are frequently the first point of contact and the main professional carers. The identification of a key worker (which will be discussed later) may also be considered central to the coordination of palliative care for a patient.

Figure 2.1 presents a model of palliative care provision. This identifies the patient and family/carers along with the designated key worker as central to high quality service provision. Primary care team members, in particular the GP, district nurse and in some cases the practice nurse, form the core services that provide generic palliative care. Adjunctive services, which include professions allied to medicine and specialist palliative care services, have greater-or-lesser-input dependant on the patient's and the primary care team's needs. Other services forming part of the greater palliative care team include hospice in-patient and day care services and other care settings such as nursing homes.

The patient's diagnosis will reflect the medical specialty involved in care. In the case of a patient with cancer this will include the oncologist, related specialist nurses and other professionals at a cancer centre or

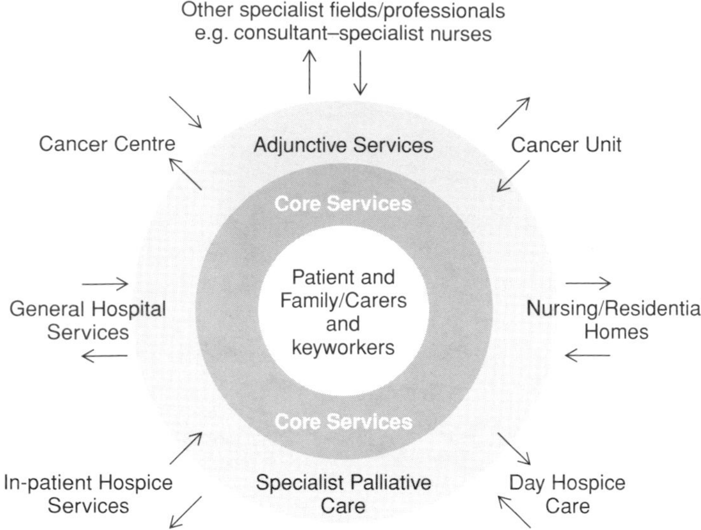

Fig. 2.1 A model for palliative care provision in the primary setting.

unit. Other life-limiting conditions will require the involvement of the medical consultant and allied staff for that specialty e.g. cardiology. Table 2.1 presents an overview of the broader palliative care team

Table 2.1 An overview of the broader palliative care team.

	Community/ Generic professionals	Specialist palliative care professionals	Other related specialties
Medical	General practitioner	Palliative medicine specialist	Medical specialist e.g. cardiology, respiratory medicine
Nursing	District nurse, practice nurse, health visitor, community psychiatric nurse	Specialist palliative care nurse e.g. Macmillan nurse, hospice home care nurse	Nurse specialist within medical field e.g. stoma care nurse, breast care nurse
		Marie Curie nurse	Nursing home staff
		Other specialist roles e.g. lymphoedema nurse	

Continued

Table 2.1 *Continued*

Adjunctive services	Social worker, occupational therapist, chiropodist, practice counselor	Specialist roles that have developed amongst professionals allied to medicine e.g. social worker, occupational therapist, physiotherapist	Pharmacist, dentist, clinical psychologist, speech therapist, dietician
Other health and social care	Meals-on-wheels, home help, nursing/ residential care home staff, private carers, day care	Hospice workers, day hospice staff	Complementary therapists, Voluntary organisations

and the potential professionals that may be involved in the care of a patient. The specific role of specialist nursing services is outlined in Table 2.2.

Table 2.2 Specialist nursing services in palliative care.

Professional	Role
Specialist palliative care nurse • Macmillan nurse • Hospice home care nurse • Community palliative care clinical nurse/specialist	Work with the primary care team and/or hospital-based professionals to enhance assessment, symptom management, emotional support and coordination of services Several levels of intervention: 1) As an educational resource 2) Consultancy and advice on individual patient cases 3) Referral of patients with complex physical and/or emotional problems Often key point of access to other specialist professionals e.g. physiotherapist, medical outpatients

Continued on p. 28

Table 2.2 Continued

Marie Curie nurses	Nurse and support patients and carers in their own homes. Staying with the patient and family overnight, or during the day, helping to prevent unwanted admission and providing respite for carers Usually accessed by the district nurse, with the level of nurse skill being matched to the patient's needs
Other nursing specialists: Lymphoedema nurse	Hospice or hospital-based. Relieve lymphoedema with massaging and bandaging techniques
Cancer site specific or disease specific nurse specialists e.g. breast care nurse, stoma care nurse, nurse specialists for multiple sclerosis	Hospital-based. Support patients with a particular diagnosis or requiring a specific treatment. May visit the patient and family at home. Play a key role in liasing between hospital and community
Hospice-at-Home	Up to 24-hour care by team of trained and/or auxiliary nurses to enable a patient to remain at home for end-of-life care. Usually additional to Marie Curie nursing care
Day hospice care	Support patients and give carers respite. Nursing and medical assessment and care and a range of therapies. Group support

Teamworking for palliative care

Effective coordination of care and teamworking has been consistently documented within palliative care literature and policy guidelines as essential elements of palliative care service delivery [1, 32–34]. However, what actually constitutes effective teamworking and how this may be achieved in practice has not always been made explicit.

There is an existing body of general knowledge describing the characteristics and functioning of a team in the delivery of health care (Box 2.1), which has been applied in the field of palliative care.

Box 2.1 General characteristics of team working

The characteristics of a team:
- members having collective responsibility for achieving shared aims and objectives
- members interacting with each other through regular meetings
- members having well defined roles which are differentiated from each other
- members having organisational identity as a work team [35]

The elements of good teamworking:
- professionals defining their role [17]
- understanding and respecting the roles of others [21, 36]
- use of communication methods: team meetings, shared records [36], and agreed protocols [37]

A number of studies have set guidelines or standards for primary palliative care practice, devised from empirical work with primary health care teams [38–40]. These standards and guidelines differ in style and the extent to which they are overtly measurable. However, they carry a number of common themes of which teamworking and patient/carer focused care are central elements. Box 2.2 highlights the common elements of a multi-disciplinary teamworking in primary palliative care.

Box 2.2 The common elements of multi-disciplinary team working in primary palliative care

Good communication within the team and between teams [29, 30, 39–42]
Assessment of patient need [9, 30, 40]
Use of a key worker/facilitator of care role [9, 12, 26, 39]
Coordinated management, regular monitoring and proactive care [9, 30, 38–40]
Agreed or shared care plan, practice protocols or guidelines [39, 41]
Good symptom control [30, 39]
Support for carer [30]
Timely and detailed referrals/appropriate timing for referral to specialists [29, 40]
Early involvement of nursing staff [39]
Joint visits between different professionals [43]
Team meetings/monthly review of care/case conferences [38, 39, 43, 44]
Practice register of palliative care patients [30, 44]
Audit and evaluation of care [40]
Multiprofessional learning [42]

Despite the publication of guidelines and standards for effective multi-disciplinary palliative care, a key issue is how professionals interpret such work to facilitate effective teamworking. What is often lacking is effective guidance as to how to implement them in practice.

It is recommended that teams devise their own guidelines or standards of care, as a means of team building and developing shared ownership of care goals [39]. This may be somewhat ambitious if the professionals are not accustomed to working as a team and may be considered a longer-term goal once teamworking practices have been developed. Existing guidelines are frequently evidence-based and provide a good point of reference, particularly when time for standard setting is at a premium. They may be then utilised to initiate the audit and evaluation of care [40].

Current guidelines for palliative care teamworking

With the increasing emphasis on evidence-based practice and developing community palliative care services, a number of national initiatives have evolved which provide guidance for palliative care teamworking.

GOLD STANDARDS FRAMEWORK FOR COMMUNITY PALLIATIVE CARE

The Gold Standards Framework (GSF) for community palliative care has been developed from a large national study involving 3000 patients across the UK [30]. This study aimed to produce a model of best practice for primary care teams to utilise in the care of patients with cancer and subsequently other non-malignant end-stage illnesses. The model of good practice on which the framework is based is achieved through three processes:

- specific identification of patients in the last months of life;
- improving the assessment of their needs, both physical and psychosocial;
- building in planning of anticipated problems and future care [30].

Seven key areas of palliative care form the basis of the framework and practical guidance is provided within the framework on each element:

- Communication—through the use of a patient register, team meetings and proactive care planning.

- Coordination—by a nominated coordinator who is responsible for maintaining the register, planning meetings etc.
- Control of symptoms—through assessment, recording, discussing and acting upon.
- Continuity of care—through transfer of information to out-of-hours service, hospital services etc.
- Continued learning—using practice-based or external teaching, a practice reference library and personal development plans.
- Carer support—including emotional, practical, bereavement and staff support.
- Care of the dying—following an agreed protocol [30].

The framework is promoted as a national initiative within the NICE guidance [12], which any primary care team may adopt. It is suggested that a coordinator be appointed to direct the implementation of the framework. This individual will have access to a variety of guidance and support provided by the local cancer network service improvement team. Implementation guidelines for the framework provide a practical and prescriptive stepwise approach for primary care teams to follow.

The benefit of the GSF is that it facilitates a validated approach to developing primary care teamworking for palliative care. Likewise, if widely adopted, it promotes equity and continuity. The principles of the framework are universally valuable for palliative care teamworking. However, it is important that teams also consider the specific local needs when developing palliative care services. The prescriptive application of guidelines should not stifle individual team initiatives.

NICE: SUPPORTIVE AND PALLIATIVE CARE GUIDELINES

NICE has developed service configuration guidance for those affected with cancer [12]. A major element of the guidelines is the coordination of care and communication between professionals and with patients and carers.

The guidelines provide a valuable framework for teamworking in the delivery of palliative care. Recommendations are provided within the guidelines for all levels of stakeholders including multi-disciplinary teams and individual practitioners. Box 2.3 outlines the elements of the NICE guidance related to the 'Coordination of Care', which has particular relevance to multi-disciplinary teamworking.

Box 2.3 NICE guidance related to the co-ordination of care [12]

- Service provision and planning level
  assess local need and current service provision
- Assessment
  individual professionals should be able to assess the care and support needs of patients/carers
  unnecessary repetition of the same assessment by different professionals should be avoided
  specific assessment tools may be employed
  assessment data should be shared between professionals
  structured assessments should be carried out at key points along the patient pathway
- Referral
  prompt referrals based on referral guidelines
- Coordination within the team
  discuss patients at multi-disciplinary team meeting
  record outcomes and communicate with patient/carer
  review this process with team to maintain effectiveness
  develop own policies and protocols in relation to communication
  identify current palliative care patients
  establish mechanisms to promote continuity e.g. key worker
- Coordination between teams
  proactive coordination to enhance continuity of care
  identify other teams/services with whom they interface and develop plans to promote coordinated care e.g. joint clinics/ward rounds, multi-disciplinary team meetings
  mechanisms for information transfer e.g. patient held records, handover forms etc.

A key recommendation with regard to the coordination of care is that each multi-disciplinary team should implement processes to ensure effective inter-professional communication and continuity of care. At an individual professional level this involves: assessing the care and support needs of each patient/carer; meeting those within the scope of the professional's knowledge, skills and competence and knowing when to refer to specialist services [12]. At a team level it also involves assessment of the local needs of the community they serve in order that services be planned appropriately. In order for care to be continuous, the NICE guidelines suggest that excellent information transfer with the patient and effective communication between professionals and services are essential [12]. Although there is little prescriptive guidance as to how this should be achieved, the guidelines do make reference to the role of a key worker as one possible method to enable this.

Implementing palliative care teamworking strategies in the primary care team

Despite the availability of literature and guidelines for multi-disciplinary teamworking in the delivery of palliative care, implementation of such strategies may still remain problematic in practice. Yet there is considerable value in developing practice and services at a local level. There can be a greater sense of ownership in implementing practice changes and strategies for good teamworking, particularly, where professionals are actively engaged in identifying solutions to practice problems, developing strategies to meet local needs and evaluating their impact. This section presents a framework for developing primary care teamworking for palliative care. The methods described are drawn from an action research study with a primary care team, which aimed to enhance multi-disciplinary teamworking in the provision of palliative care [28].

The framework adopts a two-phase approach (Table 2.3). The first phase involves a period of assessing current practice and identifying solutions to practice problems in the delivery of palliative care. The basis of this is effective teamworking and therefore the focus of this phase is the initiation of team building strategies. The second phase

Table 2.3 A two-phase approach to developing primary palliative care practice.

	Objectives	Methods
Phase One: Assessment	Team building strategies	Team meetings (use of focus group techniques and case study analysis to direct discussion)
Goal setting	Evaluation of current practice	Professional questionnaires Patient/carer questionnaires
Phase Two: Implementation	Implementing practice initiatives	Audit tools. Professional questionnaires. Patient/carer questionnaires
Evaluation	Evaluation of changes to practice	

PHASE 1
Stage:

1 Identification of professionals with responsibility for palliative care

2 Appoint coordinator/facilitator

3 Initiate regular (monthly) team meetings

4 Define individual roles and responsibilities

5 Develop a practice profile of patients with palliative care needs

6 Identify problems in the delivery of palliative care

7 Identify practice initiatives to address problems

PHASE 2
Stage

8 Case review meeting to allocate key worker for each patient

9 Implement practice initiatives

10 Utilise methods of evaluating care and practice changes

Fig. 2.2 A framework for developing primary care team working for palliative care.

involves the implementation and evaluation of changes to practice. This phase requires that team building strategies be maintained alongside the use of formal methods of audit and evaluation. Phase one requires considerable time and commitment to team building in order for phase two to be successful. This may take twelve months, particularly if the team meets only on a monthly basis [28]. Each phase involves a series of stages outlined in Figure 2.2.

Phase one

Stage one involves the *identification of primary care professionals with a responsibility for palliative care provision* (see Table 2.1). These will be the key professionals who need to meet regularly to coordinate care for patients with palliative care needs who are registered with the practice. It is essential that this group of professionals be committed to teamworking and developing palliative care practice. This would typically include: GPs, practice nurse, practice manager, district nurse, social worker and any other practice-linked professionals e.g. practice counsellor. It is important that the specialist palliative care professionals linked to the practice such as the Macmillan nurse or hospice home care nurse also attend the team meetings.

This process will require coordination and therefore **stage two** requires that the team *appoint a coordinator* with the responsibility of arranging meetings and chairing discussions. An external facilitator may be beneficial in order to prevent issues in electing a 'leader' and to enable objectivity. **Stage three** involves the initiation of regular team meetings, held at least once a month. Primarily, these are for the purpose of discussing patient care but may also be used for education sessions and initially for planning and developing services.

A period of *team building* is beneficial in order that *roles and responsibilities* for palliative care service delivery be discussed and defined. **Stage four** may be undertaken during the team meetings, in which:

- Practitioners reflect critically on their role and the provision of palliative care.
- Personal, professional and team values regarding palliative care delivery are clarified.
- Practice problems are assessed and goals and solutions identified.

A useful outcome of this process is the production of a *staff handbook*, which identifies the role profile of each professional in the delivery of palliative care and the contact and referral details of each team member.

Stage five involves identification of the patient population with palliative care needs. There is frequently no routine method for identifying patients with cancer or with palliative care needs from a practice population, apart from undertaking a hand search of patients' notes or identification of patients known to the primary health care team. Developing a practice profile of patients with palliative care needs requires the establishment of parameters for inclusion, which should be jointly agreed by the team. For example, this may be: 'all patients with a diagnosis of cancer of uncertain prognosis and uncontrolled chronically ill patients with a life-limiting condition and their families and carers' [28].

Stage six requires that some time be allocated within a team meeting to *identify problems in the delivery of palliative care services*. **Stage seven** therefore enables goals to be set and *practice initiatives* devised to provide solutions to the problems identified. A long-term outcome may be the production of locally agreed standards or protocols for care, which may be regularly audited and evaluated.

Phase two

Phase two focuses on the implementation and evaluation of the practice changes identified in phase one. Innovations in practice are supported by government recommendations for developing health care services [3]. Locally devised practice initiatives should respond to the specific needs of the patients and carers within the community. Box 2.4 outlines a number of initiatives that have relevance to any primary care team.

Box 2.4 Practice initiatives to develop primary palliative care services [28]

- A practice profile of patients with palliative care needs
- Monthly multi-disciplinary team meetings to review patient care
- The identification of a key worker for each patient
- A patient held record system
- Multi-professional education
- Auditing practice

Stage eight involves an initial *case review meeting* to assess current care provision and allocate a *key worker* for each patient. A considerable amount of time may need to be allocated for this initial meeting. However, following this a monthly team meeting to discuss new and current patient cases will be necessary, which can be limited to an hour.

Research has demonstrated that nurses are well placed to adopt the role of key worker, having the skills for patient assessment and the close, regular contact with patients and carers [28]. This may be a generic role such as the practice nurse or district nurse, with the specialist nurse taking on this role if she is intensively involved in a patient's care, or it may be taken on as a joint role. The key worker role has been evaluated as one of the most valuable elements of teamworking and patient care [28]. There are common elements described within the role of key worker or coordinator. These include: assessment, development of a care plan, referring to other agencies and on-going monitoring [29]. NICE has similarly outlined the responsibilities of the key worker role and highlighted that the professional fulfilling this role may change at transition points on the patient pathway [12].

The focus of **stage nine** is the implementation of the practice initiatives identified in phase one. This includes maintaining the monthly team meetings at which patients are discussed and the care is planned. Other initiatives may include: a patient held record system and multiprofessional education sessions. Similarly, the team may choose to implement elements of current strategies or other initiatives such as an integrated care pathway for end-stage care [45].

Patient held record systems are frequently discussed and have long been used in other fields such as obstetrics. The content of the system may vary, extending from brief medical details to a full plan of care. Ideally, this is completed by the key worker in conjunction with the patient/carer and may include: a plan of care, medication details, contact information for the patient/carer and a section for any professional to write in, following a consultation.

Considerable value is placed on professionals being involved in joint education and training. Within a primary care team, multiprofessional education sessions may take the form of a lunchtime seminar. The topics chosen should respond to an identified need. The specialist palliative care services to which the primary care team refers may be utilised as an educational resource and this may help to forge relationships between teams. Likewise, hospital professionals could be invited to speak at education sessions, with the additional bonus of facilitating working relations.

Specific practice initiatives may be developed to respond to local needs. For example the development of a surgery-based clinic for palliative care patients and their carers has been found to be beneficial to patient care and teamworking [28]. This functions as a nurse-led clinic with the practice nurse being in attendance at each clinic, and seeing each patient/carer. It is utilised by other team members to the greatest effect as a means of seeing specific patients through an appointment system. Access to a GP can also be made available for each clinic by running it alongside the routine surgery. The clinic may also provide a drop-in facility for the benefit of patients and carers, to allow them ready access to a health professional if they have a problem.

Stage ten involves utilising methods to *evaluate care and practice changes*. The evaluation of practice has become an essential element of developing evidence-based practice. This is of particular importance where changes to practice have been made. The range of evaluative methods and tools available to measure primary palliative care delivery is broad. Table 2.4 presents examples of methods and tools available to professionals for the audit and evaluation of palliative care services at both individual and community service level. Each PCT has a responsibility to demonstrate that it is providing quality palliative care services that are responsive to local needs. The collection of audit and evaluative data will facilitate this.

In particular, audit provides a structure for the case review team meetings. At each meeting a care goal is identified for each patient problem discussed and the outcome of this is assessed at the next

Table 2.4 Tools for the evaluation of palliative care service delivery.

Level of evaluation	Focus of evaluation	Examples of tools/methods
Individual patient	Measurement of individual symptoms e.g. pain, nausea, anxiety	Visual analogue/verbal descriptor scales to measure symptom intensity Pain assessment tools e.g. McGill pain questionnaire Hospital Anxiety and Depression Scale
	Multi-symptom measures Measures of Quality of Life	Rotterdam Symptom Checklist European Organisation for Research and Treatment of Cancer (EORTC QLQC30) Spitzer Quality of Life Index
	Evaluation of aspects of total patient care.	Support team assessment schedule (STAS) [46] Cambridge Palliative Care Audit Schedule (CAMPAS) [40] Palliative Care Outcome Score [48] Wishes for place of death Patient/carer views.
Primary care team	Local needs assessment	Profile of patients with palliative care needs Morbidity data
	Evaluation of services	Patient/carer views Audit of patient contacts Audit of case review meetings Use of national or local standards/guidelines to evaluate care

meeting [22]. Similarly, the team may utilise a system of audit such as the Support Team Assessment Schedule (STAS) [46], as a means of evaluating patient care. This requires the professional to use a scoring system of 0–5 to rate a number of elements of palliative care such as pain, anxiety, etc.

Developing multi-disciplinary team practice for palliative care can therefore be carried out as a stepwise approach that focuses on the establishment of teamworking strategies and professional relationships. These provide the essential building blocks for the further development of services, and a structure for the implementation of locally agreed and national standards and guidelines for practice.

The establishment of effective multi-disciplinary teamworking practice in primary palliative care is the basis of developing a seamless approach to patient care. If the key elements of care coordination and communication have been developed from the first patient contact, it will support the patient's pathway through other services and care settings. It is essential that the primary care team is proactive in developing links with secondary services and other care settings. The final section will examine the working interface between primary and secondary care.

The interface between primary care and other services

The complexity of providing community based palliative care has been acknowledged. In particular, the working interface between voluntary and statutory provision [47], and the coordination of care between different settings [12]. It is recognised that the smooth progression of care from the patient's point of view is both critical and challenging [12]. Firstly, it is important that the key worker and primary care team know which other professionals, care settings and services are involved with each patient. They also need to be aware of the referral criteria to these services and how to contact other professionals.

The use of the key worker role is invaluable in facilitating continuity of care. The key worker can take responsibility for tracking the patient through the care pathway and liasing with all other professionals involved, particularly at critical points along the pathway such as hospital/hospice admission and discharge. Patient held records and case review team meetings also assist the process of promoting continuity of care.

Other strategies may be employed to assist in the development of cohesive care. These strategies should be particularly targeted at weak areas in the care system, such as out-of-hours care and discharge planning. For example, current guidelines suggest that general medical and nursing services should have 24-hour access to specialist palliative care advice [12]. Similarly, it is recommended that there should be strategies for the transfer of information between 9–5 services and out-of-hours services and that discharge should only occur when all services are in place [12].

The use of guidelines, standards and policies for communication and coordination of care between primary and secondary services will assist the promotion of continuous care. However, such strategies will only be effective if all professionals are aware of them, agree with them and adhere to them. The importance therefore of teams from all settings collaborating in planning palliative care services is essential. The development of cancer networks was designed to enable this collaboration. It is important that this model is similarly transferred to palliative care patients with non-malignant conditions.

Conclusion

The provision of palliative care is the responsibility of a host of professionals, who may come into contact with patients and their families at differing times throughout the course of a patient's illness. Empirical evidence has shown that the coordination of such a range of professionals and services is often problematic.

The key to successful palliative care provision is effective multidisciplinary teamworking and a cohesive working interface between services and care settings. Current policy and guidelines place considerable emphasis on the development of strategies to facilitate communication and coordination within and between teams in the provision of palliative care. Simple strategies such as professionals beginning to meet regularly as a team in order to discuss patient care can go a long way to enhancing the continuity of care before other techniques, such as key worker roles and patient held records, are developed.

It is essential that the primary care teams at the centre of palliative care services are driving strategies to promote seamless care. However, all professionals involved in palliative care delivery have a responsibility to communicate, both between themselves and with the patient and their family, who must at all times be seen as the centre of teamworking.

References

1 National Council for Hospice and Specialist Palliative Care Services. *Specialist Palliative Care: A Statement of Definitions* Occasional Paper 8. London, National Council for Hospice and Specialist Palliative Care Services, 1995.

2 Doyle D. The Way Forward. Policy and Practice. In: National Council for Hospice and Specialist Palliative Care Services *Promoting Partnership: Planning and Managing Community Palliative Care*. London: National Council for Hospice and Specialist Palliative Care Services, 1998.

3 Department of Health. *Primary Care: Delivering the Future*. London: Department of Health, 1996.

4 Department of Health. *The NHS Plan*. London: Department of Health, 2000.

5 Department of Health. *'The Next Steps'*. London: Department of Health, 2002.

6 Department of Health. '*Securing Delivery.*' London: Department of Health, 2002.
7 Standing Medical Advisory Committee and Standing Nursing and Midwifery Advisory Committee. *The Principles and Provision of Palliative Care.* London: The Stationary Office, 1992.
8 Department of Health. *A Policy Framework for Commissioning Cancer Services* Report of the expert advisory group on cancer to the Chief Medical Officers of England and Wales. London: Department of Health, 1995.
9 National Council for Hospice and Specialist Palliative Care Services. *Care in the Community for People who are Terminally Ill: Guidelines for Health Authorities and Social Services Departments.* (Undated). London: National Council for Hospice and Specialist Palliative Care Services.
10 National Council for Hospice and Specialist Palliative Care Services. *Promoting Partnership: Planning and Managing Community Palliative Care.* Report of a joint conference: National Association of Health Authorities and Trusts and the National Council for Hospice and Specialist Palliative Care Services. Occasional Paper 15. London: National Council for Hospice and Specialist Palliative Care Services, 1998.
11 Department of Health. *The NHS Cancer Plan: A Plan for Investment, a Plan for Reform.* London: Department of Health, 2000.
12 National Institute for Clinical Excellence. *Guidance on Cancer services: Improving Supportive and Palliative Care for Adults with Cancer.* London: National Institute for Clinical Excellence, 2004.
13 Pringle M. *Change and Teamwork in Primary Care.* London: BMJ Publishing Group, 1994.
14 Knapman J. Teambuilding in primary care. *Primary Health Care* 1995; 5: 18–23.
15 Ovretveit J. Team decision-making. *J Interprofessional Care* 1995; 9(1): 41–51.
16 Bennett-Emslie G, McIntosh J. Promoting collaboration in the primary care team: the role of the practice meeting *J Interprofessional Care* 1995; 9(3): 251–25.
17 Barker W. Working as a team. *J Community Nurs* 1996; 10(4): 8–10.
18 Bassett P. Team care at work. *J District Nurs* 1989; 7(8): 4–6.
19 Vass N. A GP's view of teamwork. *Palliat Care Today* 1996; 5(3): 38–39.
20 McWhinney I R. Core values in a changing world. *BMJ* 1998; 316: 1807–1809.
21 Hutchinson A, Gordon S. Primary care teamwork: making it a reality *J Interprofessional Care* 1992; 6(1): 31–42.
22 Field R, West M. Teamwork in primary health care. 2. Perspectives from practices. *J Interprofessional Care* 1995; 9(2): 123–130.
23 Clarke D, Neale B. Independent hospice care in the community: two case studies. *Health and Social Care* 1994; 2: 203–212.
24 Seale C, Cartwright A. *The Year Before Death.* Aldershot: Avebury, 1994.
25 Addington-Hall J, McCarthy M. Dying from cancer: results of a national population-based investigation. *Palliat Med* 1995; 10: 66–67.
26 Grande G E, Todd C J, Barclay S I G. Symptom control issues in primary palliative care: skills and communication. *Palliat Med* 1996; 10: 66–67.
27 Millar D G, Carroll D, Grimshaw J, Watt B. Palliative care at home: an audit of cancer deaths in Grampian region. *Brit J Gen Pract* 1998; 48: 1299–1302.
28 Daniels L, Linnane J. Developing a framework for primary palliative care. *Brit J Community Nurs* 2001; 6(11): 592–600.

29 Nuffield Centre for Community Care Studies. *Palliative Cancer Care: Support in the Community Following Diagnosis and Treatment*. Based on a report by S. MacAskill and A Petch, funded by Macmillan Cancer Relief. University of Glasgow, Nuffield Centre for Community Care Studies, 1999.
30 Thomas K. *Caring for the Dying at Home*. 2003. Oxford: Radcliffe Medical Press.
31 World Health Organisation. *Cancer Pain Relief and Palliative Care. Report of a WHO Expert Committee*. WHO Technical Report Series 804. Geneva: WHO, 1990.
32 Royal College of Nursing. *Standards of Care for Palliative Nursing*. The Royal College of Nursing Palliative Nursing Group and Hospice Nurse Managers Forum. London: Royal College of Nursing, 1993.
33 Scottish Office Home and Health Department. *Palliative Care Guidelines*. Scottish Partnership Agency for Palliative and Cancer Care with the Clinical Resource and Audit Group. Edinburgh, The Stationery Office, 1994.
34 Twycross R. *Introducing Palliative Care*. Oxford: Radcliffe Medical Press, 1995.
35 West M, Poulton BC. A failure of function: teamwork in primary health care. *J Interprofessional Care* 1997; 11(2): 205–216.
36 Pearson P, Spencer J. Pointers to effective teamwork: exploring primary care. *J Interprofessional Care* 1995; 9(2): 131–138.
37 Vanclay L. Team working in primary care. *Nurs Stand* 1998; 12(20): 37–38.
38 Jones R. Primary health care: what should we do for people dying at home with cancer? *Eur J. Cancer Care* 1992; 1(4): 9–11.
39 Robinson L, Stacy R. Palliative care in the community: setting practice guidelines for primary care teams. *Br J Gen Pract* 1994; 44: 461–464.
40 Ewing G, Todd C, Rogers M, Barclay S, McCabe J, Martin A. Validation of a symptom measure suitable for use among palliative care patients in the community: CAMPAS-R. *J Pain Symptom Manage*. 2004; 27: 287–299.
41 Scott L. (1998) The National Perspective: Adjusting to Calman: Palliative Care in the Community In: National Council for Hospice and Specialist Palliative Care. *Promoting Partnership: Planning and Managing Community Palliative Care*. London: National Council for Hospice and Specialist Palliative Care, 1998.
42 Neal J. PCG's and PCT's: Their impact on palliative care services. *Palliat Care Today* 2000; 8(4): 56–57.
43 Pugsley R, Pardoe J. Community care of the terminally ill patient. In: Wilkes E, Ed, *Terminal Care Update*. Surrey: Siebert Publications, 1986.
44 Buckley D. Audit of palliative care in a general practice setting. *Palliat Care Today* 1996; 5:2.
45 Ellershaw J, Foster A, Murphy D, Shea T, Overill S. Developing an integrated care pathway for the dying patient. *Eur J Palliative Care* 1997; 4(6): 203–207.
46 Higginson I (Ed). *Clinical Audit in Palliative Care*. Oxford: Radcliffe Medical Press, 1994.
47 Robbins M A, Jackson P. Prentice. A Statutory and voluntary sector palliative care in the community setting: National Health Service professionals' perceptions of the interface. *Eur J Cancer Care* 1996; 5: 96–102.
48 Hearn J. Higginson I J. Development and validation of a core outcome measure for palliative care: the palliative care outcome scale. Palliative Care Core Audit Project Advisory Group. *Qual Health Care* 1999; 8: 219–227.

3: Rights, Needs and Social Exclusion at the End of Life

JONATHAN KOFFMAN AND IRENE HIGGINSON

Introduction: the universal right to care at the end of life

> *We emerge deserving of little credit; we who are capable of ignoring the conditions that make muted people suffer. The dissatisfied dead cannot noise abroad the negligence they have experienced* [1].

Nearly forty years ago in this statement John Hinton drew attention to the deficiencies that were evident in the care offered to many patients with advanced disease and to their families. Whilst we have witnessed a growing understanding of the palliative care needs of patients and their families and an acceptance that death is universal, which, de facto, makes it a universal public health concern, the actual provision of care has, nevertheless, remained in part, woefully inadequate.

In recent years, both in the UK and elsewhere, questions are being asked about how much palliative care do we need, by whom, where and at what cost, given that accessible and good quality care towards the end of life must be recognised as a basic human right.

> ***Everyone has the right to... security in the event of sickness, disability, widowhood, old age or other lack of livelihood in circumstances beyond his [or her] control***
>
> Article 25, United Nations Universal Declaration of Human Rights, 2001

Currently, however, we lack many of the critical pieces of information required to adequately answer all of these questions, although there is broad agreement based on local and national epidemiological surveys [2, 3], government reports and WHO data [4, 5] that the currently available palliative services from a range of providers are inadequate to meet some existing, and the rapidly growing, health and social care needs of the world's citizens with advanced disease.

In this chapter we seek to explore the concept of need in relation to palliative care, and describe the various approaches used to determine the palliative care requirements of local populations and groups within them. We draw on current evidence, primarily but not exclusively, from the UK, on how services have met the palliative care needs of some marginalised populations. These include the poor, older people, people with learning disabilities and mental health problems, black and minority ethnic communities, asylum seekers and refugees, those within the penal system and drug users. While the chapter has limited itself to these population groups, other socially excluded sectors of the population are not immune. They include those who are homeless or live in fragile accommodation, travellers and those who abuse alcohol. To date, however, little attention and therefore published research, has focused on either their met or unmet palliative care needs, a testimony to their social distance from the mainstream. We conclude by highlighting some innovative strategies that have been offered to better meet the palliative care needs of local populations.

What is need?

According to Soper, "*There can be few concepts so frequently invoked and yet so little analysed as that of human needs*" [6]. Other contributions to the definitions of need come from the fields of sociology, epidemiology, health economics, public health, as well as from clinicians. Most doctors would consider needs in terms of health care services that they can supply. Patients, however, may have different views as need incorporates the wider social and environmental determinants of health, such as deprivation, housing, diet, education and employment. This wider definition allows us to look beyond the confines of the medical model based on health services, to the wider influences on health. It is for this reason that in 1972 Bradshaw distinguished four types of need: felt need (what people want); expressed need (felt need turned into action); normative need (as defined by experts or professionals); and comparative need (arising where similar populations receive different service levels) (Box 3.1) [7]. Raised within these distinctions are the questions of: who determines need (professionals, politicians or the general public); what are the influences of education and media in raising awareness about health problems; and what are the cultural effects on need? However, perhaps the most pragmatic definition for our purpose is '*the ability to benefit from health care*', originally developed by the NHS Executive in the UK and now used in several countries [8].

Box 3.1 Need: who decides and how?

Need can be:

- What the individual feel they want (felt need)
- What the individuals demand (expressed need)
- What a professional thinks and the individual wants (normative need)
- How we compare with others' areas or situations (comparative need)

Assessing need

To assess the palliative care needs of a local population, three strategies may be adopted: epidemiological, comparative and corporate.

The epidemiological approach makes use of local cause-specific mortality in diseases that are *likely* to benefit from palliative care services, and then relates this to the type and frequency of symptoms experienced by patients suffering from these diseases. It reviews the effectiveness and cost effectiveness of care using local, national and international evidence. Lastly, it compares these with the patterns of locally available specialist and generic services to determine how well need is being met (Fig. 3.1) [9].

The incidence of patients requiring palliative care (either general and or specialist) can be estimated from death rates of common conditions. In the UK there are approximately 570,000 deaths per year, most commonly from circulatory disorders, cancer and respiratory

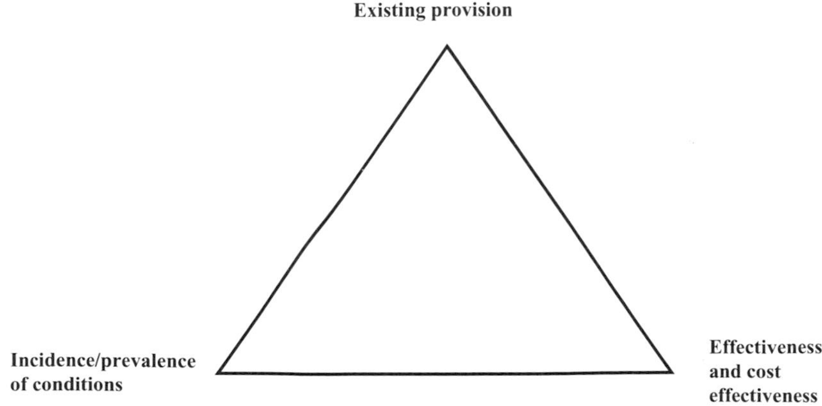

Fig. 3.1 Components of health needs assessment. Modified from Stevens and Raftery [9].

Box 3.2 Patients who may benefit from specialist and generic palliative care

1 Those whose illness progresses over time
2 Those who are relatively well, but then die suddenly
3 Those who want aggressive treatment aimed at cure whatever the benefit
4 Those who have relapses and remissions and deteriorate over time

disease. There are almost equal numbers of men and women who die and the numbers are relatively constant over time. Clearly, the illness trajectory varies between diseases and not everybody will need specialist palliative care. However, many patients die from chronic or slowly progressive conditions that could benefit from palliative care (Box 3.2). The patients and their families those who fall into groups 1 and 4, are likely to need palliative care and those who fall into groups 2 and 3 do not, although they may well need symptom control and their families will need support. Applying the likely prevalence of symptoms for different conditions to the number of people who die can provide a closer estimate of need, although it does not take into account individual wants and preferences. For example, within a population of 10,000 people (e.g. a group practice) national estimates suggest that there are approximately 28 cancer deaths per year, many of whom would have a period of advancing progressive disease, when palliative care would be appropriate. The estimates of prevalence of symptoms and problems are based on population and other studies of patients with advanced disease and their families. Applying the population estimates to the 28 patients who would die from cancer suggests that there would be 23 with pain, 13 with breathlessness, 14 with vomiting or nausea, 20 with loss of appetite and 9 where the patient and 7 where the patient's family had severe anxieties or worries that were seriously affecting their daily life and concentration. Estimates of the prevalence of symptoms and other problems can also be applied to determine the number of people with these problems in the last year of life, who die from conditions other than cancer. The number of people affected would be more than double those with cancer [10]. Primary care plays an invaluable role in the care of these patients and their families, where the pattern of dying is more uncertain and longer.

The comparative approach examines levels of service utilisation rather than disease categories. A common approach is to compare and contrast the local levels of activity against national averages so that areas of specialist practise can be examined for obvious disparities in equity of provision [2], but there are a number of difficulties in this approach. First, the main limitation of this method is that it does not assess unmet need that must then be evaluated by other methods. Second, comparing a locality with other regions does not take into consideration that districts can vary considerably in terms of demographic make-up, ethnicity and social deprivation. Lastly, the corporate approach involves the structured collection of the knowledge and views of local informants on health care services and unmet needs [9]. Valuable information is often available from a wide range of parties, for example managers in Primary Care Trusts, clinical staff, general practitioners, and importantly, patients and their families. The corporate approach is essential if policies to meet unmet needs are to be sensitive to local circumstances. There are nevertheless caveats in adopting this approach including bias and the politics of vested interests [11].

Palliative care services and unmet need

The concept of equity of access to health care is a central objective of many health care systems throughout the world. In the early 1970s, Julian Tudor Hart coined the phrase '*inverse care law*' to describe the observation that those who were in the greatest apparent need of care often had the worst access to health care provision [12]. Since that time, although a growing body of research evidence has accumulated to quantify the problem [13–16], the aspiration of making care available to all has remained elusive. This has been no less an issue for those who require care at the end of life [17–21].This may be due to palliative care services previously being developed largely based on assumptions about patient need taken from the health care professionals' points of view [22]. In recent years, the commitment to tackle health inequalities has been harnessed under the wing of 'social exclusion', a relatively new term in the UK policy debate to describe an old problem [23]. It includes poverty and low income, but is broader and addresses some of the wider causes and consequences of social deprivation. The British Government has defined social exclusion as:

> *'a shorthand term for what can happen when people or areas suffer from a combination of linked problems such as unemployment, poor skills, low incomes, poor housing, high crime, bad health and family breakdown'* [24].

Social exclusion is something that can happen to anyone. Some people from certain backgrounds are, however, more likely to suffer.

Although palliative care has become more prominent within mainstream UK's National Health Service during the last decade, it has still been very slow to meet the needs of certain patients who could benefit from it. Below we have focused on the available evidence of access to palliative care to poor and other disenfranchised population groups (Fig. 3.2). Our list of groups is admittedly restricted and we have stated that other vulnerable sectors of the society may fare as badly.

The economically deprived

Britain leads western Europe in its poverty, with twice as many poor households as Belgium, Denmark, Italy, Holland or Sweden. A quarter of men of working age were 'non-employed' in 1996, and a quarter of households existed on less than half of the national average income, after housing costs, in the early 1990s [25]. Although overall personal income rose substantially in the 1980s and 1990s, the gap between the richest and the poorest has grown dramatically [26].

Evidence from a number of studies suggests that between 50% and 70% of patients would prefer to be cared for at home for as long as possible, and would also prefer to die at home [27]. In areas of high socio-economic deprivation, however, fewer people do die at home. Further, they are more likely to die in a hospital and less likely to die in a hospice compared to other groups [28, 29]. They also die at younger ages [30], often with a poorer quality of life [31]. If specialist

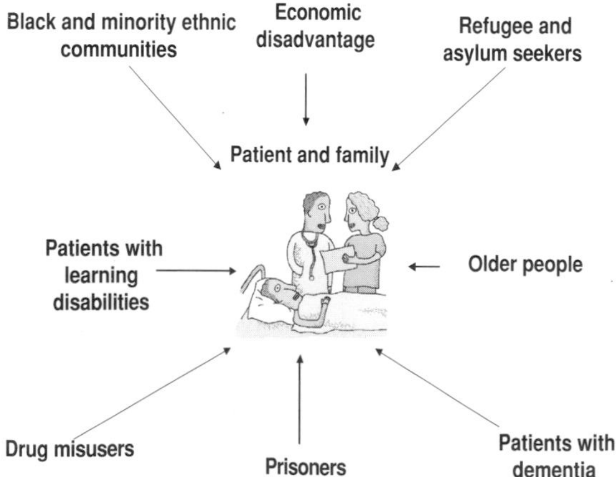

Fig. 3.2 Potential factors that influence access to palliative care provision for patients and family with advanced disease.

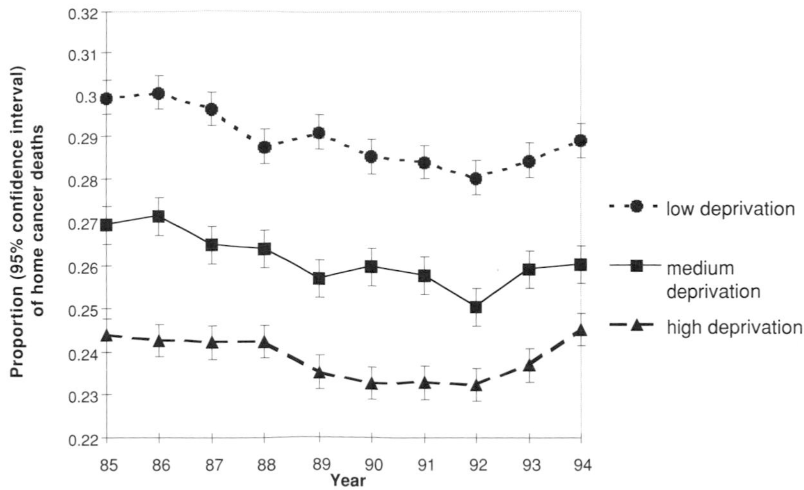

Fig. 3.3 Trends in deaths at home from cancer by deprivation band (one-third of the population sorted by score of deprivation). (Reproduced with permission from [33]).

palliative care services are available in these areas, they tend to require more resources to achieve the same level of care than in areas where deprivation is lower [32]. Figure 3.3 illustrates the wide variation in deaths at home by deprivation band [33]. It would appear that lower-occupational groups are at a disadvantage both in terms of home death and in access to cancer-related services.

Older people

The increasing elderly population presents a growing challenge to health and social care services [34]. Most people who die are old and their needs are sometimes complex as a result of multiple morbidities. While fair access lies at the heart of good public services in some areas of health and social care, older people and their carers, however, have experienced age-based discrimination in access to and availability of services [35]. Further, older people from black and minority ethnic groups can be particularly disadvantaged [36].

It has been suggested that the palliative care movement has not afforded older patients adequate care, preferring to devote more of its resources to relatively younger people [20]. Whilst some research has, in part, rebutted this accusation, an analysis of minimum dataset activity for hospices' and hospitals' palliative care services in 1997 and 1998 demonstrated that age does represent an important influence in determining which patients receive specialist palliative care [37].

In general, older people are less likely to be cared for at home and more likely to be in nursing and residential homes, where staff are often ill equipped to manage the symptoms associated with advanced disease. In an evaluation of the adequacy of pain management in nursing homes in five states in the United States of America, Bernabei et al. found that pain was prevalent among nursing home residents and was often untreated, particularly among older patients [38]. Similar concerns have been raised in the UK [39, 40].

People with dementia

In recent years dementia has become a major concern for all developed countries and greatly affects the use of primary and secondary health services and social care [41, 42]. People with severe mental illness require a range of skilled professional care, with expertise, in their management. The focus on their mental health problems can lead to the under-diagnosis of life-threatening illnesses and to the under-recognition and under-treatment of symptoms.

Dementia can legitimately be seen as a terminal illness and patients die with this mental illness [43]. Further, new variant Creutfeldt-Jacob disease (CJD) may also become a significant cause of dementia in younger people in the future. Recent research has indicated that many patients with dementia have symptoms and health needs comparable with those who have cancer, but for longer periods of time [44]. These results indicate that many patients with dementia have unmet disease-related concerns, which although can be met by generalist health and social services support, are, nevertheless, amenable to specialist palliative care.

People with learning disabilities

It has been argued that people with learning disabilities are amongst the most socially excluded and vulnerable groups in the UK today. Very few have jobs, live in their own homes, or have real choice over who cares for them. Producing precise information on the number of people with learning disabilities in the population is difficult. The Government's White Paper, *Valuing People* [45] suggests that there may be approximately 210,000 people described as having severe and profound learning disabilities and approximately 1.2 million people with mild or moderate learning disabilities in England.

Empirical knowledge of the general health needs of people with learning disabilities has increased in recent years. Research indicates that this client group has more demanding health needs than the general population and is also experiencing increased life expectancy, especially among people with Down's syndrome [46]. Increased life expectancy has in part been due to advances in medical treatments that are now available to this group of people. This, however, has resulted in the increased incidence of progressive disease, for example, myocardial and vascular disease, cancer and Alzheimer's disease [47]. Surveys have increasingly demonstrated that many people with learning disabilities have undetected conditions, which cause unnecessary suffering or reduce the quality or length of their lives [48–50].

Failure to diagnose advanced disease for this population group may mean that not only are treatment options limited, but also that the window for accessing palliative care becomes truncated. This prevents both patients and their caregivers from adequately planning and preparing for the final stages of their advanced illness [51]. Once the opportunity for palliative care presents, problems continue. Little is known about how people with learning disabilities experience pain and evidence suggests they may experience difficulties communicating its presence [52]. Other symptoms, for example nausea, fatigue or dysphagia are likewise poorly communicated by individuals or poorly understood by health care professionals, and this may result in their suboptimal assessment and management [38, 53].

People from black and minority ethnic groups

Ethnicity is difficult to define, but most definitions reflect self-identification with cultural traditions that provide both a meaningful social identity and also boundaries between groups [54]. People from minority ethnic backgrounds represent approximately 7.9% of the population in the UK. Although there is a significant lack of data about people from minority ethnic communities, the available data confirms that some groups experience disproportionate disadvantage across the board. More often they are concentrated in deprived areas and suffer all the problems that affect the other people in these places. But people from minority ethnic communities also suffer the consequences of overt and inadvertent racial discrimination—individual and institutional—and an inadequate recognition and understanding of other complexities they may experience, for example barriers like language, cultural and religious differences.

Although a number of explanations have been advanced to account for the poor up-take of services among black and minority ethnic groups, few studies have actually quantified the palliative care needs and problems of patients with advanced disease and their carers in different communities (Box 3.3). Recently, a study in an inner London health authority demonstrated that first generation black Caribbean patients with advanced disease experienced restricted access to some specialist palliative care services compared to native-born white UK patients in the same category [55], yet an analysis of local provision revealed no lack of palliative care services [56]. This is an example of under-utilisation of palliative care services by the black Caribbean community at the end-of-life supports' recent research among other minority ethnic communities [57, 58].

Box 3.3 Black and minority ethnic social exclusion at the end of life: why does it occur?

Social deprivation
Low socio-economic status has been positively linked to an increased likelihood of hospital deaths although this would apply equally to all population groups [28]

Knowledge of specialist palliative care services and poor communication
There is a growing body of evidence that black and ethnic minorities are not adequately aware of specialist palliative care services available to them [78–80]

Ethno-centralism
Demand for services may be influenced by the 'ethno-centric' outlook of palliative care services, discouraging black and minority ethnic groups from making use of relevant provisions [79]

Attitudes to palliative care
Barriers to health care that the poor and the disenfranchised have traditionally encountered may affect their receptivity to palliative care [77]

Dissatisfaction with health care
Uptake of health and social services among certain minority ethnic communities has revealed lower utilisation of services due to dissatisfaction of services [81]

Mistrust
Evidence from USA to support the contention that black and minority ethnic groups are less likely than white patients to trust the motivations of doctors who discuss end-of-life care with them [82]

Gatekeepers
Some health care professionals act as 'gatekeepers' to services among minority ethnic groups contributing to lower referral rates [83]

Refugees and asylum seekers

Estimating the total number of refugees and asylum seekers worldwide is difficult, as definitions differ widely. In the UK, refugees are defined as those who have been granted indefinite leave to remain or have permanent residence in the UK. Asylum seekers are those who have submitted an application for protection under the Geneva Convention and are waiting for the claim to be decided by the Home Office. At the time of writing there are about 230,000 people in this category living in the UK and the numbers continue to increase [59]. Refugees and asylum seekers form significant minority populations in many UK towns and cities. It is extremely difficult to obtain demographic information on refugees and asylum seekers at the local level in the UK, and this lack of information represents one of the difficulties in developing services that are accessible for these groups [60].

Although refugees and asylum seekers are often grouped together, they are not necessarily a homogenous group and have varying experiences and needs [61]. Many refugees have health problems, for example parasitic or nutritional diseases [62], and diseases such as hepatitis, tuberculosis and HIV and AIDS, which frequently overlap with problems of social deprivation. Their health problems are also amplified by family separation, hostility and racism from the host population, poverty and social isolation [60, 62, 63].

Individuals from sub-Saharan Africa, many of whom may be refugees and asylum seekers, make up the second largest group of people affected by HIV in the UK [64]. They are more likely to be socially disadvantaged and isolated, be much less aware of the health care to which they are entitled, and be more likely to present only when symptomatic. Experience has demonstrated that this patient group continues to require palliative care despite the advances made with highly active antiretroviral therapy (HAART). This is because they tend to present late with AIDS related illnesses and have higher rates of tuberculosis, both of which are linked to a poorer prognosis. For many patients, who do not have a GP and are reluctant to register with one, lack of a stable home environment and reluctance to access local services may mean that dying at home is not an option [65] (see also Chapter 14).

Drug users

In England, during the year 2000–2001, the number of drug misusers reported as receiving treatment from both drug misuse agencies and

GPs was approximately 118,500 [66]. There is very little literature on how drug misusers utilise specialist palliative care services. The paucity of literature that does exist focuses mainly on issues of pain control for this population. A single exploratory study in the USA explored the experiences of hospices providing care to intravenous HIV/AIDs drug users [67]. The survey revealed that the provision of community palliative care for these patients was frequently problematic because of patients' poor living conditions, many of which were considered unsafe to visit. Other challenges included health care professionals' concerns that patients might be resistant to hospice care if they perceived hospice as a barrier to their continued drug use.

It has been suggested that drug users require a modified health care system, which understands and considers the problems of dug users; but that initiation and maintenance of contact may require a variety of initiatives [68]. Morrison and Ruben [69] similarly argue that services need to deliver care to these groups in imaginative and innovative ways, which are not judgmental and encourage contact without reinforcing traditional stereotypes. Without appropriate services, they argue, high levels of mortality amongst drug users will continue.

Prisoners

In 2003, there were an estimated 73,500 prisoners in England and Wales of whom 5400 were serving life sentences [70]. Historically, prison health care has been organised outside the NHS. This has given rise to questions about equity, standards, professional isolation and whether the Prison Service has the capacity to carry out its health care function [71]. The Government is now committed to developing a range of proposals aimed at improving health care for prisoners. The aims include ensuring that prisoners have access to the same quality and range of health care services as the general public receives from the NHS, by promoting a closer partnership between the NHS and the Prison Service at local, regional and national levels.

To date, very little British literature has focused on the palliative care needs of prisoners and the literature available is largely descriptive or relates to single case histories [72, 73]. More research has taken place in the USA where a number of palliative care programmes have been developed for prisoners, for example, the Louisiana State Penitentiary at Angola [74]. This has been largely because in Louisiana, where the sentencing laws are tougher than of any other state in the USA and the courts hand out a disproportionate number of life sentences, few of these prisoners are granted parole. As a result an estimated 85% of Angola's 5200 inmates will grow old and die in prison [74].

There are a number of problems in introducing palliative care into prisons, not least the mutual distrust between staff and prisoners. Effective symptom control, particularly adequate pain control, can be difficult under these circumstances. Drugs to manage pain control may be used for other illicit purposes. Also visiting from family and friends can be restricted, mainly because the prison may be located at quite some distance from family and home.

Conclusions and implications for policy

Since the introduction of the National Health Service, health care has been more widely extended to sections of the population. However, universal access to care and treatment remains elusive and care provided by the modern hospice movement, with laudable aspirations to extend the right to care as widely as possible, has been shown to be inequitable on a number of fronts. This chapter has revealed that silent sections of the population are ignored or inadequately served at the end of life. Solutions to the problems come in many forms, none of which will be successful in isolation.

First, there is an urgent need to raise public awareness of palliative care services and to provide public education about the care provided to reduce any misconceptions about services that may be influencing access. Information provided to NHS Direct and Primary Care Trusts (PCTs) may also be important.

Second, health and social care professionals' knowledge and attitude towards the excluded populations must be improved [19]. Third, regional implementation groups who look after and plan palliative care services in their own areas offer the potential to explore strategy at an epidemiological and corporate level. Examples include, those published by the Welsh Office, Palliative Care in Wales: Towards Evidence Based Purchasing [75] and Palliative Care for Londoners: Needs, Experience, Outcomes and Future Strategy [76], both of which have established a framework for the development of local policies and recommended closer links between agencies involved in the provision of care. Significantly, both documents have highlighted equity of access to high quality care. Furthermore, they have recommended devoting more resources to research that explore the unmet palliative care needs of the socially excluded, given the paucity of evidence in certain areas. Without more comprehensive information moving these complex agendas forward remains challenging.

Lastly, the charitable sector is uniquely suited to support new ideas that extend care to the point where they can be integrated in society and become the social norm rather than the exception. Despite differences in the funding arrangements of care in the USA, the Robert Wood Johnson Foundation has been successful is pump-priming pilot projects to increase access to palliative care to socially deprived communities [77]. In recent years, the UK has followed suit (Box 3.4). Although palliative care cannot completely remove the impact of the advanced disease, approaches must be sought to extend its lessons to all those who stand to benefit from its increasing sophistication.

Box 3.4 Example of UK charitable sector-sponsored venture to manage social exclusion of patients with advanced cancer and their families

A '*Palliative Care Pathway*', funded through the *New Opportunities Fund*, has recently been developed in North West London focusing specifically on previously 'hard-to-access', socially excluded, patients with advanced cancer and their families. The aim of the project is to develop referral criteria, an inter-disciplinary core assessment tool, and associated documentation for use by health and social care professionals to improve end-of-life decisions for pathway patients and their caregivers.

References

1 Hinton J. *Dying*. London: Penguin, 1967.
2 Higginson IJ. Health care needs assessment: Palliative and terminal care. In: Stevens A, Raftery J eds. *Health Care Needs Assessment*. Oxford: Wessex Institute of Public Health Medicine, 1997: 183–260.
3 Ingelton C, Skilbeck J, Clark D. Needs assessment for palliative care: three projects compared. *Palliat Med* 2004; 15: 398–404.
4 WHO Expert Committee. Cancer pain relief and palliative care. Geneva: World Health Organisation Technical Report Series. World Health Organisation Technical Report Series No. 804. 1990. Geneva: World Health Organisation.
5 World Health Organisation. Report on five countries: palliative care in emerging sub Saharan Africa. 2002. Geneva: WHO.
6 Soper K. *On Human Needs*. Sussex: Harvester Press, 1981.
7 Bradshaw J. The concept of social need. *New Society*. 1972; 30: 640–643.
8 Stevens A, Raferty J. Introduction. In: Stevens A, Raftery J eds. *Health Care Needs Assessment: The Epidemiologically Based Needs Assessment Reviews* Vol 1. Oxford: Radcliffe Medical Press, 1994.

9 Franks PJ. Need for palliative care. In: Bosanquet N, Salisbury C eds. *Providing a Palliative Care Service: Towards an Evidence Base*. Oxford: Oxford University Press, 1999: 43–56.
10 Murtagh FEM, Preston M, Higginson IJ. Patterns of dying: palliative care for non-malignant disease. *Clin Med* 2004; 4(1): 39–44.
11 Clark D, Malson H. Key issues in palliative care needs assessment. *Prog Palliat Care* 1995; 3(2): 53–55.
12 Hart JT. The inverse care law. *Lancet* 1971; (1): 405–412.
13 Townsend P, Davison N. *Inequalities in Health: The Black Report*. Harmondsworth: Penguin, 1982.
14 Whitehead M. *Inequalities in Health: The Black Report and The Health Divide*. In: Townsend P, ed. Harmondsworth: Penguin, 1992.
15 Department of Health. Inequalities in Health: Report of an Independent Inquiry Chaired by Sir Donald Acheson. London: The Stationary Office, 1998.
16 Goddard M, Smith P. Equity of access to health care services: Theory and evidence from the UK. *Soc Sci Med* 2001; 53: 1149–62.
17 Addington-Hall JM. *Positive Partnerships: Palliative Care for Adults with Severe Mental Health Problems*. London: National Council for Hospices and Specialist Palliative Care Services, 2000.
18 National Council for Hospices and Specialist Palliative Care Services. *The Palliative Care Survey* 1999. London: National Council for Hospices and Specialist Palliative Care Services, 2000.
19 O'Neill J, Marconi K. Access to palliative care in the USA: why emphasize vulnerable populations? *J R Soc Med* 2001; 94: 452–454.
20 Seymour J, Clark D, Philp I. Palliative care and geriatric medicine: shared concerns, shared challenges. *Palliat Med* 2001; 15(4): 269–270.
21 Seymour J, Clark D, Marples R. Palliative care and policy in England: a review of health improvement plans for 1999–2003. *Palliat Med* 2002; 16(1): 5–11.
22 Higginson IJ, Goodwin DM. Needs assessment in day care. In: Hearn J, Myers K, eds. *Palliative Day Care in Practice*. Oxford: Oxford University Press, 2001: 12–22.
23 Barratt H. The health of the excluded. *BMJ* 2001; 323: 240.
24 Social Exclusion Unit. Preventing Social Exclusion. 2001. London: HMSO.
25 Walker E, Walker C. Britain Divided: the Growth of Social Exclusion in the 1980s and 1990s. 1997. London: Child Poverty Action Group.
26 Office for National Statistics. Social Trends. 2000. London: HMSO.
27 Sen-Gupta GJA, Higginson IJ. Home care in advanced cancer: a systematic literature review of preferences for and associated factors. *Psycho-Oncology* 1998; 7: 57–67.
28 Higginson IJ, Webb D, Lessof L. Reducing hospital beds for patients with advanced cancer. *Lancet* 1994; 344(8919): 409.
29 Sims A, Radford J, Doran K, Page H. Social class variation in place of death. *Palliat Med* 1997; 11(5): 369–373.
30 Soni Raleigh V, Kiri A. Life expectancy in England: variations and trends by gender, health authority and level of deprivation. *J Epidemiol Comm Health* 1997; 51: 649–658.
31 Cartwright A. Social class differences in health and care in the year before death. *J Epidemiol Comm Health* 1992; 46: 54–57.

32 Clark C. Social deprivation increases workload in palliative care of terminally ill patients. *BMJ* 1997; 314: 1202.
33 Higginson IJ, Jarman B, Astin P, Dolan S. Do social factors affect where patients die: an analysis of 10 years of cancer deaths in England. *J Public Health Med* 1999; 21: 22–28 1999; 21: 22–28.
34 Warnes AM. The changing elderly population: aspects of diversity. *Rev Clin Gerontol* 1991; 1: 185–194.
35 Age Concern. Turning Your Back On Us. Older People and the NHS. 1999. London: Age Concern.
36 Department of Health. They Look After Their Own, Don't They? CI (98) 2. 1998. London: Department of Health.
37 Eve A, Higginson IJ. Minium dataset activity for hospice and hospital palliative care services in the UK 1997/98. *Palliat Med* 2000; 14: 395–404.
38 Bernabei R, Gambassi G, Lapane K, Landi F, Gatsonis C, Dunlop R et al. Management of pain in elderly patients with cancer. *JAMA* 1998; 279: 1877–1882.
39 Katz J, Sidell M, Komaromy C. Understanding palliative care in residential and nursing homes. *Int J Palliat Nurs* 1999; 5(2): 58–64.
40 Komaromy C, Sidell M, Katz J. Dying in care: factors which influence the quality of terminal care given to older people in residential and nursing homes. *Int J Palliat Nurs* 2000; 6(4): 192–205.
41 Koffman J, Fulop NJ, Pashley D, Coleman K. No way out: the use of elderly mentally ill acute and assessment psychiatric beds in north and south Thames regions. *Age & Ageing* 1996; 25: 268–272.
42 Koffman J, Taylor S. The needs of caregivers. *Elderly Care* 1997; 9(6): 16–19.
43 Addington-Hall J. *Positive Partnerships: Palliative Care for Adults with Severe Mental Health Problems.* 2000. London: National Council for Hospices and Specialist Palliative Care Services.
44 McCarthy M, Addington-Hall J, Altmann D. The experience of dying from dementia: a retrospective study. *Int J Geriatric Psychiatry* 1997; 12: 404–409 1997; 12: 404–409.
45 Secretary of State for Health. Valuing People: A New Strategy for Learning Disability for the 21st Century. CM 5086. 2001. London: HMSO.
46 NHS Executive. Signpost for successful commissioning and providing health services for people with learning difficulties. 1998. London: HMSO.
47 Jancar J. Consequences of a longer life for the mentally handicapped. *Am J Ment Retard* 1993; 98(2): 285–292.
48 Tuffrey-Wijne I. Care of the terminally ill. *Learn Disabil Pract* 1998; 1(1): 8–11.
49 Howells G. Are the medical needs of mentally handicapped adults being met? *Br J Gen Pract* 1986; 36(449): 453.
50 Keenan P, McIntosh P. Learning disabilities and palliative care. *Palliat Care Today* 2000; 11–13.
51 Brown H. The service needs of people with learning disabilities who are dying. *Psychol Res* 2000; 10(2): 39–47.
52 Beirsdorff K. Pain intensity and indifference: alternative explanations for some medical catastrophes. *Ment Retard* 1991; 29(6): 359–62.
53 Tuffrey-Wijne I. Palliative care and learning disabilities. *Nurs Times* 1997; 93(31): 50–51.

54 Senior A, Bhopal R. Ethnicity as a variable in epidemiological research. *BMJ* 1994; 309: 327–330.
55 Koffman J, Higginson IJ. Accounts of satisfaction with health care at the end of life: a comparison of first generation black Caribbeans and white patients with advanced disease. *Palliat Med* 2001; 15: 337–345.
56 Eve A, Smith AM, Tebbit P. Hospice and palliative care in the UK 1994-5, including a summary of trends 1990-5. *Palliat Med* 1997; 11(1): 31–43.
57 Farrell J. Do disadvantaged and minority ethnic groups receive adequate access to palliative care services? Glasgow University., 2000.
58 Skilbeck J, Corner J, Beech N, Clark D., Hughes P, Douglas HR et al. Clinical nurse specialists in palliative care. Part 1. A description of the Macmillan Nurse caseload. *Palliat Med* 2002; 16(4): 285–296.
59 Burnett A, Peel M. What brings asylum seekers to the United Kingdom? *BMJ* 2001; 322: 485–488.
60 Bardsley M, Storkey M. Estimating the numbers of refugees in London. *J Pub Health Med* 2000; 22(3): 406–412.
61 Burnett A, Fassil Y. Meeting the Health Needs of Refugees and Asylum Seekers in the UK: An Information and Resource Pack for Health Workers. 2002. London: Department of Health.
62 Jones D, Gill PS. Refugees and primary care: tackling the inequalities. *BMJ* 1998; 317: 1444–1446.
63 Kisely S, Stevens M, Hart B, Douglas C. Health issues of asylum seekers and refugees. Australian and New Zealand *J Pub Health* 2002; 26(1): 8–10.
64 Brogan G, George R. HIV/AIDS: symptoms and the impact of new treatments. *Palliat Med* 1999; 1(4): 104–110.
65 Easterbrook P, Meadway J. The changing epidemiology of HIV infection: new challenges for HIV palliative care. *J R Soc Med* 2001; 94(442): 448.
66 Department of Health. Statistical Press Release; Statistics from the regional drug misuse databases on drug misusers in treatment in England, 2000/01. 2001. London: Department of Health.
67 Cox C. Hospice care for injection drug using AIDS patients.*The Hospice J* 1999; 14(1): 13–24.
68 Brettle RP. Injection drug use-related HIV infection. In: Adler MW, ed. *ABC of AIDS*. London: BMJ Publishing, 2001.
69 Morrison CL, Ruben SM. The development of healthcare services for drug misusers and prostitutes. *Postgrad Med J* 1995; 71: 593–597.
70 Monthly Prison Population Brief, England and Wales. 2003. London: Home Office.
71 Joint Prison Service & National Health Service Executive Working Group. The future organisation of prison health care. 1999. London: Department of Health.
72 Oliver D, Cook L. The specialist palliative care of prisoners. *Eur J Palliat Care* 1998; 5(3): 70–80.
73 Wilford T. Developing effective palliative care within a prison setting. *I J Palliat Nurs* 2001; 7(11): 528–530.
74 Project for Dying in America. Dying in prison: a growing problem emerges from behind bars. *PDIA Newsletter* 3, 1–3. 1998. Project for Dying in America.
75 Welsh Office. Palliative Care in Wales: Towards Evidence Based Purchasing. 1996. Cardiff: Welsh Office.

76 Higginson IJ. *The Palliative Care for Londoners: Needs, Experience, Outcomes and Future Strategy*. 2001. London: London Regional Strategy Group for Palliative Care.
77 Gibson R. Palliative care for the poor and disenfranchised: a view from the Robert Wood Johnson Foundation. *J R Soc Med* 2001; 94: 486–489.
78 Harron-Iqbal H, Field D, Parker H, Iqbal Z. Palliative care services in Leicester. *Int J Palliat Nurs* 1995; 1: 114–116 1995; 1: 114–116.
79 Smaje C, Field D. Absent minorities? Ethnicity and the use of palliative care services. In: Hockey J, Small N, eds. *Death, Gender and Ethnicity*. London: Routledge, 1997: 142–165.
80 Kurent JE, DesHarnais S, Jones W, Hennessy W, Levey G, Ott V et al. End-of-life decision making for patients with end-stage CHF and terminal malignancies: impact of ethnic and cultural variables. *J Palliat Med* 5(1), 1999: 2002.
81 Lindsay J, Jagger C, Hibbert M, Peet S, Moledina F. Knowledge, uptake and the availability of health and social services among Asian Gujarati and white persons. *Ethn Health* 1997; 2: 59–69.
82 Caralis PV, Davis B, Wright K, Marcial E. The influence of ethncity and race on attitudes toward advanced directives, life-prolonging treatments, and euthanasia. *J Clin Ethics* 1993; 4: 155–165.
83 Equity, ethnicity, and health care. University of Sheffield: Social Policy Association, 1995.

4: User Voices in Palliative Care

NEIL SMALL

Introduction

This chapter explores the contribution of user voices in palliative care in three areas:

- The impact user voices have on individual professionals.
- The way users can shape what organisations do.
- How national policy engages with, and reflects, user views.

'User' is a rather inelegant word to describe a person.[1] Its etymology suggests something mechanical, 'to employ for a purpose', or passive, 'to be accustomed to'. But it is also close to the more positive 'useful', 'able to produce a good result'. In this chapter 'user' will include those people who are undergoing palliative care or who have received palliative care. As palliative care offers a service wider than that of the immediate patient it also includes family and friends and the bereaved. Users do not have to join together to have influence, they do not even have to knowingly seek to effect change. But some people actively want to use their experiences to help shape what they, and others like them, experience when they need palliative care. This group might include patients, carers and those who define themselves as having been affected by terminal illness. Such people, when they join with others, constitute the collective expression of user voices.

It is possible to categorise groups as either 'user', those that engage with wider structures, or self-help/support, in which the focus is more internal. In practice, each sort of group is likely to undertake both activities—with different emphases. Even groups that are avowedly 'support groups', and who say they do not engage in consultation with outside organisations, can produce in their members the sort of enhanced knowledge, esteem and solidarity that allows people to act more effectively in their world. In what follows, I will discuss national organisations that look to influence wider structures and also offer information and support. I will consider self-help and

[1] Other words are even more problematic: patient is too narrow, consumer too passive, customer too mercantile, person with cancer too clumsy and too limiting.

support groups and will also look at user groups working with NHS organisations.

Users influence the practice of individual professionals. In the stories they tell of their experiences and in the interactions they have with care providers, users are drawing on the sense they have of their own physical, emotional and social world. This is their embodied knowledge. It shapes their subjective assessment of needs. Professionals incorporate this sort of knowing into their own structures of tacit knowledge, the 'know-how' they bring to their jobs. This interaction is a manifestation of user involvement at the level of one-to-one communication (or at most communication within a small group, a family and a professional team).

At a group level users and professionals come together in committees, working groups and the like. This level can be somewhere users experience a sense of solidarity and this can, in itself, produce benefits for users. But this level can also give a base from which they can be assertive about their needs. It is a level that interacts with organisational structures via systems of collaboration and consultation. It requires, for its success, that all involved be prepared to learn from others.

Finally there is a societal level, manifest in legislative provision and top-down directives. It can be understood using constructs including consumerism, and governmentality (explained below). In the UK the government is rhetorically committed to 'a patient centred health service' but what does this mean in practice?

I will argue that understanding the contribution of user voices in palliative care involves thinking about structures and processes. But it also involves thinking about training and support and, fundamentally, about how different ways of knowing can be combined. While many may think it a self-evident truth that we should encourage user voices to be expressed and acted upon there are far-reaching complicating factors. These include issues of equity, whose voices; of efficacy, how do we use evidence and of justice, does involvement impinge on the ability to seek redress?

Table 4.1 summarises the three levels of user voice and identifies the social processes they require and the mechanisms necessary to pursue their further utilisation.

The level of the individual: embodied and tacit knowledge

Key works in understanding the shortcomings of existing services and proposing what would better serve those near the end of their lives, have drawn heavily on the observations of individuals and on the

Table 4.1 Levels of user involvement

	Individual/couple/ family	Group	Societal
Type of social process	Embodied/tacit knowledge	Social solidarity	Consumerism/ governmentality
Level of activity	Learning from the patient	Joint working	'User at the heart'
How implemented	Education/training	Organisational structures and procedures	Legislation Inspection

reported words of patients. Much of the power of Strauss and Glasers' critique of death in hospital comes from the case history of Mrs Abel, a 54-year-old woman dying of cancer. While they illuminate the idea of dying trajectories and different forms of awareness, much of the works' impact comes from these two sociologists recording, "the lingering death of an increasingly isolated and rejected woman experiencing ever-growing pain", told over one hundred and fifty pages [1]. Mrs Abel's last words before the operation, from which she never recovered were, "I hope I die" [2–4].

In Elisabeth Kübler-Ross's, *On Death and Dying* we have transcripts of interviews with terminally ill patients. Mrs S talks of the many losses in her life; her parents' divorce and then her own divorce, the death of her daughter and of her father. Mrs C, another patient, describes how she felt she could not face her own death because of the pressure of family obligations that surrounded her [5]. Here Kübler-Ross is using the words of those interviewed to illuminate the difficulties that stand in the way of the dying communicating their wishes. She is saying that if one can listen, openly, then staff can learn and patients can be better cared for.

In the early days of the modern hospice movement, the voices of patients fundamentally shaped the emerging service. The founder of the modern hospice movement, Dame Cicely Saunders, has described the inspiration that caring for patients gave her both about the need for a new way of caring for people at the end of their lives and about the shape of services that was required. Specifically, the death of David Tasma in 1948 made her realise that what was needed was the best that science could provide, allied to somewhere a person would be listened to and helped to feel worthwhile, a coming together of the mind and the heart [6]. Other patients helped shape the identity of the hospice; Mrs G suggesting the name St Christopher's [7] and a group of long-stay patients at St Joseph's in Hackney—Alice, Terry and Louie—acted as a sounding board, today we might call this an expert patient group. The accounts of pain and then of the impact of effective pain control for Mrs M encapsulated the justification for this new way of working:

> *Before I came here the pain was so bad that if anyone came into the room I would say, "Please don't touch me, please don't come near me." But now it seems as if something has come between me and the pain, it feels like a nice thing wrapped round me* [8].

These examples of the impact of patients' voices, two from the USA and one from the UK, are illustrative of the importance of 'service users' guiding the emerging understanding of end-of-life care that developed into modern hospice, palliative care and bereavement services. They are important because they remind us that the idea of patient involvement is not new and that it does not have to have a prescribed institutional and procedural context to be influential. It requires professionals being open to different sorts of knowledge. Stories of illness and of loss have a claim to truth because they are embodied ways of knowing. Captured via narrative, they are important because they are subjective, and with that subjectivity comes the opportunity to locate the need in the context of the life. This context is vital if one is to address the 'total care for total pain' that is at the heart of hospice and palliative care [9, 10].

Recognising the importance of listening and the true claims of the subjective voice has to be continuously restated. Each new professional has to balance expert and technical, now evidence based, knowledge with embodied knowledge. The philosopher and scientist, Polyani, drew a distinction between what he terms tacit and explicit knowledge. Tacit captures the mental models, beliefs and values we have and the 'know-how' that has been transmitted through conversation and observation. Explicit knowledge is codified, formal and can be transmitted without direct person-to-person interaction. It is in the articles and books we read. Much of explicit knowledge is filtered through tacit knowledge. That is, we incorporate what we learn about the world with what we 'know' about the world [11]. But professional training and the reinforcement of work and organisational cultures can create powerful counter forces. Consequently, even with such a wealth of experience, professionals still get things wrong. They still emphasise the parts rather than the whole. They still forget the person, in the family and in the society. They still focus, just like

Glaser and Strauss observed thirty-six years ago, on the 'tumour in bed number three'. This is something exemplified in John Hoyland's 1997 newspaper account of the death of his stepfather, Jack Sutherland: "There were lots of people in charge of different parts of Jack's body, but no one was in charge of Jack" [12]. It is also evident in Jackie Stacey's cultural study of cancer, published in 1997, in which she recounts her own diagnosis of teratoma. "I am left with the news. Alone, but surrounded by strangers. I don't think they planned it this way. I don't think they planned it at all. Perhaps that's the problem" [13].

We have, in our education, training, staff development and supervision to make people realise that there are different ways of knowing. The lessons of palliative care's history is that vision and compassion, coming from working with and listening to the patient, gets things done and it gets them done well when this is allied with the analytic, with the best science.

The level of the group: solidarity and learning organisations

There are many barriers that inhibit the development of group activity amongst people who need palliative care or amongst families and friends who care for them. There is the burden of symptoms, either deteriorating health or episodic periods of great need; stigma; a reluctance to look to the future; geographic dispersal and a problem that a cause to come together does not seem apparent until needs are great. There is a barrier that comes out of a pessimism that action will not produce change and an anxiety about being with others who have a similar condition to one's own [14]. Despite these formidable barriers there are many groups made up of people with palliative care needs and their families and friends, and these groups engage with a wide range of issues and provide, or contribute to, many services.

The rise of user groups in health can be attributed to two contrasting phenomenon:

- A decision by the powerful to sponsor such groups.
- The demands of service users.

The government has moved to a position of supporting user involvement for two reasons. First, out of belief that one can think of patients as consumers of health care. This leads to an approach where consumer power can be used as a counter-balance to professional power, seen here as inherently conservative. This is the 'market' approach to change [15]. Second, and linked to 'New Labour', has been the development of governmentality. This is the move from seeing governing as something that goes on amongst a few people in centralised institutions to a way of thinking that sees it in, "a myriad of practices that proliferate throughout society" [16]. In the market the empowered consumer is the archetypal actor, in governmentality it is the active citizen.

If there has been top-down encouragement of user involvement, there has also been bottom-up demand. User involvement has been taken as well as given. It has been demanded for two reasons. First, because of a perceived failure of organisations that do not listen to users. Second, because coming together generates feelings of strength, and strength leads to action. In the 1970s and early 1980s a number of influential critiques of the shortcomings of professional knowledge in health and the damage that it can do were published [17, 18]. These sort of attacks lead to questioning of the pre-eminence of medical power. At the same time in some areas, traditionally defined as within the remit of medicine, there has been a long history of self-mobilisation and group activity that challenges definitions, generates its own information and develops independent services. Groups concerned with childbirth practices, the disability movement [19], groups of current and former mental health service users and learning disability groups provide examples [20]. In initiatives such as these we began to see the models of civil rights and 'new social movements'[2] as more appropriate paradigms for understanding what was happening than that of consumerism or governmentality [21, 22].

Closer to the remit of palliative care there have been self-help and user groups focussing on cancer, in particular breast cancer, on neurological disease, and groups linked to people with HIV and AIDS. Some of these groups grew into national organisations, the Multiple Sclerosis Society or the Terrence Higgins Trust (for HIV and AIDS) for example. Sometimes groups come together under umbrella organisations, the Neurological Alliance or Cancerlink are examples here. The latter is a nationwide service co-ordinated by the charity Macmillan Cancer Relief [23]. There are national organisations. Some offer a wide range of support and services for people with any cancer diagnosis. BACUP is an example of such a group. There are cancer site specific groups,

[2] 'New Social Movements' were typified by environmentalist groups such as the Greens, peace groups, gay rights and the womens' movement. They were seen as reacting to bureaucratisation, technocratic interference in all aspects of civic life, corporatism and sexism. They were 'new' in so far as they did not emphasise class as a defining characteristic nor party political programmes as paramount. Their values were 'non-negotiable' rather than starting points for negotiation.

OVACOME for women with ovarian cancer, six national breast cancer groups are listed in the 2003–2004 *Directory of cancer self-help and support* [24], the Roy Castle Lung Cancer Foundation has a head office and 17 branches, there are groups focusing on leukaemia, and so on. There are groups for specific sorts of people, children, adolescents, the over 50s (Action for Eileen), Gays Can, Chai Cancer Care for Jewish people, groups for black and minority ethnic communities (Black and Minority Ethnic Network and Cancer Black Care for example). Other groups have a focus on specific treatments, R.A.G.E (for radiography), colostomy groups and the urostomy association (for those who have had their bladder removed).[3] Similarly, there are national groups for people with motor neurone disease, Parkinson's disease, Huntington's disease and other conditions that may require palliative care such as Alzheimer's disease and chronic liver disease.

There are training events organised for people who belong to these groups and information packs, all designed to maximise the potential for service-user involvement and influence. For example, training developed for lay members of the Maternity Services Liaison Committee has been used to train cancer service users as part of the Cancer VOICES Project [25, 26]. Macmillan Cancer Relief offers a Cancer Support Certificate for volunteers and a Living Well with Cancer project for patients [27].

There are considerable potential benefits in this sort of group activity. The act of coming together and appreciating that they are experiencing things that others also experience can be validating, fostering solidarity and a sense of social inclusion. Additionally groups can offer specific types of help, information, assistance with specialist areas, advice on available services and welfare benefits. Groups may also be involved in collaborations with service providers. Finally, groups may organise their own services, perhaps using professionals/experts for specific inputs.

There are, however, some major challenges to groups having an impact and reflecting the views of service users. First, there are challenges at the system level. There has to be a mechanism that ensures groups have appropriate access to professionals and to the machinery of decision-making and service scrutiny. This access should afford

[3] Some of the names chosen for groups are a tonic in themselves, Bosom Pals and Bosom Buddies and, in Wakefield, Breast of Friends (breast cancer); 'Bottoms Up' a London colorectal cancer support group; About Face in Dorset, Guise and Dolls in London for head and neck cancer support; Tongue 'n'Cheek club for oral cancer and so on.

a contribution to priority setting as well as to ensure how what is decided is developed and implemented. There should be a change in professional attitude and a real sense of joint working. All of these requirements are problematic. They are also lacking in an evidence base. We know very little about how user involvement affects professional understanding, assumptions, behaviour and outcomes in terms of service priorities and delivery.

We are venturing here into the idea of teams learning together and the generation of learning organisations. There has to be a link between individual learning, team learning and organisation learning. Senge has highlighted the centrality of the team in this process [28] and Wenger describes communities of practice through which knowledge is created, information spread and identities generated [29]. Encouraging user involvement can affect two levels, one is changing the way everyone works and the second is changing the goals they are working for [30, 31]. Is having users involved essentially about effecting horizontal or vertical learning in an organisation? That is, does it impact on the way professionals understand and undertake their tasks, or does it help shape the policy and perceptions of the organisation, by having it rethink its core rationale for example?

In addition to system level uncertainties and challenges, there are problems at the service user level as well. First, are there specific kinds of people who become involved in speaking of their views as users? Does this approach attract the already advantaged and articulate [32]? Looking at patient participation with GPs, Rigge summed up a more generally applicable point: "Heartsink patients of heartsink GPs, who live on 'last resort' housing estates or in bed and breakfast accommodation, are not the obvious candidates for membership of a patient participation group, even though their views are the ones that most need to be heard" [33].

If there is a question about how socially representative 'users' are [34] there are also questions about the distribution of user groups by diagnosis. In 1998, the *Directory of Cancer Self-help and Support Groups* listed 155 specialist breast cancer groups, four testicular cancer groups, two for colorectal cancer and none specifically for lung cancer [24]. The proliferation of groups since 1998 has, in part, addressed the absolute absence of appropriate groups, although there is still a distribution that reflects the differential ability of subgroups to mobilise rather than any assessment of need. For example in 2003–2004 the Directory lists over 700 groups. If we take one area, West Yorkshire, 17 groups are listed. Eight welcome people with any cancer, five are for breast cancer, there is a group for those who have had oesophageal surgery, a throat cancer association, a laryngectomy trust and an ostomy group [27].

A further concern is the extent to which a pursuit of user voices too easily conflates the voices of the service users and their carers. The user-carer hybrid is too readily assumed. It masks many potential areas for difference, including the emphasis given to specific symptoms, the attitude towards information and the perception of the merits of planning for the future [14].

The societal level—legislating for a 'user centred' NHS

Much of the landscape of user voices in health is shaped at the societal level. We have seen that the rationale for government encouragement of user voices is complex. This section will begin by presenting the range of recent initiatives. As argued above, such initiatives arise from both a systematic plan for change and from the need to react to events, specifically the disclosure of things that have gone wrong—this is the pull and push model of policy making.

As part of continuing reform of the NHS the *NHS Plan*, in July 2000, affirmed that the new NHS would be 'designed around the patient' [36]. There would be a new statutory duty for the NHS to involve and consult the public [37]. At about the same time the public inquiry into the failure of heart surgeons at the Bristol Royal Infirmary, between 1984 and 1995, made pre-eminent amongst its 198 recommendations the need for more patient participation, involvement in decision making and better communication [38, 39].

There followed a series of new measures designed to put into place the structures and procedures that would enhance the move towards the NHS being patient-centred. Patient advice and liaison services (PALS) will be set up in every NHS Trust, including primary care trusts. These PALS can give first-line help and can also direct patients towards Independent Complaints Advocacy Support (ICAS). Each trust will have a Patient and Public Involvement Forum (PPIF), drawn from local people, with a wide range of responsibilities including monitoring PALS and identifying and making known gaps in service provision. The PPIF will be able to look at how far trusts are achieving desired and targeted health outcomes. Overseeing the new system will be a Commission for Patient and Public Involvement in Health (CPPIH).

But this linked local and national structure is not all. There will be formal requirements to survey patients' views on the services they receive. The results will be included in the performance rating system for trusts. There will be an annual Patients' Prospectus focused on how the findings of the survey are being addressed. Outside trusts, other bodies will have their own patient and public input, via a Citizens' Council into the National Institute for Clinical Excellence (NICE), for example. Networks, including cancer networks, have patient and public input. There are 51 cancer network groups or network locality groups, some with further sub-groups [27]. Research funding bodies, including the Department of Health, have user groups. For example 'Involve' has a remit to promote public involvement in NHS, public health and social care research.

Targeted at the 17.5 million people with chronic illness in the UK, there will be an 'Expert Patients' programme piloted between 2001 and 2004. This is designed around the axiom that, "the patient understands the disease better than the professional" and builds on work undertaken in the USA [40]. User-led self-management programmes will be supported. There is already some experience of this in the UK, for example training run by the Multiple Sclerosis Society and for cardiac rehabilitation based on the '*Heart Manual*'. There are also 13 specific programmes supported by the Long-Term Medical Conditions Alliance via its Living with Long-Term Illness (Lill) Project [41]. Trusts will be required to undertake expert patient programmes and their existence will inform the development of National Service Frameworks.

These policy initiatives, which impose requirements on NHS organisations, will formalise the terrain and set the climate for the expression of user voices in health care. They embrace mechanisms that will be open to people with palliative care needs. But the barriers to taking up these opportunities and to distributing this take-up equitably, as described above, remain. Formal committee structures, planning timetables and training courses may not be flexible enough to capture the contribution of those with changing palliative care needs. There are two further dangers. First that this top-down, wide ranging, structural innovation may not further the two aims of supporting the mutual listening of patient and professional, and the development of learning organisations. This will happen if instead of supporting a general cultural shift, the structural solution displaces the process changes as a focus of attention. Second, it might be that the energy and imagination of self-help groups is diverted into a narrower consultation route.

Any shift to a user centred NHS creates challenges in terms of strategic planning, the identification of new areas of concern and the harmonisation of public and patient views about priorities. Further, any user led planning has to be synergistic with financial planning frameworks, human resources and capital expenditure programmes [42].

Conclusion

Figure 4.1 summarises some of the components that would have to be in place to design a care context sensitive to user views. It would have to incorporate structure, process and attitudinal dimensions.

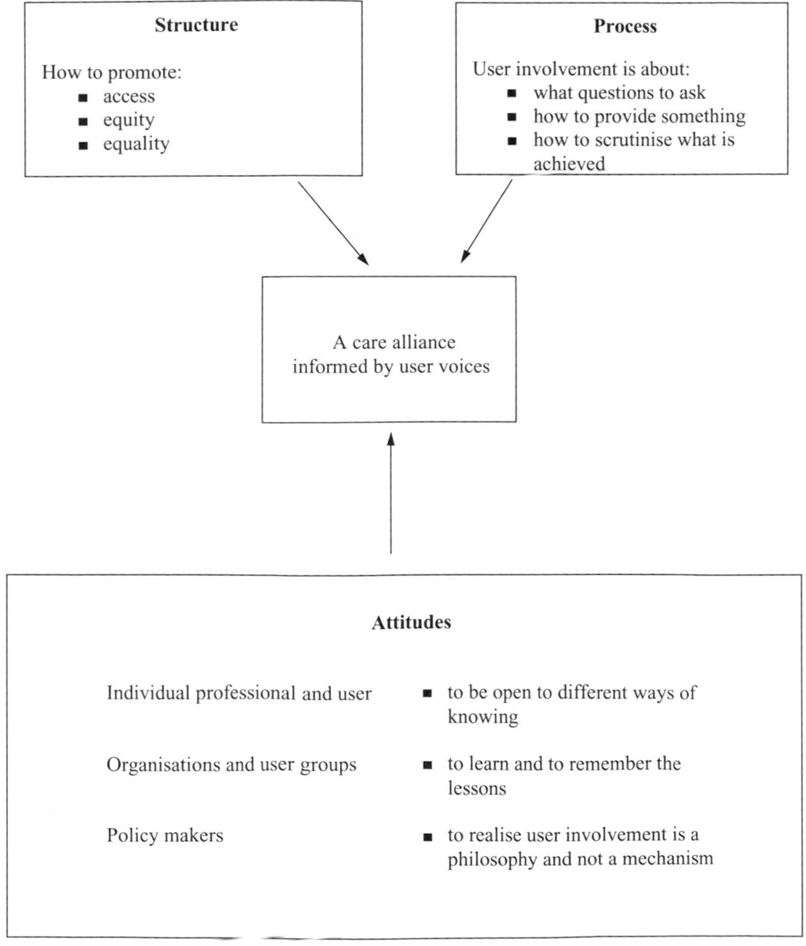

Fig. 4.1 What would make a care context informed by user voices.

Each area of activity requires staff to address possibilities and overcome barriers to enhanced user involvement. For example in relation to structure, how can people access user groups and how do such groups access professional systems? How do we reconcile a wish to redress inequalities and a wish to treat all equally—the equity-equality dilemma. In relation to process concerns, how do we help user groups frame agendas and not just react to externally set questions? How can we help people join in providing services and how can we involve them in auditing what has been achieved? In Figure 4.1 these areas of concern exist above a foundation of attitudinal change. That change has to occur and should be maintained in each of the levels of activity addressed in this chapter.

If we wish to promote the use and usefulness of user voices in palliative care we need to help systems of decision-making and of education change so that users are made more skilful at engaging with technical knowledge, and professionals are made more susceptible to embodied knowledge. We have to understand how bringing together users and a range of professionals creates an organisational structure that learns and changes together. Further, we have to devise a civic discourse than can embrace the potentially conflicting views of users and the public and that builds on, rather than diverts, the energy of user groups.

References

1 Plummer K.. *Documents of Life*. London: Sage, 2001: 132.
2 Strauss A, Glaser BG. *Anguish: A Case History of a Dying Trajectory*. Oxford: Martin Robertson, 1977: 21.
3 Glaser BG, Strauss A. *Awareness of Dying*, London: Weidenfeld and Nicolson, 1967.
4 Glaser BG, Strauss A. *Time for Dying*. Chicago: Aldine, 1968.
5 Kübler-Ross E. *On Death and Dying*. Chapter 10. London: Routledge, 1970.
6 Saunders, Dame Cicely. An Omega Interview. *Omega*, 1993; 27(94): 263–269.
7 Saunders. C. A patient .... *Nursing Times*, 1961; 31 March: 394–397.
8 Saunders, Dame Cicely.. A voice for the voiceless. In: Monroe B, Oliviere D. eds. *Patient Participation in Palliative Care*. Oxford: Oxford University Press, 2003: 3–8. Extracts from the interview with Mrs M were first broadcast on BBC Radio in February 1964 as part of a Good Cause Appeal.
9 Saunders C. The symptomatic treatment of incurable malignant disease. *Prescribers' J*, 1964; 4(4): 68–73.
10 Clark D, Seymour J. *Reflections on Palliative Care*. Buckingham: Open University Press, 1999.
11 Polanyi M. *The Tacit Dimension*. London: Routledge and Kegan Paul, 1967.
12 Hoyland J. Thanks, NHS, for a rotten way to die. *The Independent Tabloid*. 22 April 1997. Quoted in, Wilkie, P. The person, the patient and their carers. In:

Faull C, Carter Y, Woof R, eds. *Handbook of Palliative Care*. Oxford: Blackwell Science, 1998: 55–63.
13 Stacey J. *Teratologies*. London: Routledge, 1997: 105.
14 Small N, Rhodes P. *Too Ill to Talk? User Involvement in Palliative Care*. London: Routledge, 2000.
15 Small N. The changing National Health Service, user involvement and palliative care. In: Monroe B, Oliviere D. eds. *Patient Participation in Palliative Care*. Oxford: Oxford University Press, 2003: 9–22.
16 Marinetto M. Who wants to be an active citizen? *Sociology*, 2003; 37(1): 103–120.
17 Illich I.. *Medical Nemesis: The expropriation of Health*. London: Marion Boyars, 1975.
18 Kennedy I.. *The Unmasking of Medicine*. London: George Allen and Unwin, 1981.
19 Oliver M. *The Politics of Disablement*. London: Macmillan. See also, Campbell J, Oliver M. *Disability Politics: Understanding our Past, Changing our Future*. London: Routledge, 1996.
20 Goodley D. *Self-advocacy in the Lives of People with Learning Difficulties*. Buckingham: Open University Press, 2000.
21 Beresford P. Researching citizen-involvement: a collaborative or colonising enterprise? In: Barnes M, Wistow G. eds. *Researching User Involvement*. Leeds:Nuffield Institute for Health Service Studies, 1992.
22 Offe C. New social movements: challenging the boundaries of institutional politics. *Social Research*, 1985; 52(4): 833–834.
23 Bradburn J. Developments in user organizations. In: Monroe B, Oliviere D. eds. *Patient Participation in Palliative Care*. Oxford: Oxford University Press, 2003: 23–38.
24 Cancerlink. *Directory of Cancer Self-help and Support*. London: Cancerlink, 1998.
25 Bradburn J. Listening to the voices of experience. *Prof Nurse*, 2001; 16 No 5 (Supplement) 53–54.
26 Gott M, Stevens T, Small N Ahmedzai SH. *User Involvement in Cancer Care*. Bristol: Policy Press, 2000.
27 Macmillan Cancer Relief. *Directory of Cancer Self-help and Support Groups*. London: Macmillan Cancer Relief, 2004.
28 Senge P. *The Fifth Discipline: The Art and Practice of the Learning Organisation*. London: Century Business, 1990.
29 Wenger E. *Communities of Practice: Learning, Meaning and Identity*. Cambridge: Cambridge University Press, 1998.
30 Braye S. Participation and involvement in social care: an overview. In: Kemshall H, Littlechild R eds. *User Involvement and Participation in Social Care*. London: Jessica Kingsley, 2000.
31 Peck E, Barker P. Users as partners in mental health – Ten years of experience. *J Interprofessional Care*. 1997; 11(3): 269–277.
32 Harrison S, Barnes M, Mort M. Praise and damnation: mental health user groups and the construction of organisational legitimacy. *Public Policy Adm*. 1997; 12: 14–16.
33 Rigge M. Sharing power.*Health Serv J: Health Manage Guide*. 1993; October: 1–3.

34 Beresford P, Campbell J. Disabled people, service users, user involvement and representation. *Disabil Soc.* 1994; 9: 315–325.
35 Department of Health. *The NHS Plan. A Plan for Investment – A Plan for Reform* Cm 4818. London: The Stationary Office, 2000.
36 Department of Health *Health and Social Care Act.* Section 11. London: Department of Health, 2001.
37 Bristol Royal Infirmary Inquiry. *Learning from Bristol: the report of the public inquiry into children's heart surgery at the Bristol Royal Infirmary 1984–1995.* Command Paper: CM 5207, 2001.
38 Department of Health. *Learning from Bristol: The DH Response to the report of the public inquiry into children's heart surgery at the Bristol Royal Infirmary 1984 –1995.* London: Department of Health, 2002.
39 Lorig KR, Mazonson PD, Holman HR. Evidence suggesting that health education for self-management in patients with chronic arthritis has sustained health benefits while reducing health care costs. *Arthritis Rheum.* 1993; 36(4): 439–446.
40 Department of Health. *The Expert Patient.* London: Department of Health, 2001.
41 Felce D, Grant G. *Towards a Full Life.* Oxford: Butterworth Heinemann, 1998.

5: Ethical Issues in Palliative Care

DEREK WILLIS

'I will not administer a poisonous drug, even if asked'

The Hippocratic Oath

Introduction

Why bother?

Why bother at all with ethics? It could be argued that ethics is just a series of circular arguments that are of little help to those involved in the real clinical care of patients. I do not hold this view! In the first part of the chapter I will argue that ethics has great practical value and I will then attempt to show how this can be applied specifically to palliative care. My arguments can be distilled down into two main points:

- Patients need to trust health care professionals and ethics is concerned with defining moral practice.
- Ethics should make practitioners more aware of the need to respect a patient's autonomy.

Ethics, simply defined, is the study of what we may classify as a good or a bad action and provides a framework for us to weigh that action. Are there actions that are always inherently wrong or is there ever a case for justifying a bad action for a good outcome? Ethics also concerns itself with what the character of a 'moral person' should be. So in the case of medical ethics, what would we class as a good action for a health care professional and who would we class as a good medical practitioner?

What about the case of palliative care? Surely no one could doubt that those involved in hospice work are altruistic through and through and good moral people! Whether we choose to admit it or not, our relationships with patients always have a power imbalance. Even more so for patients with palliative care needs who are particularly dependent on their doctors, nurses and allied specialists. We provide advice, therapy and often the very basics of care to people at a very vulnerable time of their lives. Such dependence and vulnerability requires patients to place a great deal of trust in their health care provider.

The fiduciary relationship

The term for such a professional relationship founded on trust is a *fiduciary relationship*. If the patient cannot guarantee to himself or herself the ethical nature of the health care providers' practice, they will not trust them and a fiduciary relationship therefore cannot exist.

This argument can be looked at in another way. Palliative care involves a differing mindset to that of other areas of medicine. The focus of attention is not solely on the patient's cure and often involves withdrawing treatment rather than just starting it. It also can involve using drugs that are potentially life threatening, that are controlled drugs and often used outside of licence. A success in palliative care is not a patient 'cured' but a patient who has had a good end to his or her life. This differing focus can make people feel uncomfortable and is often a particular struggle for those who do not work in the speciality full time. Perhaps also those who do work full time in the speciality may also become too blasé about the issues involved. To work within an ethical framework in palliative care ensures that we act in the patient's, society's and our profession's interest whilst maintaining transparency in our actions.

Ethics is at the heart of how health care personnel treat their patients and stemming from this is the reason that a relationship can exist between therapist and patient. It is therefore at the heart of every clinical decision made and is particularly relevant within the palliative care setting, which involves caring for very vulnerable people and providing symptom control rather than cure. Have I laboured the point? If you still remain unconvinced the reductivist argument might sway you—if you do not understand ethics you may get sued!

Autonomy—'to self-govern'

The patient's autonomy has not always been viewed as an important factor in the clinical setting. A few decades ago, it could be argued, it was felt by the medical profession that responsibility for ethical decisions regarding health care rested with health care professionals solely. The health care professionals made this decision based on what they felt was appropriate for their profession to practice. This is part of what is termed *professional autonomy*, i.e. a particular job can decide what its role is and police and discipline its own members independently. However, our present day society would recognise the individual as having more say in what is done to them i.e. *individual autonomy*. In other words my ability to make my own decisions for my life and my treatment and to be assisted, rather than instructed, in this by a professional.

Difficulties often arise where the autonomy of one of these groups is given prominence to the detriment of the other. Perhaps like many things in life the 'truth' is that the middle ground between these two often-polarised viewpoints is the most helpful. Doctors should have some freedom and right to decide how they practice, but patients should also have a say in what is done to them.

Additional perspectives

In no sense am I trying to suggest that the whole of ethical thought can be summarised in the short statements above. Nor am I suggesting that ethics should be solely concerned with autonomy and fiduciary relationships. However, in the clinical arena, ensuring that autonomy is respected and that practitioners can be trusted is, in my opinion, a priority. Various other models of ethics concentrate on the morality of actions (deontology and utilitarianism), the character of a moral agent (virtue theory), or the duties owed to another person (non-maleficence, beneficence). There is not enough space in one chapter to cover all these. If the reader wishes to look at other ethical models there is a list of further suggested reading at the close of this chapter.

I will now go on to look at particular clinical situations and discuss what role a fiduciary relationship and autonomy may have to say concerning these. Unless otherwise stated, the scenarios are fictitious. Where the example is a legal case, the case reference is provided. Please refer to the end of the chapter for an explanation of legal referencing, if required.

Truth or dare

> *Mrs Taylor's daughter, who is also your patient, asks to see you before you visit her mother at home. She states that she knows her mother has breast cancer. However, she insists that you do not inform her mother of this diagnosis, as she knows that her mother will not cope with the information. You meet Mrs Taylor later that day, who asks you what the tests showed when she was in hospital.*

This can be a fairly common situation. It is tricky to deal with as one does not wish to alienate or disregard the relatives of the patient. Furthermore, part of the holistic mindset that palliative care encourages involves caring for the family as well as the patient. However, if one considers the fiduciary relationship of doctor and patient and the right of people to make autonomous decisions, it can change the emphasis of such ethical dilemmas. If I tell a lie that is well meaning, even if it is meant to protect a patient from what I may perceive to be harmful information, I may potentially harm the relationship that I have with that patient in the future. If I have lied to them why should they trust me in the future? It may be that their loss of faith in me may mean that they can no longer form a therapeutic relationship with me.

Who does this information belong to in the first place? Obviously the answer is to the patient and therefore it is for them to decide who does and does not know their diagnosis and also how much of that diagnosis they wish to know about. The control of the information should rest with the patient. Therefore, if Mrs Taylor asks me what her diagnosis is, I am duty-bound to respect her question, despite what her daughter might say to the contrary.

Two provisos to what may seem like a fairly strident position. We have to respect both a patient's right to know and right not to know. If patients do not wish to know their diagnosis and I inform them of this, I have not respected their autonomy. The guide must be patients themselves in how much and in what way their information is presented to them.

Such a position is easier if the patient is well known to the health care professional. In these circumstances you may have already gained insights into how your patients want their information given to them. Sometimes health care professionals meet a patient for the first time and have no idea of how this particular person may want their information given to them. A relative may be able to help guide you in this decision. This is not to say that the relative has a right of veto over what you tell the patient but can act as an aid in doing this. The General Medical Council (GMC) guidelines are clear on this point. In their opinion, it is the patient who ultimately decides on treatment and on how much information is given, but that it is good practice to involve relatives in this process:

- The patient has the right to know the truth if they ask for it
- The best guide for how much information to give is the patient themselves
- The relatives can assist with this but do not have a right of veto.

Withdrawing and withholding treatment

> *Ms B was a social worker who was tetraplegic and eventually required ventilation. The lady no longer wished to have the ventilator sustain her and requested that the ventilator be turned off. She had her case heard at the high court in order to decide that she was competent to make this decision. She was found to be competent and the ventilator was switched off.*
>
> *Ms B vs. An NHS Hospital Trust* (2002) All ER 449

Consent must first be obtained from a patient for any procedure to occur. For us to respect a patient's autonomy we have to provide sufficient information for the patient to make this decision. We also have to be sure that the patient is not pressurised into making the decision that we feel is the correct one. It is important to note that under the English legal system we are not duty bound to tell the patient absolutely everything—just the information that the patient needs in order to make the decision. This is what is meant in England by 'informed consent'. This still allows the patients to say that they do not want to know all the side effects or consequences but still be consenting. In this country the benchmark as to what is adequate information for consent is still the average practitioner 'Bolam'.[1] This is in contrast to America where it is the average patient who is taken to be the guide in law. Bolam therefore states that it is what the 'reasonable medical practitioner' would have done in similar circumstances, which is taken as standard practice.

If a patient does not give consent for a medical intervention to happen, and a medical practitioner performs this despite the patient's wishes, then in law 'battery' has occurred. Or, to put this in ethical terms, a patient's autonomy has not been respected. For example, if a person who is a Jehovah's Witness wishes not to have blood, then that decision must be respected. Therefore, before we proceed with interventions we are duty-bound to gain consent from the patient, having provided the level and amount of information that the patient has asked for. A patient does have the ethical and legal right to refuse treatment provided that they do not have reduced competence to do so.

[1] *Bolam v Friern Hospital Management Committee.* [1957] 2 All ER 118 is a land-mark case were a doctor was acquitted for causing harm to a patient through not using muscle relaxants whilst administering ECT. His defence, now known as the Bolam test, was that he was acting in a similar way as a body of reasonable and ordinary practitioners would have done in similar circumstances at that time.

Competence is legally defined as when patients can:

1. understand and retain the information;
2. they believe this information;
3. they can weigh the information presented to them.[2]

It is not enough to say that a patient suffers from a medical condition and therefore is incompetent to make a decision. Rather it must be proved that the medical condition inhibits the patient's ability to satisfy the three-pronged test described above. It is therefore conceivable that a patient may competently request for a treatment not to occur or to be withdrawn even if this treatment or procedure may result in their death. In the above case Ms B was deemed to be competent to make an informed decision, therefore her ventilation was discontinued.

This is all very well if patients are able to communicate their wishes to us, but very often patients may be deeply unconscious or confused, particularly in the last days of their life. How is it possible to know what to do in these circumstances? In this situation a living will (advanced directive) can be used to direct the care that is to take place. A living will can state what a person wants to happen or not happen to them if they become unable to take part in their discussions. This has legal weight. It is therefore a medical practitioners duty to respect the patient's wishes if they do not, for example, wish to have antibiotics should they have a large stroke. Failure to do this could be viewed as battery.

If a patient refuses to continue with treatment then there is strong legal and ethical argument supporting the patient's stance. However, this does not mean that the medical professional is duty-bound to always provide the treatment that a patient requests. Patients cannot demand that a doctor or nurse does exactly as they wish them to do. This highlights one of the tensions that can often exist in health care situations. Not only does the patient have autonomy that should be respected but to some extent the professional also has some amount of autonomy. Or to put this in a different way, a job that is termed professional does have some right to limit what the people involved in that job can do. The GMC supports this standpoint and recognises that there may be times when active therapeutic intervention in a patient's care may be inappropriate, but this standpoint has recently been legally challenged and a decision is pending in the appeal court. The GMC

[2] *Re C* is a legal case listed in 1 All ER 819 where a gentleman with a mental illness refused to have his leg amputated. The case rested on whether he was competent or not to make the decision. He was found to be competent and the case produced the precedent for assessment of competence outlined above.

recognises that life has a natural end. Their guidelines on good practice state that:

> *'doctors should not strive to prolong the dying process with no regard to the patient's wishes, where known, or an up-to-date assessment of the benefits or burdens of treatment or non-treatment'* [1].

It is recognised by the GMC that sometimes there may be conflict between the opinion of doctors (for whom the guidelines are expressly written) and patients. To use the terms that we have been using, sometimes the autonomy of the patient and the autonomy of the doctor may clash. It is recommended by the GMC that in such circumstances legal help should be sought.

It is difficult to give a definitive answer to all the eventualities that could occur in practice because there isn't one! Life or even death is never that simple. However we have seen that some general guidelines are as follows:

- Competent patients have the right to refuse treatments
- Living Wills have some legal standing
- Health Care Professionals also have some level of autonomy.

Live and let die

> *Diane Pretty was a lady who suffered from Motor Neurone Disease. She was concerned that she had become so incapacitated that she was not [have been] able to take her own life. She went to the UK and then the European Courts to ensure that should her husband assist her in trying to take her own life that he would not be prosecuted. Her case and subsequent appeal were turned down, the court deciding that if this were to happen, then a criminal act would have occurred.*
>
> *R. vs. Director of Public Prosecutions* (2002) 1 All ER 1

The English law is clear that a person assisting someone in an act of euthanasia would be prosecuted for murder. This is so even if the patient is competent and is expressing this wish as part of an autonomous choice. There is therefore a definite limit to how much a patient may dictate as to what happens during their care. The RCN's General Secretary stated:

> *'The RCN is opposed to the introduction of legislation that would place the responsible nurses and other medical staff to respond to a demand for termination of life from any patient'* [2].

Space does not allow a full discussion of this area but let us consider the fiduciary relationship and autonomy. If my relationship with my health care professional depends on my trusting them, will that trust be eroded if I know they can harm me? If doctors specifically develop the power to prematurely end someone's life, will this reduce a patient's trust and faith in their doctor? At the moment a patient can guarantee that their doctor will never give them something intentionally that will kill them. This is a powerful guarantee and legalising euthanasia could destroy that.

We have seen how the patient-carer relationship is one where there is a balance of autonomy between patient and caregiver. The patient cannot demand everything they want of the carer and the carer cannot expect the patient to do everything that they want either. There is a balance to be negotiated in the relationship. A profession can decide for itself what its absolute limits are. For a group of people dedicated to caring it would seem sensible that this absolute would be not taking a life. It would therefore limit a caring profession's autonomy if they were expected to perform actions that would harm their patient.

A further argument used is that if euthanasia becomes an acceptable practice then it may cease to become a choice. If euthanasia became available it may be that patients would choose this rather than be a burden to the family. This may be something that the patients may not themselves want, but do as it is expected of them:

- The voluntary taking of someone's life is illegal
- Arguments against this can be put forward using autonomy
- Aiding someone with euthanasia is also illegal.

Double effect

> *Dr Cox was a hospital physician responsible for the care of a lady who was suffering from rheumatoid arthritis. This lady was in intractable pain from her medical condition. Dr Cox felt that he had tried everything to help this lady become pain free. He therefore decided that, in his opinion, the most compassionate thing to do was to give this lady a lethal dose of potassium chloride. He did this and the lady died. He was later taken to court and was tried for murder. He had his sentence reduced to manslaughter, and was sent to prison.*
>
> *R vs. Cox* (1992) BMLR 38

The law as it stands has a fairly strong position concerning euthanasia. Such a strong position can often make health care professionals quite circumspect about performing or prescribing certain therapeutic procedures. For example, in palliative care morphine is commonly given for the treatment of pain. It could be that in giving morphine, in a dose, to control very severe and complex pain, that a person's life is prematurely shortened. In other words, in trying to make a good action occur, one may cause a bad action to happen. In these circumstances one would know that such consequences are possible. There is an ethical and legal phrase—'*the doctrine of double effect*' that recognises that this dilemma exists. The doctrine can be broken down into the following elements:

1. The original action intended is a good one in itself
2. The sole intention of the action is good
3. The good effect is not produced as a consequence of the bad effect
4. The required outcome is significant enough to permit the bad outcome occurring.

What does all that actually mean? Let us use the example of the patient who is in pain. The relief of pain particularly in the terminal stages of life is a good action and also one that is significant enough, it could and is argued, to justify the possibility of premature and unintentional shortening of life. However, what cannot be justified is that causing someone's death as a method of pain control. The intention has to be, to fit with the doctrine, not to kill the patients but to make them pain free. The intention must not be to make them pain free by terminating their life. Dr Cox could not justify his actions using the doctrine of double effect, as he intended to end the patient's suffering by terminating life. The only possible use of potassium chloride in the dose under the circumstances used was to end the patient's life.

This may seem just complicated semantics but the law and ethics recognise that intention is important. One large proviso—this doctrine does not excuse malpractice. Guidelines and agreed standards of practice should be followed. Morphine and other opioids must be used at the correct dose for the circumstances.

The reason for the doctrine existing is to reassure medical personnel that if they treat their patients correctly and with good practice, then they have no reason to fear prosecution. It would be unethical for a patient to be left in pain with a medical person unable or unwilling to give them pain control. One of the largest factors that can return a patient's autonomy is giving them the necessary medication to allow them to be pain free.

- Patients have a basic human right to be pain free
- Some medications may cause harmful effects
- The doctrine of double effects can be used in these circumstances

- This has four elements, all four of which must apply for the doctrine to be used
- To intend to cause death is illegal in most countries.

Summary

I started this chapter by emphasising how important ethics is in everyday practice. What I have tried to do is show how ethics, at the heart of it, is about preserving the relationship between clinician and patient. This relationship is vital not only for individual therapeutic relationships but also for the standing of health care professionals in the community. This chapter cannot hope to act as either a philosophical or legal textbook and space does not allow for the details required to fully explore the issues involved. Further reading is suggested below. Indemnity organisations and/or professional bodies are helpful in clarifying specific legal situations.

Legal references and standard abbreviations

In this chapter citation has been made of several legal cases. Standard practice for a legal reference is that the title in italics refers to the actual case name whilst the title in bold refers to the year and name of legal report where the case can be found.

All E R All England Law Reports

BMLR Butterworth's Medico-Legal Reports

The number before the legal report title is the volume number and the number after the legal report is the page number.

The legal cases are annotated at more length and discussed in more depth in *Law and Medical Ethics* (listed in further reading).

References

1 http://www.gmc-uk.org/standards/default.htm '*Withholding and Withdrawing Life-prolonging Treatments: Good Practice in Decision Making.*' Section 12 2002

2 http://www.rcn.org.uk/news/ '*The Royal College Nursing General Secretary, Dr Beverly Malone Comments on Today's Debate on Euthanasia*' June 6th 2003

Further reading and useful resources

General Medical Council Guidance on Good Practice http://www.gmc-uk.org/standards

Lawtel gives details of all case and statutory law in this country and Europe http://www.lawtel.com (subscription required)

Mason JK, McCall Smith RA, Laurie GT. *Law and Medical Ethics.* 6th edition. London: Butterworths, 2002.

Gillon R. *Philosophical Medical Ethics.* 7th edition. Chester, UK: Wiley Publications, 1994.

Glover J. *Causing Death and Saving Lives.* 2nd edition. (Harmondsworth: Penguin Books, 1990.

Midgley M. *The Myths We Live By.* 1st edition. London: Routledge, 2003.

Morra J, Robson M, Smith M (eds). To die laughing by Critchly S. *The Limits of Death* Chapter 1. 1st edition. Manchester: Manchester University Press, 2000.

Warnock M. *An Intelligent Persons Guide to Ethics.* 1st edition, Chapter 1, London: Duckbacks Publishers, 2001.

Boyd KM. Mrs Pretty and Ms B. *J Med Ethics* 2002; 28: 211–212.

6: Communication Skills in Palliative Care

CANDY M COOLEY

Introduction

Many patients and families can give an extremely detailed account of receiving serious news, even years after the experience. This communication between the health professional and the patient and their family may significantly influence the subsequent relationship and have a considerable effect on their quality of life and end of life care.

Everyone is able to communicate in some form. From the very young to the very old, the sick of mind and body—all find some way of communicating their needs, desire, anger, sadness and happiness. So why is communication with people who have a life-threatening disease and their families considered so difficult? This is a conversation I have regularly within the classroom with a range of health professionals and personnel. The general consensus is that communication in palliative care is difficult for two major reasons—it brings home our own mortality and we have an almost desperate desire to get it right.

Maybe one of the most important skills in ensuring good communication in palliative care is a sound understanding of how we feel about our own mortality and a realistic view of what the patient actually expects from us. In many situations we do not question our ability to communicate; we take it for granted like breathing or blinking [1]. However, it is one of the most vital aspects of health care [2] and worrying about what we may say could lead to us forgetting to ask how the patient actually feels [3]. Sheila Cassidy makes a wonderful observation that: *Patients know we are not God; all they ask is that we do not abandon them* [4].

It is important to always remember the individuality of each patient and their families as this will enable the health professional to realise that listening, sensitivity and intuition are essential skills in the art of communication. Patients need to be able to make decisions based on their own personal values and beliefs; they need to receive relevant information and be supported to make plans that enable them to live within the context of their disease [5].

The purpose of good communication is to achieve a two-way process of trust and honesty between the patient and the health professional [1]. It can also reduce uncertainty, avoid unrealistic expectations and prevent the collusion of silence rather than open dialogue [6]. The following sections look at the issues which can affect the process of communication, and consider strategies to support the health professional dealing with palliative care patients in their care.

Barriers to communication

Poor communication and information giving is one of the commonest causes of complaint to the NHS Ombudsman [7]. However, when one considers that the health professionals only have a desire to impart information and to do their best for their patients and the families, why can it all go wrong?

Language barriers

We live in a multicultural society in which for both the patient and the health professional English may not be the first language [8]. This may be exacerbated in areas with a strong local accent. For example, it has been reported that the strong accent and dialect of the 'Black country' has caused much confusion for overseas nurses working within Dudley in the West Midlands.

Similarly, within the health profession we have our own language, which we feel confident to use. We understand it and it makes sense to us. But like the colloquialism of a regional accent the patient may not always understand our jargon. One of the most important skills in communication is remembering that it is not what we say that is important, but what the patient hears and understands.

Language must be simple but not condescending. It should be ensured that at the end of a conversation:

- you understand the concerns and requirements of the patient;
- you are confident that the patient understands what information you have given them.

Without ensuring this, mistakes occur, messages get confused, patients feel let down, angry and lose confidence in the health professional [1]. At the end of each meeting it is important to ask more than just 'do you have any questions?' or 'do you understand?' These will usually be answered in the way the patient thinks you would like to hear. You must ask appropriate questions to ensure confusion is limited. These questions could be specific such as 'Just to ensure that there has been no confusion can you just quickly tell me what you understand about the information I have just given you.' It may be necessary to use an interpreter or language line. Using an interpreter has potential problems and pitfalls, but it is usually better not to use family members as interpreters, as they may only tell the patient part of the story, to minimise distress or because they are embarrassed by the conversation. If however, there is no option, then you must explain the importance of good information and at a more appropriate time get a professional interpreter to assess the level of understanding.

Physical barriers

Both disease and age can affect the communication process [8,1]. For example, patients with cognitive dysfunction and patients in severe pain can find it problematic to understand too much information. Co-occurring disorders may also limit good communication. Find out if the patient has a hearing loss or reduction. Sometimes people, especially older people, may act as though they have heard and understood rather than admit to being hard of hearing, or to seem foolish, or to be wasting your time. Beware the smiling, nodding older person; this may be 'deafness' but it is never 'daftness' [9].

Also beware that just because people are old does not mean that they are deaf or of limited cognitive ability. One of the common reasons for the older person not questioning or asking for clarity is the respect and awe in which they perceive the health professional. Ensuring that the patient feels confident that you are interested in them personally and in what they wish to discuss is imperative to ensuring effective communication.

Short-term memory loss may mean that the patient is constantly asking the same questions. This situation needs careful handling and sometimes written information or a tape may be of benefit. Patients and professionals can become irritated by this situation and a managed plan between the patient, the carers and the health professionals may be of benefit. The impact of pain or other symptoms on an individual's ability to concentrate and communicate may be fairly apparent. In some situations it is necessary to deal with the physical concern before moving on to the psychological support.

Distraction and noise

One of the reasons that patients may be reticent in their disclosure of concerns may be the environment in which the discussion takes place. Much has been written over the years about inappropriate places that patients and their relatives have received bad news [1,10]. However, whilst the lack of sound-proofing made by curtains is never in question, just having a separate room does not solve all the issues.

Working within the patient's own home can have other distractions. Asking for the television to be turned off, for some private time for the patient and health professional, and for pets to perhaps be moved out of the room, can be difficult. But these issues can be negotiated if the importance of good communication is explained to the patient and family. Having a growling dog, talkative parrot or afternoon television will hinder the opportunity for good communication. But the health professional is always a guest in the home of the patient and their family, and trust and the opportunity for negotiation may only come over a period of time.

One of the commonest reasons for distraction is when the health professional (and patient) knows that they have many other jobs to do. Interruptions by other staff, bleeps, mobile phones and glancing at watches all lead the patient to perceive that time is of essence and there is a need to 'get on with it'. Most health professionals would state that lack of time is a common reason for poor communication. However, what often matters is the quality of interaction rather than the length of time. Giving a few moments of time, which are totally focussed on the patient's communication needs, can often limit the amount of time spent communicating later when further explanation and/or clarity are required.

Make sure colleagues are aware that you are not to be disturbed. Ensure you work as a team when information is being imparted. One-to-one communication is fine as long as the team is included in the action plans. Patients may want to be able to have confidential discussions. Clarity of how much can be disclosed to colleagues to ensure continuity of care needs to be established. It is important that patient care is not compromised by a lack of sharing information.

Fear

Emotions play an important part in the clarity of communication. Fear, especially, can be a potent communication barrier influencing both what the patient hears and is prepared to accept and what the health professional says. Health professionals will often describe a fear of saying the wrong thing, saying too much or contradicting their colleagues [5].

For the patient, fear can make it difficult to hear and connect with what is being said. Comments such as—'I heard the word cancer and nothing after that'—are common [10]. Preparing the patient with 'warning shots' and allowing time for the initial panic to subside may be of help. Some patients, though, need time and space to think through what they have been told. Running on into discussions surrounding treatment choices and decisions will be unproductive.

Ensuring good communication between health professionals can reduce the fear associated with passing on information incorrectly. It also ensures that there is an openness and honesty between the team, which will improve the confidence of the patient in those giving care.

Facilitators of communication

There are two main tasks of communication: to find out what the problems are and what the patient needs and to give patient information to address the problems. Both of these tasks require particular skills to achieve a two-way process of trust and honesty between the patient and the health professional.

Listening

One of the most important skills required for communication in palliative care is to listen and hear. This is the type of listening in which you demonstrate to patients that you have really heard what they are saying, asking and feeling. It is all too easy to hear the first thing that the patient says and then whilst you are considering your response you do not hear what is said next [11].

Listening does not mean not responding. You should use body language, eye contact and simple sounds, such as 'hmm' or 'yes', to show that you are listening. When the patient stops talking, allow a little time. Checking with the patient that what you have heard is what the individual meant is an important way of demonstrating you are really listening. So too is asking if they have any other concerns prior to your response. This offers them an opportunity to raise an issue that they may have found difficult, but now that they have started talking find a little easier to discuss.

Listening is an art and those who do it well will focus on the patient's agenda rather than on the agenda that the health professional perceives as important. We are aware that many complaints to the NHS Ombudsman surrounding communication are made because patients do not feel that anyone is listening to them [7]. They also can feel that their agenda is not what the health professional perceives. Research does demonstrate that the concerns of patients are sometimes different from those identified by the people caring for them [12]. For example, the patient is often concerned with wider issues such as family support, coping and emotional worries. Whereas the health professionals may be more likely to identify physical health issues, factors which they felt they could 'do something about'.

Therefore, to ensure good communication occurs it is important to:

- really listen to what the patient is saying about their concerns;
- repeat your understanding of what they have said back to them and have it confirmed that that is what they are really saying.

Do not ever assume that you think you know what would be a patient's worry. That would be your worry and will probably not be theirs.

Getting across the information

Whilst listening is key within communication, in health care, information giving can be equally important [13]. Patients and relatives will be able to give graphic accounts of when and how bad news was given to them and so some thought needs to influence your practice.

- Will you be distracted?
- Should you give the news alone?
- Do the patients want someone there with them?
- Do you have all the possible answers that this news may require?
- Are you the most appropriate person to give this information? If not, why not?

These questions will take only seconds in your head but may make a significant impact on the way the news is given and received. Many patients, but not all, wish to have a family member there with them. Ensuring that you have the time and the correct information will ensure that the patient does not feel hurried or of little importance. Often, having another appropriate health professional with you will ensure a team approach to information giving and can also ensure that there is a dissemination within the team of what was said and how it was received.

Making sure that the patient has taken in and assimilated the information can take much longer than may be available to one health professional. A team approach can give more time for an evaluation of understanding. This will also ensure that the patient has time to question and consider the many options that are often available.

It is important to remember that there are many methods of giving information, other than verbal communication. The professional has a responsibility to assess the appropriate sources of information and to direct the patient to these. Box 6.1 highlights a number of different sources of information available to patients, carers and professionals.

Box 6.1 Sources of information

Patient level
Information directly from professionals involved in care
Written information e.g. booklets and leaflets
Internet web sites which you may want to recommend
Expert patients
Self-help groups
NHS Direct
Internet access

Local community level
Information on local services
Local support groups

National level
Department of Health guidelines and strategies
Books/journals
National organisations e.g. Cancer Bacup, Macmillan Cancer Relief

Coping with emotion

Patients and relatives will respond to news in a variety of ways that may vary over the time you see the patient. The most important thing is to be non-judgemental and prepared for all emotions [11]. Those emotions can be wide ranging, come in no predictable sequence and may include:

- *Fear*: This may be shown as denial, anger or anxiety, sometimes in the form of a panic attack.

- *Anger*: Blame of health professionals, God, their lifestyle. Or it may be just anger as to why them or their loved one.
- *Despair*: A sense of helplessness and hopelessness that can limit the ability to think or speak.
- *Isolation*: Feeling a need to withdraw from family and friends, looking for personal time and space.
- *Faith*: May be positive that God has a purpose or can make people question their faith and beliefs.
- *Depression*: Sadness is common, but this can become clinical depression if it becomes overwhelming [5].

Acknowledging emotion and enabling the person to talk through powerful emotions can be very therapeutic. But the health professionals must be cognisant of their personal limitations and be able to identify when the patient's need has become greater than their skill [14]. A multidisciplinary approach can ensure that the most appropriate health professional can offer support. Sometimes a psychologist or psychiatrist will be far more appropriate in enabling the patient's to make sense of their emotions and to develop a strategy to deal with powerful emotional responses.

The angry patient or relative is commonly identified as a concern for health professionals [5]. One of the most important things to remember is that the anger is very rarely about you as an individual. This thought should prevent you from getting drawn into an unhelpful spiral of reflected anger, raised voices and reduced chances of communication. It is important to:

- acknowledge the anger and respect the cause of the anger;
- offer the patient or relative the opportunity to articulate the cause of the anger, which may include guilt, blame of self or another individual, and fear of the consequences of the news.

Do not get drawn into a discussion of who is to blame but see your role as helping to move the individual through their anger to a degree of acceptance [5, 10, 11].

Breaking bad news

Breaking bad news is considered to be one of the most fraught communication encounters. Breaking bad news has had more comment and written word than any other patient/professional encounter and is still considered by health professionals to be the most difficult scenario [1, 10, 11]. The key starting points have already been mentioned—making the place, person and time appropriate and being prepared to deal with a range of emotions. Some patients surprise us by their lack of emotion or by displaying what may be considered inappropriate emotion. Remember the importance of being non-judgemental and working with the patient's agenda.

Another important issue is who is told the information. Patient information is confidential to the patient and therefore any information should only be given to the patient, unless, it is the expressed wish of the patient not to be told the results of their investigations. Pressure on busy health professionals or a desire to minimise the distress to the patient are reasons why relatives are given information either before the patient or instead of the patient [11]. However, consider how you would feel if information was given and decisions made about you without your involvement. Relatives do not have a right to demand the silence of a health professional. It is therefore, very important that a conversation takes place and is documented prior to the results being available as to the patients wishes [1]. Patients know if they have tests they will get results, and empowering them to state who they wish involved in the information derived from the test will reduce confusion, collusion and ensure trust between the patient and the health professional is maintained.

When you are about to give 'bad news' it is recommended that you deliver a 'warning shot', leading the patient towards a sense of knowing [10]. Something like, "You know we are here to discuss the results of your test . . . (pause) . . . Well they have shown that you have a serious problem" or ". . . they have shown that things are not going as well as we had hoped." You may find that the patient then clearly articulates their expectations, "Is it fatal?", "Is it cancer?", "I'm dying aren't I?" This then allows the health professional to deal with the patient's questions and move the individual forward. If, however, the patient says nothing then the reality of what the results mean will need to be delivered in small jargon-free sentences. Pause regularly for confirmation of whether the patient has understood or has a question, and knows how to deal with the emotion. Try to avoid 'don'ts' such as "don't cry" and "don't worry". Crying is a good coping strategy and they *will* worry [1]. Acknowledge their distress, suggest some time to collect themselves, offer a tissue and show you understand and respect their emotions. It is important that they know that the health professional believes that their feelings are significant, important and reasonable.

Box 6.2 outlines the 10 step process to breaking bad news as recommended by Kaye, a consultant in palliative medicine [6]. Utilising these steps as a framework will ensure that you feel a degree of confidence that you have thought through this communication. However, the individuality of each encounter needs to be remembered. What might work very well in one situation may not be so successful in another, maintaining a degree of flexibility within the framework will ensure that the patients and their families feel that their particular needs are being considered.

Box 6.2 Ten steps for breaking bad news (Kaye [6])

1 Preparation
2 What does the patient know?
3 Is more information wanted?
4 Give a warning
5 Allow denial
6 Explain
7 Listen to concerns
8 Encourage feelings
9 Summary and plan
10 Offer continual support and availability

Communication between health professionals

One of the commonest causes of stress within multidisciplinary teamwork is a perceived lack of communication, most evident when the team is caring for an individual during the end stages of life. This can be particularly problematic in the community setting when the opportunities for dialogue between professionals may be limited. Without good communication individuals within the team may not understand treatment decisions, patient and relative knowledge levels or patients' choices. This may lead to feelings of inadequacy and fear of saying or doing the wrong thing. Open and honest communication with an opportunity for each individual's concerns to be articulated and respected will limit the stresses within the team, thereby improving patient care and morale. Chapter 2 has explored ways to establish good team communication.

Ensuring good communication between places of care is important in continuity of care. This is particularly relevant towards the end of life when things need to happen quickly especially, for instance, if a very sick patient wishes to go home. Some of the major complaints from relatives following the death of their loved one relates to breakdown in the communication of final wishes. Recent government guidance on ensuring the patient has greater choice in their preferred place of death should lead to patients' final wishes being achieved [15]. Close contact with colleagues in other care settings and good documentation can make all the difference to the patient's care.

It is healthy and good clinical governance for the team to allow time, following any difficult situation, for some structured reflection and an opportunity to discuss possible ways of handling the situation in the future. This may include organisational strategies to minimise conflict for the future and offers an opportunity for concerns to be aired and respected. This degree of communication within the team will maximise the team's potential in developing most effective care strategies.

Conclusion

Communication is one of the most important aspects in the care and management of the patient requiring palliative care. Poor communication is a major cause of distress to patients, their families and the caring team. It is therefore imperative that health professionals consider the implications of any interaction and think through the possible results of their actions. This should not cause the health professionals alarm or fear but should encourage them to recognise that it is not just what they do to a patient that ensures care but how they do it. The good communicator who looks into the patient's agenda will find that care delivery is enhanced and professional, patient and carer satisfaction increased.

References

1 Cooley CM. Communication skills in palliative care. *Prof Nurse* 2000; 15(9): 603–605.
2 Burnard P. *Communicate: A Communication Skills Guide for Health-Care Workers* 1992: London: Arnold.
3 Penson J. Psychological needs of people with cancer. *Sr Nurse* 1991; 3: 37–41.
4 Cassidy S. *Sharing the Darkness.* London: Darton, Longman and Todd, 1988.
5 Jeffery D. Communication skills in palliative care. In: Faull C, Carter Y, Woof R. eds. *Handbook of Palliative Care.* Oxford: Blackwell Science, 1988.
6 Kaye P. *Breaking Bad News: A Ten Step Approach.* Northampton: EPL Publications 1996: 3–25.
7 Department of Health. *Organisation with a Memory.* London: DOH, 1999.

8 Becker R. Teaching communication skills across cultural boundaries. *Br J Nurs.* 1999; 8(14): 938–942.
9 Cooley C, Coventry G. Cancer and older people. *Nursing the Older Person.*2003; 15(2): 22–26.
10 Buckman R. *How to Break Bad News.* London: Papermac, 1992.
11 Maguire P, Booth K, Elliot C, Jones B. Helping health professionals involved in cancer care acquire key interviewing skills—the impact of workshops. *Eur J Cancer.* 1996; 32A(9): 1486–1489.
12 Heaven C, Maguire P. Training hospice nurses to elicit patients concerns. *J Adv Nurs.*1996; 23: 280–286.
13 Fallowfield L, Jenkins V. Effective communication skills are the key to good cancer care. *Eur J Cancer.* 1999; 35(11): 1592–1597.
14 Baile WF, Kudelka AP et al. Communication skills training in Oncology. *Cancer.*1999; 86(5): 887–897.
15 National Institute for Clinical Excellence *Guidance on Cancer Services: Improving Supportive and Palliative Care for Adults with Cancer.* National Institute for Clinical Excellence, 2004.

7: Adapting to Death, Dying and Bereavement

BRIAN NYATANGA

Introduction

Our fear of death and the loss of a loved one are two of the most monumental emotional challenges of human existence. This anxiety is usually suppressed and is only exposed when the reality of a possible death is confronted. Fear of death stems from different sources, for example, the thought of our non-existence [1] and the fear of the unknown of what lies beyond death [2].

Palliative care has recognised the power of this suffering and is concerned with helping people cope and adapt. This is incorporated into a philosophy of care that has resulted in the principles of palliative care [3].

This chapter will review literature that has improved the understanding of the processes involved, the damaging consequences that can occur and the role of health professionals in caring for the dying and the bereaved.

Fear of death in society

Humanity's fear of death has interested artists and scientists alike. Philosophers have considered death in terms of fear of extinction and insignificance; psychologists have devised models that explain death-related emotion [4]; and sociologists have observed how death anxiety can bind groups (e.g. societies, religions, armies). Freud claimed that social life was formed and preserved out of fear of death. In industrialised and technological societies, death has been removed from the family home into institutions with care provided by professionals. This has resulted in a lack of familiarity with the dying process, which may contribute to a fear of death and dying within society.

In day-to-day life individuals contain such fears; however, death anxiety can be seen as hugely influential on behaviour. Factors such as those illustrated in Table 7.1 highlight the potency of death anxiety and help explain how people react when faced with death.

Table 7.1 Factors that induce fear of death.

Drivers of death anxiety affecting males and females (Nayatanga [5])	Factors affecting the general public (Diggory and Ruthman [6])	Death fears as advocated by (Chonnon [7])
• Dependency • Pain in dying process • Isolation • Indignity of dying process • Afterlife concerns • Leaving loved ones • Fate of the body • Rejection • Separation	Grief of relatives & friends End of all plans and projects Dying process being painful One can no longer have experiences Can no longer care for dependents Fear of what happens if there is life after death Fear of what happens to one's body	Fear of what happens after death Fear of the act of dying (e.g. pain, loss of control and rejection) Fear of ceasing to be

People differ in how they respond to the prospect of death. In caring for the dying and bereaved, it is useful to try to understand the different factors that influence this behaviour. Although personal factors are very important (e.g. gender, nature of disease and treatment, coping mechanisms, social support, personality, etc.), these partly relate to what is known as the 'death system' in a society. This phenomenon varies between societies and depends on the following four factors [8]:

1 Exposure to death—prior experience of death has a strong influence on the approach to subsequent deaths, including our own.

2 Life expectancy—society holds an estimate for what is considered a reasonable life span, based on observations of the community.

3 Perceived control over the forces of nature—beliefs about the ability to influence destiny (fate vs. control) will affect perceptions of death.

4 Perception of what it means to be human—'meaning' in this context relates to a variety of belief systems that constitute spirituality. The clarity and conviction with which a society holds these views will influence the death system.

Each death will be influenced to varying degrees by a combination of personal factors within a particular cultural death system. For instance, an elderly Indian widow who sees illness in a religious sense will respond differently from the young Western atheist who has never experienced death and believes in their own ability to control life events.

Personal spirituality

Spirituality is concerned with how individuals understand the purpose and meaning of their existence within the universe. It requires individuals to develop a harmonious intellectual connection between themselves and their spiritual thought. For some there may be a strong religious component to this aspect of their life, and it must be emphasised that religion and spirituality are separate entities. However, for others such cultural norms are less relevant. These differences are readily seen in pluralistic Western societies such as the UK and may have a profound effect on how individuals view death and dying.

Death poses a challenge to these personally held belief systems. Some individuals possess a set of beliefs that adequately answer this challenge, but others can suffer as they strive to attain an inner peace. It is clear that a patient's individual spirituality can never be assumed. Carers must remain aware of this when considering the spiritual needs of patients. Spiritual health can be encouraged in several ways:

- eliminate the distraction of physical suffering;
- encourage the expression of repressed emotion;
- assist patients to attain spiritual growth, either by personal reflection or with the help of an adviser (professional or lay);
- respect the individuals and their cultures in all interactions.

The spiritual component of health is an important theme in the philosophy of palliative care [9], and is recognised as one of the four components of holistic assessment in palliative care [10]. The Trent Hospice Audit Group has developed a standard for the assessment, delivery and evaluation of spiritual care, which includes three levels of assessment; routine assessment: for all patients, multidisciplinary assessment particularly sensitive to spiritual issues, and specialist assessment, e.g. undertaken by a chaplain [10]. Such initiatives provide a framework for practitioners to address what is often a neglected area of palliative care.

Adapting to dying

By understanding how societies deal with death, it is possible to explore the more specific issues of how patients cope, the problems that can arise and how carers should respond. This includes care of both the patient and those important to them (significant others). This whole topic area has been termed, 'anticipatory grief' which requires adjustment and adaptation. The adjustment and adaptation can be at both physical and psychological level, to ensure that people are functioning within the realms of the new reality.

Psychosocial theories

Various psychological models have been developed which provide insight into patients' responses to their impending death. The most celebrated work was performed by Kubler-Ross [11], who described a five-stage model of dying: denial, anger, bargaining, depression and acceptance. Other authors have proposed different models that also contribute to our understanding [12–17]. The main advantage of these theories is that they allow us to make sense of people's behaviour more constructively. Parkes sums it all up succinctly:

> *It is not enough for us to stay close and open our hearts to another person's suffering: valuable as this sympathy may be, we must have some way for stepping aside from the maze of emotion and sensation if we are to make sense of it* [18].

However, these models have their limitations. They should only be used to assist in the understanding of patients and allow the carer not to be overwhelmed by the emotions observed. Too rigid application of such models may prevent the individual needs of the patient and carers being assessed and met.

Particular problems in adapting to dying

The extent of the distress experienced by patients depends on a wide variety of factors. In many cases, the psychosocial needs of the patient and carers are met with honest information given sensitively. But in more complex instances, the debilitating effects of the adaptive process require more intense professional support. Physical symptoms can be influenced by the emotional state of patients. Concepts such as 'total pain' are at the core of the palliative care philosophy. Consequently, emotional distress can be an important component in physical suffering and therefore in its management.

There is an array of emotional responses that can occur when facing death, which can be difficult for patients to bear. These include anger, anxiety, guilt and depression. As patients grapple with all these emotions and the changing nature of their illness, feelings of isolation can also occur. This alienation compounds the many other losses that are experienced at this time.

Not surprisingly, the enormity of the adaptive process can be overwhelming and result in psychiatric morbidity. Although research has found it difficult to confirm, it is said that there is an increased prevalence of depression, anxiety, panic and suicidal behaviour [18].

Although some patients do undoubtedly suffer in this way, it is important to remember that many adapt healthily. Research has revealed that patients achieve this by using techniques such as 'positive reappraisal' and 'cognitive avoidance strategies' [19]. To the professional observer, some of these strategies may seem like distortions or misinterpretations of the facts, but to the patient they insure against emotional overload. It is important not to dismantle individual adaptive processes.

The debilitating effect of the emotional consequences of a terminal illness compounds the physical deterioration to produce significant social costs. Social losses are closely related to quality of life issues and include such things as employment, recreation, relationships and family.

The demands of caring for a terminally ill patient should not be ignored by professionals. Indeed, in some cases the multidisciplinary team's focus is more appropriately directed not so much at the patient but at the patient's family and friends. The need for constant nursing care at home can be physically draining and occasionally result in injury or illness to the carer. In addition, family and friends are subjected to a series of actual and potential losses that demand considerable emotional strength. Examples of these challenges include the following:

- loss of a certain future;
- loss of role within the family and the outside world;
- concerns about the burden of caring;
- issues about sexuality;
- loss of financial security.

In many cases these questions provoke emotions in carers that are similar to those experienced by their dying loved one. Such emotional strain can result in significant levels of sleeplessness, anxiety and weight loss.

The social consequences of caring for a terminally ill loved one can be far-reaching. The time and energy required can impinge on employment, recreation and relationships. Although society recognises this in terms of respect for altruism, the economic burden can be considerable and only partially compensated for by statutory government allowances.

The multidisciplinary team has an important role in recognising the potential dangers of caring for a loved one and should endeavour to intervene to prevent problems.

Managing the adaptation process

Assessing the emotional needs of dying patients and significant others requires an empathic attitude complemented by adept communication skills and familiarity with the issues surrounding the subject. Research suggests certain factors may be inherently influential on the process of adaptation (age, gender, interpersonal relationships, the nature of disease, past experience and culture) [21]. However, given the diversity of emotional responses, it is usually necessary to make a detailed individual assessment. In order to get an accurate picture of the patient, it may be necessary to meet on a series of occasions and incorporate the opinions of the multi-disciplinary team.

Symptom control. Unremitting physical symptoms can be 'soul destroying', therefore symptom management is a key requirement of the adaptation process. This will then facilitate the management of emotional needs.

Communication. Skills in communication are pivotal to effective and sensitive care (see Chapter 6).

Counselling and therapy. Counselling is concerned with enabling individuals to attain solutions to an emotional challenge by using particular techniques. This approach can be especially helpful in unusually difficult situations. This intervention can be achieved either through one-to-one work or as part of group therapy [22], and often needs the involvement of specialist help.

Maintaining hope. Patients require hope to be sustained. This is achieved either by setting achievable goals or by the use of intermittent or persistent denial. What is important here is that the hope should reflect or be based in the reality of the situation, otherwise the goals may not be achieved.

Drugs. Appropriate use of psychotropic medicines (antidepressants, anxiolytics or antipsychotics) is occasionally useful in palliative medicine. In some cases it is difficult to differentiate between clinical psychiatric morbidity, which may respond to pharmacological intervention, and the normal emotions of dying. In this circumstance a trial of medication is a reasonable approach.

Complementary therapies. Various complementary modalities can be helpful in relieving emotional distress (see Chapter 23).

Emotional crises

This subject cannot be discussed in sufficient depth here to do justice to the importance of this area. The reader is referred to Stedford [23], Vachon [19], Stevens [24] and Lloyd-Williams [25].

Emotional crises do not arise without a trigger and pre-morbid factors of vulnerability. Understanding both of these for patient and family will help in management of the distress. Vulnerable patients and families should be identified in order to try to prevent crises through proactive access to additional support.

Various risk factors have been identified:

- pre-morbid factors in the family at diagnosis;
- strong dependency issues; hostility, ambivalence;
- other stresses within the family, e.g. relationship problems, poor housing, debts;
- illness and bereavement history—previous experiences of death and loss are important both in the quantity and quality of experience and coping mechanisms developed (or not developed) with previous distress;
- poor coping mechanisms;
- psychiatric history;
- for the family, poor patient adjustment compounds their risk of distress;
- nature of illness—families of older male patients dying from lung cancer and of young women dying from cancer of the cervix are more at risk of becoming overwhelmed and distressed [26].

MANAGEMENT OF EMOTIONAL CRISES

It is important to have a team approach, with more than one professional available to a family in acute distress, although one professional should take the lead role and act as the patient's key worker during the episode of care (see Chapter 2). The distress needs to be acknowledged and space must be given for the patient and/or family to regain control. In order to facilitate this, the cause of the distress should be explored. The 'cues' to this may need to be picked up from the patient.

Once the background and the triggers have been understood a plan can be negotiated. Many crises arise because the patient and/or family feel trapped, with no control and with no choices and options. Any physical and practical input required should be provided in order to reduce concerns and facilitate a sense of control over the situation. Discussing options that they have not perceived can diminish distress. Follow-up is essential to review the situation and plan, to modify the plan when necessary, and to explore any unresolved issues. A sense of security for the patient and family, and also trust in the professional team are important therapeutic components.

Adapting to bereavement

Although many people possess sufficient resources to cope with bereavement, for some the emotional challenge can be exacting and a risk to health. This observation has encouraged some health workers to develop patterns of care for the bereaved, most noticeably within the hospice movement [27] and voluntary sector.

Bereavement support of some kind has become a fundamental aspect of palliative care, although there is a view that it continues to be a marginalised service [28], with reports of inequitable distribution of services [29].

Currently, NHS Trusts are encouraging the development of bereavement support services. In part this has been prompted by public airing of concerns surrounding post mortems, organ retention [30] and the impact of delays on the carrying out of rituals by the family and community.

Psychological theories on bereavement

It might be tempting to view bereavement as a variant of depression and anxiety, but doing so would ignore a wealth of literature that enables us to understand more clearly the processes and emotions involved.

Freud's influential work [31] described grief as a period of time where the reality of a death is repeatedly tested until attachment is withdrawn from the deceased. Although complete withdrawal is advocated by Freud, in reality individuals find means of coping with their loss by, for example, finding an inner place to 'shelf' their attachment or memories while attending to other business. From observations made of bereaved people, Lindemann [32] describes five sub-groups of grief symptoms: somatic distress, preoccupation with images of the deceased, guilt, hostility and activity that appears restless and meaningless.

Bowlby, building on his psychoanalytical theories on attachment and loss, interpreted previous publications to devise a four-stage model for bereavement [33]. Although individuals can move back and forth between stages, there tends to be a progression through the following phases:

1 Phase of numbing
2 Phase of yearning and searching
3 Phase of disorganisation and despair
4 Phase of reorganisation.

The suggestion from Bowlby's theory is that only where there is an attachment bond will loss be experienced. It is also correct to suggest that the deeper or stronger the bond is, the more intense the loss that is felt.

Stroebe [34] has developed an idea, first discussed by Parkes [35], and has proposed the Dual Process Model of Coping with Grief. This theory describes a process where the bereaved oscillate from time to time between two psychological orientations (see Figure 7.1). Individuals choose to change orientation to achieve relief from the emotional pain of the other.

Drawing from empirical and anthropological observations, Walter [36] has proposed that the bereaved need to talk about the deceased in order to construct a biography that they can integrate into their ongoing lives. This allows the creation of a new identity that includes the persistent and usually unobtrusive memory of the deceased.

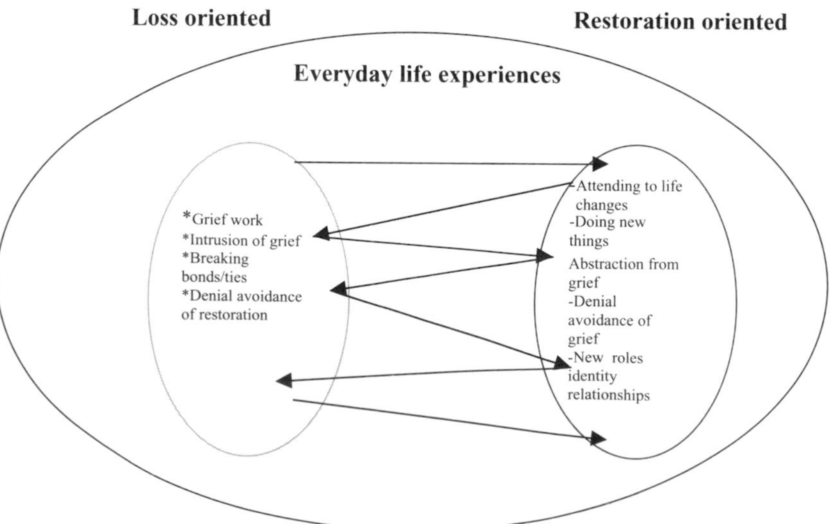

Fig. 7.1 A Dual Process Model of Coping with Grief [34].

While theories and models can guide us, we have to accept the individuality of each bereaved person. Grief creates chaos in the bereaved world and people will try and bring some order to their own chaos in their own time. It is not always helpful for us as professionals to put time frames on this process.

Consequences of bereavement

There has been considerable research into the adverse health consequences of bereavement [37, 38]. Studies have attempted to confirm the lay theory that patients can die of a 'broken heart'. In fact this has been very hard to prove, but it is probably true that the bereaved are at greater risk of death themselves, although this risk remains low in absolute terms. Other work has examined the psychiatric morbidity following bereavement. This research has been difficult to perform, but it seems to suggest that the bereaved are at risk of the following complications [37, 38]:

- depression;
- anxiety;
- alcohol abuse;
- increased use of prescribed drugs;
- suicidal tendencies and behaviour.

The evidence for an increase in physical morbidity is less conclusive, as research has failed to confirm any association between grief and physical disease.

PATHOLOGICAL BEREAVEMENT

The boundary between the normal emotions of grief and those exaggerated responses that would constitute abnormality, has been the subject of considerable debate. For severe psychiatric disease, the notion of abnormality is straightforward (like suicidal activity, alcohol abuse). However, for more minor affective disorders (e.g. depression, anxiety), it could be said that the symptoms represent normal bereavement. Various authors have proposed means to differentiate the normal from the abnormal. Time has been suggested as a useful, if arbitrary, discriminator. Unfortunately, no consensus appears to have been agreed upon and times ranging from 2 to over 12 months have been suggested [37, 38]. It is important to remember that individuals may differ with bereavement periods falling outside prescribed ranges.

Table 7.2 Examples of abnormal bereavement reactions.

Absent Individuals show no evidence of the emotions of grief developing, in spite of the reality of the death. This can appear as an automatic reaction or the result of active blocking.
Delayed This initially presents in a similar way to absent grief. However, this avoidance is always a conscious effort and the full emotions of grief are eventually expressed after a particular trigger. This may be seen in more compulsively self-reliant individuals.
Chronic In this instance, the normal emotions of grief persist without any diminution over time. It is postulated that this is most often seen in relationships that were particularly dependent.

Other research has concerned itself with describing symptoms that combine to produce particular bereavement syndromes. It is hoped that in defining new conditions in this way, clinicians will be able to develop care for those bereaved individuals who present with particular problems. Consequently, an array of terms has been devised leading to some confusion. Recently, an attempt to reach some international consensus was made, and three conditions seem to have achieved some recognition as pathological bereavement reactions (see Table 7.2) [39].

Assessment of bereavement needs

As in other aspects of palliative care, accurate assessment is a necessary part of management. This could be performed by any member of the multi-disciplinary team and is best achieved by someone with the following attributes:

- Good communication skills to facilitate expression of emotion.
- An ability to screen for psychiatric disease (e.g. depression, anxiety, suicidal intent).
- Familiarity with events surrounding death.
- An understanding of the social background.
- An awareness of risk factors of pathological grief (see Box 7.1).

Melliar-Smith describes the development and practical use of a risk assessment tool for bereavement, which is adaptable to a variety of palliative care settings [40].

Box 7.1 Risk factors for pathological bereavement

- Younger age
- Poor social support
- Sudden death
- Previous poor physical health
- Previous mental illness
- Poor coping strategies
- Multiple losses
- Stigmatised death
- Economic difficulties
- Previous unresolved grief

Other needs should also be considered when assessing the bereaved. These include social needs, i.e. the social consequences of a bereavement that may need attention, and occasionally the assistance of a social worker (e.g. re-housing benefits, day care). In some circumstances there are also physical needs; for example where a death results in unmet nursing needs in the bereaved. This may occur in the case of an elderly couple and may require the input of district nursing services or the geriatric health visitor.

The development of bereavement assessment skills is essential especially as there seems to be no measurement tools available specifically to evaluate the bereavement process. The closest tool measures death depression and was developed by Templer and others [41] in 1990. The only drawback is that this tool requires the bereaved person to self-assess by answering 17 questions on a Likert-scale format, and these questions may provoke unwanted emotions at such a sensitive time.

Management of bereavement needs

Although there are known adverse health consequences of bereavement, many bereaved individuals adapt to their loss with minimal assistance from health care professionals. Indeed, there are potential dangers in overmedicating grief. For instance, a bereavement can promote emotional growth within individuals and families. However, accurate assessment of risk remains the key component of appropriate bereavement management [42].

The recently developed Supportive and Palliative Care Guidelines outlines a three-component model of bereavement support, which it recommends should be implemented in each Cancer Network (Box 7.2). Similarly, the Standards for Bereavement Care in the UK may be applied to enable the development and evaluation of local bereavement services [43].

Box 7.2 Elements of the three-component model of bereavement support [30]

Component 1:	Grief is normal after bereavement and most people manage without professional intervention. All bereaved people should be offered information about the experience of bereavement and how to access other forms of support, e.g. leaflet.
Component 2:	Some people may require a more formal opportunity to review and reflect on their loss experience. Volunteer bereavement support workers, self-help groups, faith groups and community groups provide much of the support at this level.
Component 3:	A minority of people will require specialist interventions. This will involve mental health services, psychological support services, specialist counselling/psychotherapy services, specialist palliative care services, and general bereavement services.

BEREAVEMENT SERVICES

As a result of the assessment it may be necessary to provide some emotional support. This could involve brief intervention by the professional making the assessment or by using the array of bereavement services available. The services listed below do not include the very important help provided by religious advisers, but focus more on the work of health professionals and allied workers. Besides the bereavement services, various communities have developed social groups designed to overcome loneliness.

Written information

For those with low risk, providing written information may be all that is needed. This could range from pamphlets on where to get help should problems arise, to practical guides on what to do after a death and self-help books that normalise the bereavement process, (see useful web sites). There are some useful books that can be particularly helpful when explaining death to children.

Primary care team

The fact that patients are registered with personal general practitioners (GPs) promotes continuity of care and encourages primary care involvement in bereavement support. Although bereavement visits are made, GP input tends to be variable and in many cases is only reactive to requests for help. GP bereavement care could include such things as a bereavement visit, brief emotional support, referral to practice counsellor, use of psychotropic drugs or the involvement of other services. The key worker may have an ongoing supportive role for some time and should assess the need for referral to other agencies.

Specialist palliative care services

The hospice movement has seen bereavement care as integral to its service and has adopted a proactive approach. In some instances, these teams are considered as specialists within this field. They can provide an array of services, including: one-to-one support; telephone contact; written information; anniversary letters; social activities; group work; and memorial services [27]. In general, trained volunteers who are supervised by hospice staff perform this work.

Voluntary services

In the UK the main voluntary service is CRUSE Bereavement Care. This national organisation takes referrals from any source and can provide one-to-one or group work. It is staffed by trained volunteers and functions with a system of formal supervision. They prefer to take self-referrals and are contactable by phone (see Useful Addresses). The experience of some volunteers makes them able to tackle complex bereavement reactions.

Other organisations can provide support for parents who have lost a child (e.g. Compassionate Friends), see Useful Addresses.

Hospital-based services

Most hospitals have bereavement officers to assist with certain aspects of the arrangements following the death of an in-patient.

Some departments provide other aspects of support for particular bereavements:

- Some casualty departments have a role following sudden deaths brought to them.
- Midwives or maternity units may provide support to their patients who suffer loss.

In addition, psychiatric teams are involved in the more damaging bereavement reactions, particularly those resulting in major psychiatric illness.

Funeral directors

Some funeral directors are beginning to consider bereavement support as part of their service.

BEREAVEMENT COUNSELLING/THERAPY

Supporting the bereaved involves the application of the communication skills outlined elsewhere in this book (e.g. active listening, empathy, setting limits, clarification). Specialist authors have gone further and formulated approaches that provide greater guidance on bereavement counselling, either as general principles or in particular situations. Generally these have been based on the concept of 'grief work', of which Worden's book has been the most influential [44]. He suggests that it is helpful to separate counselling (helping people facilitate normal grief) from therapy (specialist techniques that help with abnormal grief). Central to his approach is the need for the bereaved to work through the four 'tasks of mourning' (see Table 7.3).

This model has recently been criticised for not allowing denial, lacking evidence of effectiveness, and inconsistencies with cross-cultural or historical perspectives. While this theoretical controversy continues, readers may find some of Worden's suggestions helpful.

Table 7.3 Worden's four tasks of mourning.

Task 1
To accept the reality of the loss
Task 2
To work through the pain of grief
Task 3
To adjust to the environment in which the deceased is missing
Task 4
To emotionally relocate the deceased and move on with life

Summary

Death, dying and bereavement challenges the fundamental values and meaning of the human experience. Such a threat has the potential to provoke considerable distress and has therefore interested health professionals. As a consequence, it has been possible to identify maladaptations and formulate responsive patterns of care. This has considerable implications for the work of health care professionals. Likewise, current guidelines for supportive and palliative care specify the development of bereavement services which require Trusts and professionals to ensure that resources are available to meet these guidelines [29].

It is important while providing care that we do not lose sight of the individual patient involved and the individuality of each experience of dying, death and bereavement. This chapter has detailed some of the literature on this subject with an aim to improve understanding of the process involved and the role of professionals in providing care.

References

1 Heidegger M. *Being and Time.* New York: Harper & Row, 1927.
2 Parkes CM. Bereavement as a psychosocial transition: process adaptation and change. In: Dickinson D, Johnson M, eds. *Death, Dying and Bereavement.* London: Sage, 1978.
3 World Health Organisation, *Cancer Pain Relief and Palliative Care: Report of the WHO Expert Committee*, Geneva: WHO, 1990.
4 Kastenbaum R, Aisenberg R. *The Psychology of Death.* New York: Springer Publishing Company, 1972.
5 Nyatanga B. *Why is it so Difficult to Die?* Wiltshire: Quay Books, 2001.
6 Diggory J, Rothman D. Values destroyed by death. *J Abnorm Soc Psychol* 1961; 63(1): 205–210.
7 Chonon J. *Death and the Modern Man.* New York: Macmillan, 1974.
8 Pattison EM. The living-dying process. In: Garfield CA, ed. *Psychological Care of the Dying Patient.* New York: McGraw-Hill, 1978.
9 Narayanasamy B. *Spiritual Care: A Resource Guide.* Nottingham: BKT Information Services, 1991.
10 Hunt J, Cobb M, Keeley VL, Ahmedzai SH. The quality of spiritual care-developing a standard. *Int J Palliat Nurs* 2003; 9(5): 208–215.
11 Kubler-Ross E. *On Death and Dying.* New York: Macmillan, 1969.
12 Glaser BG, Strauss AL. *Awareness of Dying.* Chicago: Adeline, 1965.
13 Timmermans S. Dying awareness: the theory of awareness revisited. *Sociol Health Ill* 1994; 16: 322–337.
14 Glaser BG, Strauss AL. *Time for Dying.* Chicago: Adeline, 1968.
15 Greer S. Psychological response to cancer and survival. *Pyschol Med* 1991; 21: 43–49.
16 Copp G. Facing impending death: the experiences of patients and their nurses in

a hospice setting. In: *Conference Proceedings—Palliative Care Research Forum UK*. Coventry: Palliative Care Research Forum, 1996.
17 Noyes R, Clancy J. The dying role: its relevance to improved patient care. In: Corr CA, Corr D, eds. *Hospice Care—Principles and Practice*. London: Faber & Faber, 1983.
18 Parkes CM. Bereavement as a psychosocial transition: process adaptation and change. In: Dickinson D, Johnson M, eds. *Death, Dying and Bereavement*. London: Sage, 1993.
19 Vachon MLS. Emotional problems in palliative medicine: patient, family and professional. In: Doyle D, Hanks G, MacDonald N, eds. *The Oxford Textbook of Palliative Medicine*. Oxford: Oxford University Press, 1993: 577–605.
20 Jarrett SR, Ramirez AJ, Richards MA et al. Measuring coping in breast cancer. *J Psychosom Res* 1992; 36: 593–602.
21 Neimyer RA, Van Brunt D. Death anxiety. In: Wass H, Neimyer RA, eds. *Dying—Facing the Facts*. Washington: Taylor & Francis, 1995.
22 Kirk M, McManus M. Containing families' grief: therapeutic group work in a hospice setting. *Int J Palliat Nurs* 2002; 8(10): 470–480.
23 Stedford A. *Facing Death*. Oxford: Heinemann Medical Books, 1984.
24 Stevens MM. Family adjustment and support. In: Doyle D, Hanks GWC, Macdonald N, eds. *Oxford Textbook of Palliative Medicine*. Oxford: Oxford University Press, 1993: 707–717.
25 Lloyd-Williams M. *Psychosocial Issues in Palliative Care*. Oxford. Oxford University Press 2003.
26 Wellisch DK, Fawzy F, Landsverk J, Pasnau RO, Wolcott DL. Evaluation of psychosocial problems of the homebound cancer patient: the relationship of the disease and the sociodemographic variables of patients to family problems. *J Psychosoc Oncol* 1983; 1: 1–15.
27 Payne S, Relf M. The assessment of need for bereavement follow up in palliative and hospice care. *Palliat Med* 1994; 8: 291–297.
28 Payne S. Bereavement support: something for everyone. *Int J Palliat Nurs* 2001; 7(3):108.
29 National Institute for Clinical Excellence. *Guidance on Cancer services: Improving Supportive and Palliative Care for Adults with Cancer*. London, National Institute for Clinical Excellence, 2004.
30 Derrick G. Lessons we can learn from organ retention. *Brit Med J* 2003; 327: 996.
31 Freud S. Mourning and melancholia. In: *Collected Papers Vol IV*. London: Hogarth Press, 1925.
32 Lindemann E. Symptomatology and the management of acute grief. *Am J Psych* 1944; 101: 141–148.
33 Bowlby J. *Loss: Sadness and Depression (Attachment and Loss)*, Vol. 3. New York: Basic Books, 1980.
34 Stroebe M. Helping the bereaved come to terms with loss. In: *Bereavement and Counselling-Conference Proceedings*. London: St George's Mental Health Sciences, 1994.
35 Parkes CM. *Bereavement Studies of Grief in Adult Life*. London: Tavistock Publications, 1972.
36 Walter T. A new model for grief: bereavement and biography. *Mortality* 1996; 1: 7–25.

37 Woof WR, Carter YH. The grieving adult and the general practitioner; a literature review in two parts (part 1). *Br J Gen Pract* 1997; 47: 443–448.
38 Woof WR, Carter YH. The grieving adult and the general practitioners: a literature review in two parts (part 2). *Br J Gen Pract* 1997; 47: 509–514.
39 Middleton W, Moylan A, Raphael B et al. An international perspective on bereavement and related concepts. *Aus NZ J Psych* 1993; 27: 457–463.
40 Melliar-Smith C. The risk assessment of bereavement in a palliative care setting. *Int J Palliat Nurs* 2002; 8(6): 281–287.
41 Templer, D. La Voie, M. Chalgujian, H. Thomas-Dodson, S. The measurement of death depression. *J Clin Psychol* 1990; 46: 834–839.
42 Parkes CM. Bereavement counselling—does it work? *BMJ* 1980; 281: 3–10.
43 Bereavement Care Standards UK Project. *Standards for Bereavement Care in the UK*. October 2001. Accessible at: http://www.bereavement.org.uk/standards/index.asp
44 Worden JW *Grief Counselling and Grief Therapy*. London: Routledge, 1992.

8: The Principles of Pain Management

MIKE BENNETT, KAREN FORBES
AND CHRISTINA FAULL

Introduction

The successful management of pain requires careful assessment of the nature of the pain, an understanding of different types and patterns of pain and knowledge of how best to treat it. Good initial pain assessment will act as a baseline against which subsequent interventions can be judged. The multi-dimensional nature of pain means that the use of analgesics may be only part of a multi-professional team strategy addressing physical, psychological, social and spiritual distress, and, at times, the need for behavioural change. Negotiation of a management plan is a vital part of the process and requires good communication with patients and their carers.

Pain occurs in up to 75% of patients with advanced cancer [1] and in about 65% of patients dying from all other causes [2]. Of patients dying from heart disease, 78% are reported as having pain in the last year of life [3]. Despite considerable scientific and pharmacological progress, pain continues to be substantially undertreated [4–6]. The use of opioids remains an area of major concern for many clinicians, and the increasing variety of available formulations may compound this. This chapter will discuss the nature and experience of pain for patients, particularly those with cancer. A framework for the effective use of drugs and other interventional techniques in pain management will be discussed.

The nature of pain

Pain is an unpleasant sensory *and* emotional experience. Pain is essentially subjective since it can only be identified and quantified as 'what the patient says hurts' and is individual to the person experiencing it. Observation of behaviour and physical signs may provide some additional information but it must be recognised that the correlation between observer- and patient-reported pain may be poor. One person's response to the same painful stimulus will differ from another's according to a variety of circumstances. The observation of behavioural responses to pain is, however, particularly important where language is limited or absent, for example in neonates, infants, the mentally incompetent and those deprived of language (e.g. following a stroke).

The concept of total pain

The experience of pain is influenced by physical, emotional, social and spiritual factors. The concept of total pain acknowledges the importance of all of these dimensions of a person's suffering, and that good pain relief is unlikely without attention to all of these areas [7] (Figure 8.1).

Patients with chronic or advanced disease face many losses: loss of normality; loss of health; and potential loss of the future. Pain imposes limitations on lifestyle, particularly in terms of mobility and endurance. In addition, the pain can be interpreted as a reminder of the underlying disease and its present and possible consequences. The significance of pain for patients with advanced disease will vary

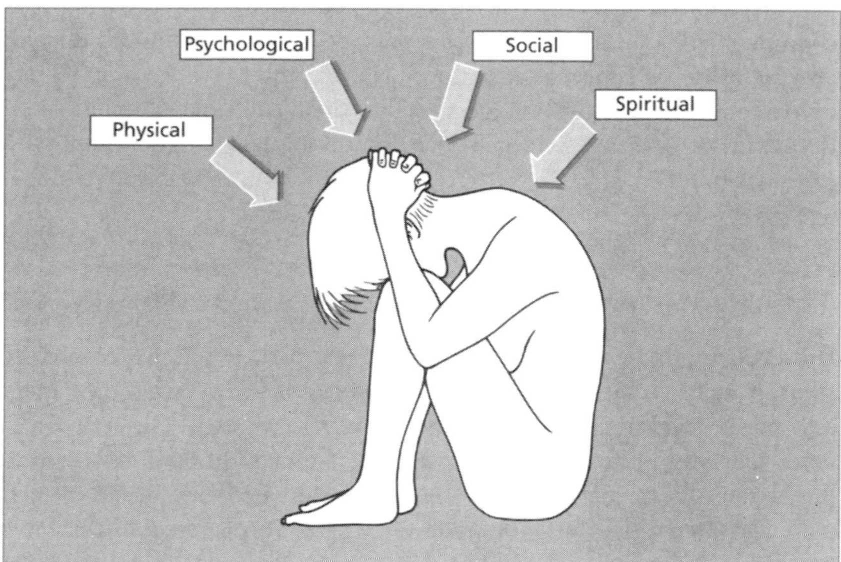

Fig. 8.1 The concept of total pain.

according to the person, their circumstances and the illness. Pain due to muscle spasm in chronic degenerative neurological disorder may be distressing and frustrating; however, a patient with ischaemic heart disease may believe each episode of chest pain signifies imminent death.

Many people feel that severe pain is inevitable in cancer, and this may lead to fear, suffering and reluctance to ask for help. Pain may be erroneously interpreted by patients as an indication of progression of their cancer and therefore a signal of their approaching death.

Neuroanatomy and neurophysiology of nociception and analgesia

Nociception is the detection of noxious stimuli by specialised nerve endings known as nociceptors. Activation of nociceptors by mechanical, thermal or chemical stimuli leads to the perception of so-called nociceptive pain. An understanding of the physiology that underlies this will allow improved pain assessment and management. A simplified schema of the neuroanatomy and site of action of a variety of analgesic modalities is shown in Figure 8.2.

Nerve fibres are classified as A, B or C fibres, with alpha, beta, delta and gamma subcategories. A-beta, A-delta and C are sensory fibres and therefore have a role in pain perception. A-delta nociceptors respond to pricking, squeezing or pinching and lead to the 'fast', sharp pain of an injury. They are involved in the analgesia produced by acupuncture-like transcutaneous electrical nerve stimulation—(TENS) (see below). 'Polymodal' C fibres respond to many noxious stimuli to produce 'slow', throbbing, more diffuse pain. These nociceptive afferent fibres synapse with neurones within the dorsal horn of the spinal cord; these project on, via interneurones, to the thalamus and cortex. A-beta and other sensory afferent nerve fibres also synapse with these dorsal horn neurones and may inhibit the transmission of the painful stimulus to the thalamus and cortex. This is known as gate control and is the mechanism of action of conventional TENS (see below).

Normal activation of nociceptive pathways (that is, a noxious stimulus triggers nociceptor firing) is known as nociceptive pain. Abnormal activation of nociceptive pathways is known as neuropathic pain (see below). Descending inhibitory neural pathways from the brain to the spinal cord also modulate incoming nociceptive information. The major neurotransmitters involved in these descending inhibitory

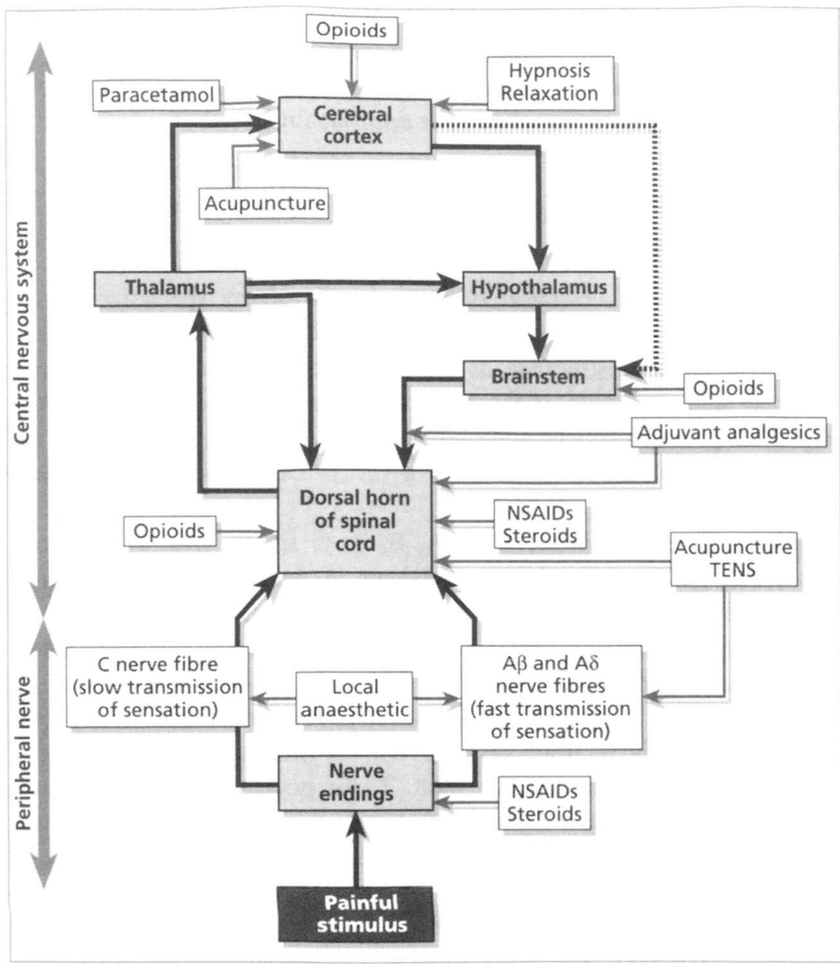

Fig. 8.2 A schema of the neuroanatomy of pain and the sites of action of different analgesic modalities.

pathways are serotonin and noradrenaline. This is the probable site of action of many adjuvant analgesics.

Opioid receptors occur throughout the spinal cord and in many areas of the brain. There are at least three types of opioid receptor that subserve opioid analgesia (see Box 8.1). The analgesia produced by acupuncture is thought to be due to the release of endogenous opioids (endorphins, dynorphins and enkephalins) in the spinal cord.

Box 8.1 Opioid receptors

Opioid receptor subtype:	Effect of agonist
Mu	Analgesia, respiratory depression, reduced gastrointestinal motility, hypotension
Kappa	Analgesia, sedation, psychomimetic effects; some respiratory depression
Delta	Analgesia, respiratory depression

Patterns and types of pain

The classification of pain is not an esoteric exercise, since the type of pain may suggest its underlying cause and guide treatment decisions.

Acute and chronic pain

Whilst acute pain provokes a 'fight or flight' (sympathetic) response with tachycardia, hypertension and pupillary changes, chronic pain allows adaptation to this. Many patients mount this physiological response only during acute exacerbations of pain, with few if any such signs at other times.

Chronic pain is not simply prolonged acute pain. Repeated noxious stimulation leads to a variety of changes within the central nervous system (CNS). For example, repeated C-fibre stimulation leads to accentuated neuronal responses in the dorsal horn of the spinal cord, leading to increased and prolonged pain perception. This is termed 'wind up', which is thought to be mediated via the action of glutamate at the N-methyl-D-aspartate (NMDA) receptor.

SOMATIC AND VISCERAL PAIN

Somatic and visceral pain are both nociceptive pains. Somatic pain arises from damage to the skin and deep tissues. It is usually localised and of an aching quality. Visceral pain arises from the abdominal and thoracic viscera. It is poorly localised and described as 'deep' and 'pressure'. Visceral pain is sometimes 'referred' and is felt in a part of the body distant to the site of noxious stimulation—for example, the visceral pain of diaphragmatic irritation is felt in the shoulder tip, and the pain of ischaemic heart disease radiates into the neck and arms. Visceral pain is often associated with other symptoms such as nausea and vomiting. Both types of pain usually respond well to the non-opioid or opioid analgesics (see section on WHO analgesic ladder).

Neuropathic pain

Neuropathic pain arises as a consequence of a disturbance of function or pathological change in a nerve or the nervous system [8]. It may arise from a lesion within the peripheral or central nervous system, and may follow nerve damage due to trauma, infection, ischaemia, degenerative disease, compression, tumour invasion or chemical- or radiation-induced injury. The primary injury may sometimes be trivial. Neuropathic pain often occurs in an area of abnormal or absent sensation [9].

Deafferentation pain is a type of neuropathic pain, for example following brachial or lumbosacral plexus avulsion injuries. Phantom limb pain is the classic example of deafferentation pain. Central pain is neuropathic pain following damage to the CNS, for example pain following stroke. Complex Regional Pain Syndromes (CPRS) are pains that are associated with autonomic dysfunction and for this reason are classified as neuropathic pains. Autonomic dysfunction can occur either after tissue injury (for instance Colle's fracture) but no clear nerve injury (CRPS I) or it can occur with clear nerve injury (CRPS II, previously known as causalgia). Symptoms common to both types of CRPS include swelling, changes in sweating and temperature, and trophic changes such as thinning of tissues, loss of hair and abnormal nail growth.

Neuropathic pain may be improved but is often not completely relieved by non-opioid or opioid analgesics. Adjuvant analgesic drugs are often required (see p. 143).

ABNORMAL SENSATIONS IN NEUROPATHIC PAIN

Various abnormal sensations are associated with neuropathic pain. Spontaneous pains (pains that arise in the absence of a stimulus)

> continuous (dysaethesias)
> paroxysmal.

Evoked pains (abnormal responses to a stimulus)

> Allodynia: painful response to a non-painful stimulus.
> Hyperalgesia: increased painful response to painful stimulus.
> Hyperpathia: delayed and prolonged response to stimulus.

Breakthrough or incident pain

Pain that occurs intermittently or is only associated with specific movements is often called breakthrough pain, incident pain or more recently, episodic pain [10]. There is increasing recognition that this type of pain is more common and more severe than previously thought. Patients with uncontrolled incident pain are also more likely to be depressed and have a poorer quality of life [11].

The assessment of pain

Successful pain management relies on careful assessment to elucidate possible underlying causes and the effect the pain is having on the patient's life, plus the psychosocial and spiritual factors that might be influencing the pain and its impact on the patient. A full pain history (see Box 8.2) and a clinical examination are vital, and laboratory or radiographic investigations may then be necessary. It may be useful to use a specific assessment and monitoring tool.

Pain is a uniquely personal experience. There is no standard language of pain. Descriptions of pain will vary within families and cultural groups. It may be extremely difficult for a patient with advanced disease to find the language to describe his pain since it may be unlike anything he has previously experienced not least because of its emotional, social and spiritual components.

Box 8.2 Taking a pain history

1. When did the pain start?
2. Where is it, and does it go anywhere else?
3. What does it feel like (nature and severity)?
4. Is it constant or does it come and go?
5. Does anything make it better or worse?
6. Are there any associated symptoms?
7. Is it limiting the patient's activities?
8. What does the patient think the pain is due to?
9. What does the patient feel about the pain (emotional impact)?
10. Which analgesics have been tried and what effect did they have?
11. What are the patient's expectations of treatment?
12. What are the patient's fears?
13. What is the patient's previous experience of pain and illness?

Pain and behaviour

Pain impinges on and alters people's lives, turning their focus inwards and potentially isolating them. This behavioural response may be graded by an observer—for example, grimacing or crying in a child—or reported by the patient—for example, alterations in behaviour such as:

- pain at rest, but pain can be ignored;
- in pain, but can carry out tasks;
- in pain, but with concentration can carry out tasks;
- pain overwhelming, dominating everything.

Pain assessment tools

Pain assessment tools will aid initial understanding of the nature of pain for the individual and will allow clear assessment of the effect of analgesics and other interventions. A report that the pain is 'better' is ambiguous and without such records may mean either improved or cured. Most patients can grade their pain out of 10. If this concept is difficult, a simpler categorical scale can be chosen in discussion with the patient (see Box 8.3).

Box 8.3 Simple verbal and numerical scales for pain assessment

- Present/absent
- Good/bad
- None/mild/moderate/severe
- None/mild/moderate/severe/excruciating
- Graded out of 10, where 0 = no pain and 10 = worst pain ever

VISUAL ANALOGUE SCALES

A visual analogue scale (VAS) is a 10 cm line labelled at each end to denote the minimum and maximum extremes of whatever is being measured (in this case pain). The line is usually horizontal but some patients find vertical lines more understandable.

Least possible pain ———————————————— Worst possible pain

The patient puts a mark on the line corresponding to the intensity of the pain and the observer then measures its position. VASs are simple, reproducible and reliable and correlate well with scores derived from categorical scales. They can be used in both clinical and research settings.

BODY CHARTS

Body charts can be used to evaluate the site and nature of pain. Body charts may emphasise that a patient has pain at several sites, possibly of different aetiologies and therefore requiring different treatments.

PAIN QUESTIONNAIRES

There are numerous pain questionnaires but many are suitable for research only. The McGill Pain Questionnaire (Figure 8.3) is used extensively in pain research [12] and can be a useful clinical tool for patients with difficult pain management in a specialist setting. The LANSS (Leeds Assessment of Neuropathic Symptoms and Signs) pain scale is a validated measure for identifying patients in whom neuropathic mechanisms dominate their pain experience [13].

USEFUL TOOLS FOR CHILDREN

Children may be more comfortable drawing their pain on a body chart than describing it. Their use of colour at various sites can be discussed and related to the nature and severity of each pain. A pain thermometer can be used in the same way as a VAS, i.e. the child marks the intensity of the pain on the thermometer and the observer then measures the position of the mark. The shading of the thermometer from blue to red provides visual cues for children, who may not grasp the concept of a VAS.

Face scales have been developed for the assessment of pain in children. Children rank their pain against a series of drawings or photographs of faces showing varying facial expressions of pain. They may also be useful when language presents a barrier between patient and professional.

Management of cancer-related pain

The remainder of this chapter will concentrate largely on pain due to cancer although many of the principles can be extrapolated to the

McGill pain questionnaire

Patient's name .... Date .... Time .... am/pm

PRI: S............... A............... E............... M............... PRI(T)............... PPI.........................

(1–10) (11–15) (16) (17–20) (1–20)

1 Flickering, Quivering, Pulsing, Throbbing, Beating, Pounding

2 Jumping, Flashing, Shooting

3 Pricking, Boring, Drilling, Stabbing, Lancinating

4 Sharp, Cutting, Lacerating

5 Pinching, Pressing, Gnawing, Cramping, Crushing

6 Tugging, Pulling, Wrenching

7 Hot, Burning, Scalding, Searing

8 Tingling, Itchy, Smarting, Stinging

9 Dull, Sore, Hurting, Aching, Heavy

10 Tender, Taut, Rasping, Splitting

11 Tiring, Exhausting

12 Sickening, Suffocating

13 Fearful, Frightful, Terrifying

14 Punishing, Gruelling, Cruel, Vicious, Killing

15 Wretched, Blinding

16 Annoying, Troublesome, Miserable, Intense, Unbearable

17 Spreading, Radiating, Penetrating, Piercing

18 Tight, Numb, Drawing, Squeezing, Tearing

19 Cool, Cold, Freezing

20 Nagging, Nauseating, Agonizing, Dreadful, Torturing

PPI

0 No pain
1 Mild
2 Discomforting
3 Distressing
4 Horrible
5 Excruciating

Brief
Momentary
Transient

Rhythmic
Periodic
Intermittent

Continuous
Steady
Constant

E = External
I = Internal

Comments:

Fig. 8.3 The Mcgill pain questionnaire.

management of chronic pain in other illnesses. It should not be assumed that cancer will lead inevitably to pain; some patients with cancer do not experience pain, and not every pain experienced by a patient with cancer is due to the cancer itself (see Box 8.4).

Box 8.4 Pain due to cancer

Thirty percent of people with cancer do not develop pain. Those with pain may have four or more different types:
- related to the cancer
- related to the treatment
- related to consequent disability
- due to a concurrent disorder

Principles of pain management in patients with cancer

The management of pain in cancer patients should be undertaken in a systematic manner, based on certain principles. Firstly, assess each pain separately, and ascertain if the pain is related to the cancer. If so, consider three main types of cancer-related pain.
- Somatic/visceral pain: usually opioid sensitive; use the WHO analgesic ladder (see below).
- Bone pain: usually NSAID sensitive; may be poorly opioid sensitive; radiotherapy often helps.
- Neuropathic pain: may respond poorly to opioids; co-analgesics have a key role; often difficult pain to manage; may need *early* specialist referral for best results.

It is also important to consider if the pain is incident pain, which is best managed by treating the underlying cause where possible. Different analgesic doses are required for rest pain and movement-related pain to avoid excess sedation at rest, i.e. give extra analgesics before movement in anticipation of pain. Spinal routes of analgesic delivery may be useful (see the section on World Health Organization (WHO) analgesic ladder for cancer pain).

Treatment modalities

There are seven well described approaches in the management of all pain. The first five of these are commonly used whereas the last two are interventions that are only required by a few patients.
(i) *Explanation.* A patient who understands the cause of their pain and the nature and expectations of the treatment is likely to cope better.

(ii) *Raise pain threshold.* Pain tolerance threshold (the maximum level pain can be tolerated rather than perception threshold—the minimum level pain can be perceived) can be influenced by a number of factors. Most important of these are social support, activity, increased mood including hope and the absence of helplessness and adequate sleep. A depressed, socially isolated, bored patient who sleeps badly is unlikely to cope well with their pain in this situation.
(iii) *Modify lifestyle.* Assess the need for aids and adaptations and plan ahead to reduce painful situations.
(iv) *Modify the pathological process.* For some patients it may be possible to treat the underlying cancer and thus reduce pain. This is based on the rationale that good disease control usually results in good symptom control. There are three main treatment approaches. One is chemotherapy: for example, palliative chemotherapy may reduce liver capsule pain by shrinking hepatic metastases. Another is radiotherapy; for example, a single fraction of radiotherapy for bone metastases provides good pain relief in up to 80% of patients. The third approach is hormone therapy: for example, bone pain related to metastatic prostatic cancer may be reduced by the commencement of antiandrogen treatment.

For other patients an orthopaedic procedure to stabilise a fracture or decompress the spinal cord, whilst not affecting the cancer, may relieve pain, particularly incident pain. For example, pain in the thigh due to a femoral metastasis may be relieved by internal fixation.
(v) *Modify pain perception.* Pain perception can be modified largely through drug treatments but also through non-drug treatments such as acupuncture (discussed in Chapter 10). To better understand the effects of treatments, it is useful to clarify some definitions. *Antinociceptive* refers to the ability of an agent to reduce the reception of noxious stimuli at the level of the sensory organ e.g. the action of aspirin in reducing inflammatory activation of cutaneous nociceptors at nerve endings. *Antalgesic* or *analgesic* refers to the action of an agent in modulating the neural pathways that transmit pain.

Some patients may seek other approaches such as complementary medicine to control their pain. In most patients, but especially in those that are anxious, relaxation techniques may improve pain. Patients may be helped by visualising their pain to be decreasing. Hypnotherapy can also be a powerful analgesic tool. Some patients find that aromatherapy massage decreases pain by relieving muscle spasm and producing relaxation. Homeopathic remedies may also be helpful. More detailed descriptions of analgesics are given below.

(vi) *Interrupt pain pathways.* In a patient with pain that is not responding to drug treatment, which is localised or appears to be within the distribution of a single nerve root, referral for consideration of a nerve block may be indicated. Nerve blocks are usually carried out initially with local anaesthetic to assess response. Injection of local anaesthetic plus steroid may then provide pain relief for some weeks. Neuroablation using phenol, cryotherapy or radiofrequency lesions is indicated when pain improves initially but recurs.
Nerve blocks commonly used include:

- intercostal nerve blocks for chest wall pain (rib metastases or pleural infiltration);
- lumbar/caudal epidural for low back or sacral root pain;
- coeliac plexus or splanchnic nerve block for the pain of carcinoma of the pancreas, liver metastases or chronic pancreatitis;
- femoral nerve block for fracture of the femur;
- brachial plexus block for pain, particularly with axillary recurrence of breast cancer. It may be necessary to infuse local anaesthetic via a fine catheter;
- dorsal root ganglion blocks may help local or radicular back pain, particularly the acute, severe pain of an osteoporotic crush fracture;
- patients with advanced disease may have coexisting osteoarthritis, and facet joint injections and injections into painful sacroiliac joints or shoulders may provide relief;
- lumbar sympathectomy for tenesmus and pelvic visceral pain;
- cordotomy is occasionally useful for unilateral body pain.

(vii) *Psychological intervention.* In a small number of patients with chronic pain, referral to a clinical psychologist can be helpful. These situations are usually characterised by patients with exaggerated or irrational beliefs about their pain, or pain experience dominated by cognitions, emotions and behaviours that are unpleasant for the patient.

The World Health Organization (WHO) analgesic ladder for cancer pain

The Cancer Pain Relief Programme of the WHO advocates a three-step 'analgesic ladder' in an attempt to improve the management of pain due to cancer worldwide [14, 15] (Figure 8.4). The underlying principle is that, following good pain assessment and with a thorough knowledge of a small number of analgesics, a simple approach should produce safe and effective pain relief in the majority of patients.

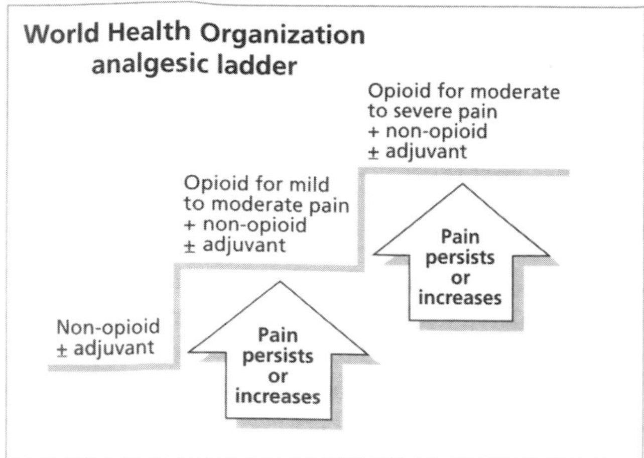

Fig. 8.4 The WHO analgesic ladder. The ladder has no 'top rung' as there is no maximum dose for strong opioids. If pain is still a problem with doses of morphine >300 mg/day reconsider the underlying cause of the pain and/or seek specialist advice. (Adapted from [15].)

Although the WHO analgesic ladder was developed for use in cancer pain, a stepwise approach using a limited number of drugs is equally applicable to the management of chronic pain due to other causes and has the potential to simplify prescribing. Pain which is judged to be mild is treated with a step one analgesic. Pain that is mild to moderate in intensity, or pain that has not responded to a step one analgesic is treated with a step two analgesic. Similarly, moderate to severe pain or pain that has not responded to a step two analgesic is treated with a step three analgesic. The ladder design means that the patient's pain determines the initial and subsequent analgesic to be used. It does not mean that all patients should be treated with a step one analgesic before commencing to step two or three analgesia.

Opiates, opioids and non-opioids: terminology

An *opiate* is a drug derived or synthesised from the opium poppy, such as morphine. The term *opioid* includes naturally occurring, semisynthetic and synthetic drugs which, like morphine, combine with opioid receptors to produce their effects. These effects are antagonised by naloxone.

The *non-opioid* analgesics available in the UK are paracetamol and the non-steroidal anti-inflammatory drugs (NSAIDs), which include the salicylate, aspirin.

Step 1: Non-opioid analgesics

NON-STEROIDAL ANTI-INFLAMMATORY DRUGS (NSAIDS)

The NSAIDs are a group of chemically unrelated drugs which have analgesic, anti-inflammatory and antipyretic properties through inhibition of the enzyme cyclo-oxygenase (COX), involved in prostaglandin synthesis (Table 8.1)

Table 8.1 Types and recommended doses of NSAIDs.

	Recommended dose			
NSAID	Oral i.r.	Oral m.r.	Rectal	Parenteral
Salicylates				
Aspirin	600 mg q.d.s.	–	600 mg q.d.s.	–
Diflunisal	500 mg t.d.s.	–	–	–
Acetates				
Diclofenac	50 mg t.d.s.	75–100 mg b.d.	50 mg t.d.s.	75 mg b.d.
Indometacin	50 mg t.d.s.	75 mg b.d.	100 mg b.d.	–
Sulindac	200 mg b.d.	–	–	–
Propionates				
Flurbiprofen	50 mg t.d.s./q.d.s.		200 mg o.d.	100 mg b.d.
Ibuprofen	600 mg t.d.s.	–	–	–
Naproxen	500 mg b.d.	–	500 mg b.d.	–
Ketorolac	10 mg q.d.s.	–	–	30–90 mg S.C.
Fenamates				
Mefenamic acid	500 mg t.d.s.	–	–	–
Oxicams				
Piroxicam	10–30 mg o.d.	–	–	–
Pyrazolanes				
Phenylbutazone	Ankylosing spondylitis only			
Butazones				
Nabumetone	1 g nocte	–	–	–
COX-2 inhibitors				
Rofecoxib	12.5–25 mg o.d.			
Celecoxib	100–200 mg b.d.			

Key: i.r. = normal-release preparation; m.r. = modified-release preparation.

There are two forms of COX. COX-1 is involved in normal prostaglandin synthesis, including the protective effect of prostaglandins in the gastrointestinal tract. COX-2 is only found in normal tissues in the presence of inflammation and thus the anti-inflammatory and analgesic effects of NSAIDs are related to inhibition of COX-2. NSAIDs that are relatively COX-2-specific, such as rofecoxib and celecoxib, do have fewer gastrointestinal side-effects [16].

NSAIDs are analgesic in their own right and can be used in conjunction with analgesics from all three steps of the WHO analgesic ladder. They are used in the following situations:

- for pain due to bony metastases, which may respond poorly to opioids;
- where pain has an inflammatory aetiology, e.g. pleuritic chest pain;
- for musculoskeletal pain, rheumatoid arthritis and osteoarthritis;
- for the pain of soft-tissue injuries and fractures and for dysmenorrhoea, dental pain and headache.

Side-effects of NSAIDs

NSAID prescriptions are numerous and it is estimated that there are 3000 NSAID-related deaths in the UK each year. NSAIDs and aspirin will precipitate symptomatic bronchospasm in 5% of asthmatic patients, and a few individuals develop allergic reactions such as anaphylaxis, rashes and urticaria.

Gastrointestinal effects. Up to 20% of people given any particular NSAID will develop dyspepsia, nausea or vomiting, and some will develop peptic ulceration, haemorrhage or perforation. Various steps can be taken to avoid or reduce these side-effects. Patients at high risk of ulceration are those with a history of dyspepsia or ulceration, smokers, those aged over 60, and those taking both NSAIDs and steroids. Patients with advanced disease, whatever the aetiology, are likely to be at increased risk of peptic ulceration. It is common practice to prescribe either a COX-2 NSAID alone or a standard NSAID plus a proton pump inhibitor (e.g. lansoprazole) in these situations. Some centres prescribe COX-2 plus a proton pump inhibitor.

Renal effects. NSAIDs increase sodium and water retention and can lead to oedema and even congestive cardiac failure. NSAID-mediated reduction of renal prostaglandins may lead to acute renal failure, particularly in the elderly, those on diuretics and antihypertensives, and those with impaired renal function. Renal function should be monitored in those at risk. Sulindac is relatively safe for those with impaired renal function.

Haematological effects. Aspirin and the NSAIDS inhibit platelet aggregation. This is clinically significant only if patients are also taking anticoagulants. Patients on anticoagulants who require an NSAID should be treated with a COX-2 NSAID and a proton pump inhibitor.

Parenteral NSAIDs

Diclofenac and other NSAIDs are available for deep intramuscular injection. Due to injection site problems the subcutaneous route should generally not be used.

Ketorolac may be delivered by the subcutaneous route when diluted with water, but has a high risk of gastrointestinal side-effects. A loading dose of 30 mg can be given intravenously or intramuscularly prior to commencing a subcutaneous infusion. The patient should be commenced on 30 mg over 24 h, increasing to 60 mg and 90 mg if necessary. If pain does not respond within 48 h the infusion should be stopped.

PARACETAMOL

Paracetamol is a relatively safe and effective step one analgesic with similar indications for use as for NSAIDs. It has antipyretic and analgesic properties but no peripheral anti-inflammatory effects. It is thought to work via central nervous system prostaglandin inhibition. In overdose, paracetamol can cause hepatic damage leading to hepatic failure and this can occur with doses of 10 g per 24 h.

Cochrane reviews of research compare analgesics using the denominator 'number needed to treat' or NNT. This represents the number of patients who need to be treated with the analgesic for one patient to experience 50% pain relief. The lower the NNT, the more effective the analgesic. On this basis, clinical trials in acute pain (i.e., not in cancer pain) suggest that ibuprofen 800 mg, a relatively safe NSAID, has a NNT of 1.6, rofecoxib 50 mg has a NNT of 2.3 and paracetamol 1 g has a NNT of 3.8 [17]. Although paracetamol is less effective, it is safer than NSAIDs. Other NSAIDS have higher NNTs (i.e. less effective) than ibuprofen and are less safe. This indicates that if a patient's pain does not improve with either ibuprofen, rofecoxib or paracetamol as first line choices, a step two analgesic is required.

Step 2: Opioids for mild to moderate pain

Opioids commonly used for mild to moderate pain include codeine, dihydrocodeine dextropropoxyphene and tramadol. The first three are available in combination with step 1 analgesics (see Box 8.5). Codeine probably has 10% of the potency of morphine. A maximum daily dose of codeine (60 mg four times daily = 240 mg) is therefore equivalent to about 24 mg of morphine. This means that if the patient's pain is not improving on this dose of codeine (either alone or as cocodamol 30/500 for example), the starting dose of morphine per 24 h needs to be at least 40 mg before an improvement in analgesia can be expected.

Box 8.5 Useful step 2 analgesics

Co-codamol 30/500	Codeine 30 mg + paracetamol 500 mg per tablet Dose: 2 tablets 6-hourly
Co-proxamol	Dextropropoxyphene 32.5 mg + paracetamol 325 mg per tablet Dose: 2 tablets 4–6 hourly
Dihydrocodeine	Dose: 30–60 mg 4–6 hourly
Tramadol	Dose: 50–100 mg 4–6 hourly (relatively high potency; see Table 8.2)

Step 3: Opioids for moderate to severe pain

Medicines used in this category are often referred to as 'strong opioids' and there are many preparations available.

Their relative potencies and potential areas of use are shown in Table 8.2. In the UK, morphine is the drug of choice for oral administration, and diamorphine for parenteral administration. The legal requirements governing the prescription of morphine and its availability in different countries vary, sometimes making prescribing problematic (see Chapter 1). Diamorphine is not available in some countries, such as the USA.

MORPHINE

Morphine is a natural derivative of the opium poppy. It is readily absorbed after oral administration, mainly in the upper small bowel, and is metabolised in the liver and at other sites to morphine-3-glucuronide (M3G) and morphine-6-glucuronide (M6G). M6G is an

Table 8.2 The relative potencies of opioids.

Drug	Approximate equivalence to repeated doses of 10 mg of oral morphine sulphate: Oral dose	s.c./i.m. dose	Indication
Morphine	10 mg	5 mg	Oral strong opioid of choice in the UK
Diamorphine	10 mg	3–5 mg	Strong opioid of choice in the UK
Hydromorphone	1.3 mg	0.5 mg	As for morphine
Methadone (chronic use)	3 mg	2 mg	Specialist use
Oxycodone	5 mg	2.5 mg	As for morphine
Buprenorphine	0.2 mg (s.l.)	–	Possible alternative to low dose morphine (has a ceiling effect)
Tramadol	70 mg	100 mg	Potent step 2 –(analgesic)
Pethidine	160 mg	40 mg	Unsuitable for chronic pain
Codeine	120 mg	80 mg	WHO step 2 (analgesic)
Dihydrocodeine	100 mg	–	WHO step 2 (analgesic)
Dextropropoxyphene	100 mg	–	WHO step 2 analgesic

The reader may find slight variations in equivalence in other texts. However, the table is designed to be useful in clinical practice.

active metabolite, and is a more potent analgesic than morphine. Morphine and its glucuronides are excreted renally and so may accumulate with impaired renal function.

Regular administration by any route (determined by the duration of action of the preparation) is necessary to achieve constant, therapeutic blood concentrations.

Morphine preparations available in the UK

Various preparations of morphine are available in the UK.
Oral preparations. For oral normal-release administration there is a choice of either tablets or liquid, while for oral modified-release the alternatives are: 12-hourly modified-release tablets or capsules;

12-hourly modified-release suspension; and 24-hourly modified-release capsules.

Rectal suppositories. These may be useful in the short term in a patient who cannot take oral morphine because of vomiting or a decreased level of consciousness. Absorption from the rectum can be variable, although the same dose and a 4-hourly dosing interval are recommended. Normal- and modified-release oral preparations of morphine are not suitable for rectal use.

Injection. Morphine has poor solubility, which results in large-volume, and therefore uncomfortable, intramuscular or subcutaneous injections. Diamorphine is the preferred drug in those countries where it is available.

Commencing oral morphine

The European Association for Palliative Care published guidelines on the use of morphine in cancer pain in 1996, which expanded the principles of the WHO analgesic ladder [18]. The guidelines recommended the use of normal release morphine preparations during titration in order to achieve steady state quickly. However, this is not always practical in a community setting and significant nursing time is required to dispense controlled drugs every 4 hours on an inpatient unit. A recent study examined hospitalised cancer patients taking step two analgesics who were then randomised to normal or modified release morphine for their pain [19]. Time to achieve pain control was 1.7 days for the modified release group and 2.1 days for the normal release group. In addition, the normal release group reported more tiredness. Other studies undertaken on cancer outpatients with pain report similar findings.

In all, this suggests that modified release preparations of morphine are an effective alternative to normal release preparations when commencing step three analgesia in a significant proportion of cancer patients with pain. In some patients however, normal release preparations are recommended. These include frail elderly patients, patients with renal impairment and patients in whom the previous analgesic intake is not known. The dose and its effect should be monitored very closely in this group.

Patients who are not pain controlled on a step-two analgesic should be commenced on 5–10 mg oral normal-release morphine scheduled 4-hourly or 20–30 mg 12-hourly of modified release morphine. Pain occurring between regular doses of morphine is termed breakthrough pain. Patients should have 'rescue' normal-release morphine for breakthrough pain, at a dose equivalent to one sixth of their 24 h total dose. After 24–48 h at the starting dose, the dose (not the frequency of administration) should be increased if the patient's pain is not under control. The new dose can be calculated by adding up the patient's oral morphine requirement over the last 24 h (regular plus breakthrough doses) and dividing this by six for 4-hourly administration or two for 12-hourly administration. In the majority of patients this will result in a safe and clinically effective dose increase of 30–50% of the current dose. The rescue doses for breakthrough pain should be increased by the same proportion.

If patients are treated with 4-hourly morphine, it is better to wake them at night to maintain their dosing schedule rather than give a double dose at bedtime as suggested in the EAPC guidelines. Recent research shows that the latter approach results in less effective pain control, more breakthrough analgesia and no difference in sleep disturbance than patients woken for their dose during the night [20]. In general, modified release preparations are superior to both approaches ensuring sustained pain control without sleep disturbance.

Several important practical points must be borne in mind. Firstly, patients must be given very clear instructions (preferably orally and in writing) about the use of modified-release and normal-release preparations. Particular note should be made of the following:

- prescribing modified-release preparations by time interval not frequency (e.g. '12-hourly' not 'b.d.');
- the use of rescue normal-release medication for breakthrough pain;
- the need to continue regular medication even if breakthrough medication has been used.

Rescue normal-release morphine (or occasionally other normal-release opioid) at a dose equivalent to the 4-hourly dose should always be available. If rescue medication is required regularly, the total 24 h opioid requirement should be calculated and the dose of the modified-release preparation and rescue medication increased accordingly.

Patients should never be prescribed more than one modified-release opioid preparation at a time.

Patients with cancer-related pain require regular review. If further pain develops, the cause and treatment should be assessed as above. It is unwise to assume that any new pain is also cancer related and/or that opioids are necessarily the most appropriate form of management for the new pain.

ALTERNATIVES TO ORAL MORPHINE

In general, morphine is no less and no more effective an analgesic than its alternatives. Differences lie in the side effect profiles of each drug. For example, fewer patients report constipation when taking fentanyl than when taking morphine. Others report less sedation on oxycodone than morphine, allowing dose increases to control pain that would not be acceptable on morphine. However, a significant proportion of cancer patients with pain are effectively treated with morphine and do not require an alternative opioid.

Oxycodone

Oxycodone preparations are similar to morphine: modified release 12-hourly tablets, normal release tablets and solution, and injections are available. They are used for the same indications as morphine. Oxycodone pectinate suppositories may be used as an alternative to morphine suppositories because of their longer duration of action (6–8 h). In the USA, oxycodone is available in combination with paracetamol and has proved a very useful drug for both cancer and non-malignant chronic pain.

Hydromorphone

Hydromorphone is pharmacologically similar to morphine. It is available for oral (both normal- and modified-release preparations), rectal and parenteral use in the USA and Ireland; and for normal and modified-release oral use in the UK and many other European countries. The concentrated injection is useful where high-dose opioids need to be given to cachectic patients. As for other strong opioids, in some patients it may have a preferential side-effect profile when compared with morphine.

Methadone

Methadone is well absorbed by mouth. Its average half-life is 24 h, although this may vary between 8 and 80 hours in different individuals. Methadone should be used with extreme caution, particularly in the elderly, because its unpredictable half-life means that accumulation may occur. Patients may require up to six doses per day initially, but the dosing interval will subsequently be more prolonged so that one or two doses per day may be sufficient for maintenance.

Methadone may be useful in some patients who do not respond to or are intolerant of morphine (i.e. as a second line opioid). Specialist advice should usually be sought because of its complex pharmacokinetics and its use in patients with complicated pain.

PARENTERAL OPIOIDS

Diamorphine injections and infusion

Diamorphine is highly soluble. It is a prodrug and its analgesic effect depends on metabolism to morphine and M6G. Diamorphine should be given 4-hourly by injection or by continuous infusion. Administration by injection is more potent than oral morphine. A dose of 1 mg parenteral diamorphine is equivalent to 3 mg of oral morphine. Diamorphine is not a more effective analgesic. Pain not controlled on oral morphine will not be improved by conversion to an equivalent dose of injectable diamorphine. Diamorphine mixes with many other drugs, such as antiemetics, and therefore useful in a syringe driver if parenteral use is necessary (see Chapter 20).

Oxycodone injection and infusion

Oxycodone is also available for use as 4-hourly injection or by infusion. This allows continuity of analgesic effect for patients treated with oral oxycodone who are no longer able to take oral medicine.

TRANSDERMAL PATCHES

There are two preparations of opioids currently available as transdermal patches; fentanyl and buprenorphine. The availability of transdermal preparations has offered a new option for pain-control for patients. However, as with all modified-release opioids, transdermal patches present potential problems when prescribed by those unfamiliar with their use or when insufficient information is given to patients. For this reason, the indications, practicalities and difficulties in their use will be discussed in some detail.

The use of transdermal patches may be considered for patients with stable, opioid-responsive pain as an alternative to morphine (i.e. as a second-line opioid for moderate to severe pain). They are most appropriate in the following situations:

1 Where the patient is: unable to tolerate morphine (i.e. a patient who has intolerable side-effects, including constipation); unable to take oral medication (e.g. dysphagia); is requesting an alternative method of drug delivery, *or*

2 Where pain control might be improved by reliable administration. This might be useful in patients with cognitive impairment or those who for other reasons are not able to regularly self-medicate with their analgesia.

Transdermal patches are not suitable for acute pain, where rapid dose titration is required, nor is it suitable for patients whose total daily requirement of opioid is equivalent to < 30 mg/24 h of oral morphine.

Starting transdermal patches

The following description is a general guide to using transdermal patches but readers are referred to the manufacturer's guidance for further details. It takes 24–48 h to reach steady state of analgesia using transdermal patches so that additional analgesics are required until steady state is reached. Converting from oral opioids:

- Calculate patch strength from manufacturer's guidelines (see Table 8.3).
- Apply patch and continue oral medication for the next 12 h (i.e. give last dose of 12-hourly morphine or three further doses of 4-hourly morphine).
- Ensure breakthrough doses are available.
- Patients should be warned that they may experience more breakthrough pain than usual in the first 1–3 days.

Table 8.3 Guidance for the relative doses of morphine, transdermal buprenorphine, transdermal fentanyl and diamorphine.

4-hourly oral morphine (mg)	5	10	15	20	25	30	35	40
24-hourly oral morphine (mg)	30	60	90	120	150	180	210	240
Buprenorphine patch* (mg/h)	35	35	52.5	70	87.5	105	122.5	140
Fentanyl patch (μg/h)	N/A	25	25	25	50	50	50	75
24-h s.c. diamorphine (mg)	10	20	30	40	50	60	70	80

* maximum dose: 140 μg/h.

The dose of the patch should not be changed within the first 2 days of the first application or of any change in dose. Adequate analgesia should be achieved using breakthrough medication as needed. Subsequent dose changes should be made according to the patient's requirement for breakthrough analgesics or follow the '30–50%' rule—the patch strength as near to this increase as possible should be selected.

Practicalities when using transdermal patches

Fentanyl and buprenorphine transdermal patches are designed to give 72 h of analgesia. They should be replaced at the same time every 3 days, although the site of application should be varied with each patch change. In a small number of patients analgesia decreases on the third day and patches need to be changed every 48 h. The patches should be stuck to a flat, clean, dry area of hairless skin, usually on the trunk or back or on the upper outer arm. Men may need to cut, not shave, body hair, but the skin integrity must be preserved. The patches should not be cut.

Patients are able to shower with the patches in place, but hot baths and directly applied heat will rapidly increase absorption, as will raised body temperature from pyrexia. Used patches should be folded sticky side together, and disposed of safely or returned to a pharmacist.

In 10% of patients a physical and/or depressive opioid withdrawal syndrome occurs on changing from morphine to transdermal fentanyl. This is short lived (usually a few days) and easily treated by the use of normal-release morphine when symptoms occur.

Discontinuing transdermal patches

Transdermal patches may need to be discontinued because a patient has rapidly changing pain or because of side-effects. A therapeutic subcutaneous depot of drug remains for at least 12 h, and can last up to 24 h after the patch has been removed. This usually means that no additional analgesia is required during the first 12 h after removing the patch but regular analgesia is required in the subsequent 12 h period. Different strategies are adopted depending on whether or not a patient's pain is under control.

Discontinuation in a patient whose pain is controlled. When discontinuing patches in a patient whose pain is controlled, two options can be considered:

1 Changing to 12-hourly modified-release morphine:
- calculate the 24 h dose of morphine required from manufacturers' guidelines;
- remove patches 12 h before the first modified-release morphine dose;
- ensure an adequate dose of normal-release oral morphine is available for breakthrough pain.

4 Changing to subcutaneous diamorphine infusion:
- calculate the equivalent 24 h dose of oral morphine from manufacturers' guidelines and divide this dose by 3 to establish 24 h dose of diamorphine;
- set up the syringe driver about 12 h after removing the transdermal patches; ensure an adequate dose of normal-release oral morphine or parenteral diamorphine is available for breakthrough pain.

Discontinuation in a patient whose pain is not controlled. In a patient whose pain is not controlled, the steps of patch discontinuation are to:
- calculate the equivalent dose of oral morphine or parenteral diamorphine required (using calculation in step two above);
- increase this dose by 30%;
- administer a 4-hourly equivalent dose of normal release morphine or diamorphine as needed;
- give modified release morphine or set up a diamorphine syringe driver 12 h after removing the transdermal patch based on the calculated dose increase.

It is vital to review the patient regularly during this changeover period.

SIDE-EFFECTS OF MORPHINE AND OTHER OPIOIDS

Side-effects should be discussed with patients before they decide to commence opioids. The majority of patients experience initial mild sedation on starting opioids or for 2–3 days after increasing the dose. All opioids can cause nausea (30–60% of patients), vomiting (10% of patients) and constipation (95% of patients). All patients commenced on opioids should be prescribed softening and stimulant laxatives and have access to an antiemetic (see Chapter 10).

Other well-recognised side-effects are dry mouth, itching, sweating, myoclonic jerks and occasionally hypotension.

FEARS ABOUT MORPHINE AND OTHER OPIOIDS

Both professionals and patients have fears about the use of strong opioids, particularly morphine (see Box 8.6). These fears are largely unfounded and with careful, knowledgeable use there are few problems. However, since these fears are common and may lead to poor pain management, the professional will need to discuss these issues with the patient when commencing strong opioids.

Box 8.6 Fears about opioid use

Professional's fears:	**Patient's fears:**
Addiction	Addiction
Respiratory depression	Side-effects
Excess sedation	Impending death
Confusion	Tolerance
	Decreased options for future pain relief

Addiction

Addiction does not occur when opioids are used for the management of pain. If the cause of the pain is removed (e.g. by a nerve block or radiotherapy) then opioids can generally be reduced or withdrawn with no psychological problems. Occasionally there is a degree of *physical* dependence, with a physical withdrawal syndrome apparent upon withdrawal of the drug. However, with withdrawal of opioid in staged decrements this is easily managed.

Respiratory depression

Respiratory depression is unusual but may occur in opioid-naive patients given a large dose of an opioid for acute pain, or due to a drug error or accumulation of morphine metabolites in renal failure. In chronic use, tolerance to the respiratory depressant effects occurs rapidly and provided the dose is titrated against the patient's pain, morphine can be used safely, even in patients with chronic lung disease.

Sedation and cognitive effects

Mild sedation is common when commencing morphine and after the dose has been increased. It usually wears off after 2–3 days at the same dose, and patients on stable doses of morphine can be allowed to drive. Hallucinations, confusion and vivid dreams may necessitate a dose reduction or a change to an alternative opioid; alternatively they can be managed with a small dose of haloperidol (1.5–3 mg) at night.

Tolerance

'If I take it now, it won't work later, when I really need it.' This fear is unfounded. An increase in analgesic requirement is usually due to an increase in pain due to advancing disease rather than to tolerance. Increasing experience of the use of opioids in both cancer and non-cancer-related pain confirms that tolerance is rare. There is much topical debate about tolerance and its apparent mechanisms, and specialist advice should be sought about a patient who appears to have tolerance to the effects of opioids.

Management of neuropathic pain

Combining the WHO ladder with co-analgesics

The presence of neuropathic pain mechanisms can result in pain with reduced sensitivity to opioids compared with nociceptive mechanisms. This does not mean that opioids are ineffective; merely that the pain may not be effectively controlled with opioids alone, or the patient may experience opioid side effects before analgesia. In these situations, additional medicines, called adjuvant drugs or co-analgesics, are required that have been shown to be effective in controlling neuropathic pain.

Large observational studies demonstrate the effectiveness of combining standard analgesics from the WHO ladder with additional measures. In one study, around 36% of patients with cancer presenting to a pain clinic had neuropathic pain mechanisms [21]. Using the WHO ladder together with selected co-analgesics, mean pain score in this neuropathic pain group fell from 71 mm to 28 mm on a visual analogue scale over a four-week period.

Selecting a co-analgesic

There is no evidence to support the concept that certain neuropathic pain symptoms respond to certain classes of co-analgesic. In fact, large trials and meta-analyses suggest that the most commonly used co-analgesics are equally effective for a range of symptoms. There is good evidence to support the use of the following co-analgesics [22] (Box 8.7):

Box 8.7 Commonly used co-analgesics in neuropathic pain

Co-analgesic	Usual starting dose	Usual maximum dose	Common side effects
Amitriptyline	10–25 mg at night	50–100 mg	Dry mouth, drowsiness
Gabapentin	100 mg t.d.s.	600–900 mg t.d.s.	Drowsiness, dizziness
Carbamazepine	100 mg b.d.	200–400 mg t.d.s.	Nausea, drowsiness,
Ketamine	10–25 mg q.d.s. orally 50–100 mg/24 h subcut infusion	50–100 mg q.d.s. orally 500 mg/24 h subcut infusion	Drowsiness, hallucinations
Baclofen	5–10 mg t.d.s.	20 mg t.d.s.	Drowsiness, muscle hypotonia

Other co-analgesics have been described as effective but the evidence to support such claims is more limited. Treating neuropathic pain often requires combining drugs with care to achieve a balance of benefit over burden of side effects. Advice should be sought early from an experienced palliative medicine or pain management service doctor to ensure effective prescribing in this context.

Management of bone pain

See also Chapter 10 on management of complications of cancer.

Patients with bone metastases often present with pain that is difficult to control, particularly because it manifests as incident pain. The same principles apply as for neuropathic pain and include titrating analgesics using the WHO ladder. Additional measures are usually necessary and include radiotherapy, intravenous bisphosphonate treatment (with pamidronate or zoledronate) and the use of rapidly acting opioids. For example, transmucosal fentanyl is a rapidly-acting opioid which is effective within several minutes and has a half life similar to normal release morphine. For many patients, this results in a rapid onset of analgesia that wears off after a few hours—a profile that matches their incident pain. However, for some patients the duration of analgesia is longer.

Spinal analgesia

Spinal analgesia encompasses the epidural and intrathecal delivery of drugs for pain relief. Spinal catheters are usually sited by pain clinic anaesthetists. Various factors influence the suitability of a particular patient for spinal analgesia. Firstly, the likely candidate will have pain that is not controlled by escalating doses of opioids, or will have intolerable side-effects from opioids. Secondly, other possible measures to produce pain relief, for example surgery and radiotherapy, will have been explored. Thirdly, the patient's major sites of pain will generally be in the lower half of the body.

If the patient can be at home, facilities must be available in the community setting for care of the spinal catheter and for replenishing the syringe driver or pump. Specialist advice must be available for problems outside normal working hours.

Suitable drugs

Opioids, local anaesthetics and other adjuvant drugs such as clonidine (which augments the action of opioids and local anaesthetic) can be given spinally. The choice of epidural or intrathecal route depends usually on operator preference, though intrathecal routes are generally more reliable and are associated with lower rates of infection. Intrathecal infusions can be administered via external pumps or implanted computer programmed devices.

Opioids can be given spinally, usually as diamorphine (100 mg diamorphine s.c. = 10 mg epidurally = 1 mg intrathecally). Patients should have normal-release oral opioids available for breakthrough pain or an 'on demand' spinal route delivery system (i.e. patient-controlled analgesia). Other opioids, apart from rescue medication, should be stopped.

The local anaesthetic bupivacaine can be given spinally for neuropathic pain. Concentrations of 0.125%and 0.25% usually produce pain relief. Concentrations of 0.375% and 0.5% often produce sensory change and then motor block. If the dermatomal spread of pain relief is inadequate then the rate of infusion is increased. Intrathecal infusions run at 0.5–2 ml/h, the epidural range generally is 2–6 ml/h. Patients should be monitored for side-effects after a dose change or an increase in the rate of the infusion. Side-effects are sedation, respiratory depression, hypotension, sensory loss, weakness and itch. Spinal analgesia may mask spinal cord compression.

Transcutaneous electrical nerve stimulation (TENS)

TENS was originally used to select patients who were suitable for implantation of dorsal column stimulators for pain relief. It has since been used widely to relieve pain in its own right.

Electrical stimulation is achieved by attaching a TENS machine to electrodes on the skin. For conventional TENS, the waveform of the stimulator is set so as to stimulate large myelinated afferent (A-beta) fibres. This reduces the input from nociceptors via C fibres to the spinal cord and brain (gate control of pain). For acupuncture-like TENS, high-intensity, low-frequency stimulation produces muscle twitching. The A-delta fibres so stimulated induce pain relief by releasing endogenous opioids in the spinal cord (see Figure 8.2).

In patients with chronic pain 70% respond to TENS initially. However, only 30% still find TENS effective after one year. Electrodes may be placed over the painful site, but greater pain relief is usually gained by stimulating over the nerve proximal to the area. Successful use of TENS requires a thorough explanation of the principles of TENS and a patient's willingness to experiment with pad positions and stimulation waveforms and intensities.

Severe pain as an emergency

Usually this arises in an acute or chronic pattern: there is usually a warning as pain builds up over days and also an understanding of the underlying aetiology of the pain.

Acute, unanticipated pain may be due to:

- fracture;
- haemorrhage (e.g. haemorrhage into liver tumours);
- infarction or thrombosis;
- perforation of a viscous;
- nerve compression or inflammation;
- obstruction with colic.

Assessment of the likely cause of the pain is essential in management. Severe pain is an emergency which requires constant attention until the pain is controlled. Specialist referral and inpatient admission are often needed to provide sufficient observation and intervention for the patient.

Immediate management

The immediate management of severe pain is strong opioid analgesia, usually given parenterally for fast effect: for example, diamorphine i.m. s.c. equivalent to the 4-hourly dose or 10 mg in an opioid-naive patient. This is repeated after 30 minutes if the effect is insufficient. There may be added benefit from sedation with diazepam (5–20 mg p.r. or titrated i.v.) or midazolam (2.5–10 mg s.c. or titrated i.v.).

Ketamine 20–100 mg (0.5–2 mg/kg) i.v. or i.m. may be useful as a rapidly acting (minutes), analgesic and sedative, especially in severe nerve-related pain (e.g. haemorrhage into the spinal canal). It may require co-administration of midazolam or other benzodiazepine to avoid dysphoric side-effects. It is available in the community only on a named patient basis.

Simple nerve blocks with lidocaine 2% or bupivacaine 0.5 % may be useful for fracture-related pain: a femoral nerve block can be used for a fractured femur, and an intercostal nerve block for a fractured rib.

Nitrous oxide (carried in ambulances) may have some role in fracture- or movement-related pain. Hyoscine butylbromide 20–40 mg s.c. or i.m. may be useful for colic.

Conclusion

In patients with advanced disease, successful management of pain requires evaluation to assess the likely cause of the pain and the impact that pain is having on the patient's physical and emotional life. A thorough knowledge of a small number of drugs and a simple stepwise approach to their use will improve pain in the majority of patients. Continued reassessment and re-evaluation will allow a treatment regimen to be modified according to side-effects or changing circumstances. A minority of patients will have more difficult pain. Co-analgesic drugs can then be introduced according to the probable cause of the pain. In patients whose pain persists despite these measures, referral for specialist advice is indicated.

References

1 Bonica JJ. Cancer pain: current status and future needs. In: Bonica JJ, ed. *The Management of Pain*, 2nd edition. Philadelphia: Lea & Febiger, 1990: 400–445.
2 Seale C. Death from cancer and death from other causes: the relevance of the hospice approach. *Palliat Med* 1991; 5: 12–19.
3 McCarthy M, Lay M, Addington-Hall J. Dying from heart disease. *J Roy Coll Phys* 1996; 30:325–328.
4 Larue F, Collequ SM, Brasser L, Cleeland CS. Multicentre study of cancer pain and its treatment in France. *BMJ* 1995; 310: 1034–1037.
5 Cleeland CS, Gonin R, Hatfield AK et al. Pain and its treatment in outpatients with metastatic cancer. *New Engl J Med* 1994; 330: 592–596.
6 Addington-Hall J, McCarthy M. Dying from cancer: results of a national population-based investigation. *Palliat Med* 1995; 9: 295–305.
7 Saunders CM. *The Management of Terminal Illness*. London: Hospital Medicine Publications, 1967.
8 International Association for the Study of Pain Subcommittee on Taxonomy. Classification of chronic pain. *Pain* 1986; Suppl. 3: 216–221.
9 Glynn C. An approach to the management of the patient with deafferentation pain. *Palliat Med* 1989; 3: 13–21.
10 Mercadante S. Radbruch L. Caraceni A. Cherny N. Kaasa S. Nauck F et al. Episodic (breakthrough) pain: consensus conference of an expert working group of the European Association for Palliative Care. *Cancer* 2002; 94(3): 832–839.
11 Portenoy R, Payne D, Jacobsen P. Breakthrough pain: characteristics and impact in patients with cancer pain. *Pain* 1999; 81: 129–134.
12 Melzack R. The McGill Pain Questionnaire. In: Melzack R, ed. *Pain Measurement and Assessment*. New York: Raven Press, 1983: 41–48.
13 Bennett MI. The LANSS pain scale—the leeds assessment of neuropathic symptoms and signs. *Pain* 2001; 92: 147–157.
14 World Health Organization. *Cancer Pain Relief*. Geneva: WHO, 1986.
15 World Health Organization. *Cancer Pain Relief*. Geneva: WHO, 1996.
16 Hawkey CJ. Laine L. Simon T. Quan H. Shingo S. Evans J. Rofecoxib Rheumatoid Arthritis Endoscopy Study Group. Incidence of gastroduodenal ulcers in patients with rheumatoid arthritis after 12 weeks of rofecoxib, naproxen, or placebo: a multicentre, randomised, double blind study. *Gut* 2003. 52(6): 820–826.
17 Oxford league table of analgesics in acute pain. (www.jr2.ox.ac.uk/bandolier)
18 Hanks GW de Conno F, Ripamonti C et al. Morphine in cancer pain: modes of administration. *BMJ* 1996; 312: 823–826.
19 Klepstad P, Kaasa S, Jystad A, Hval B, Borchgrevink PC. Normal release or sustained release morphine for dose finding during start of morphine to cancer patients: a randomised double blind trial. *Pain* 2003; 101: 193–198.
20 Todd J, Rees E, Gwilliam B, Davies A. An assessment of the efficacy and tolerability of a 'double dose' of normal-release morphine sulphate at bedtime. *Palliat Mede* 2002; 16(6): 507–512.
21 Grond S, Radbruch L, Meuser T, Sabatowski R, Loick G, Lehmann K. Assessment and treatment of neuropathic cancer pain following WHO guidelines. *Pain* 1999; 79: 15–20.

22 Sindrup SH, Jensen TS. Efficacy of pharmacological treatments of neuropathic pain: an update and effect related to mechanism of drug action. *Pain* 1999; 83: 389–400.

Further reading

Section 8.2. The management of pain. In: Doyle D, Hanks GW, Cherny N, Calman K, eds. *Oxford Textbook of Palliative Medicine*, 3rd edition. Oxford: Oxford University Press, 2003.

McGrath PA. *Pain in Children: Nature, Assessment and Treatment*. New York: The Guildford Press, 1990.

Twycross RG. *Pain Relief in Advanced Cancer*. Edinburgh: Churchill Livingstone, 1994.

9: The Management of Gastrointestinal Symptoms and Advanced Liver Disease

ANDREW CHILTON AND CHRISTINA FAULL

Introduction

Patients with advanced disease, of whatever nature, commonly have symptoms related to the gastrointestinal tract and all such patients should be specifically asked about dry and sore mouth problems, eating, nausea and constipation. Unrelenting nausea can be more disabling than pain, and effective management requires a logical, systematic and persistent approach. Constipation is often neglected and can be prevented for most patients. Cancer may obstruct the gastrointestinal tract causing well-defined syndromes and the options for palliation of these symptoms are described in detail in this chapter.

Eating and defecating can be a major point of reference for patients and their carers about their health, and their dysfunction may carry enormous significance about sustaining life and the approach of death. The importance of this in caring for patients should never be underestimated.

The palliative care needs of patients with advanced liver disease are now more recognised [1]. As patients become less well, most of the palliative care is provided by the primary care team. However, crises and therapeutic interventions are generally dealt with by acute hospital services and most patients die in hospital. A small number of patients access specialist palliative care services and this model of care will undoubtedly develop further. At present there is no evidence base to compare clinical cost or quality-of-life outcomes.

Cachexia, anorexia and nutrition

Cachexia and anorexia are commonly experienced symptoms of advanced malignant and non-malignant disease and up to 10% of patients with cancer in the community will have a body mass index of less than 20 m^2/kg. The associated distress can be marked, especially in terms of body image and quality of life. Cachexia has been found to be associated with a shorter prognosis for many diseases including cancer [2], chronic obstructive airways disease [3], heart failure [4], liver disease [5] and the 'wasting disease' AIDS [6].

Detailed discussion of pathophysiology is beyond the scope of this book but might include:

- Unresolved nausea
- Mechanical effects of tumours and ascites
- Cytokines (e.g. Tumour Necrosis Factor) causing: increased basal metabolic rate; increased hepato-gluconogenesis, using protein as substrate; increased glucose intolerance; altered lipid metabolism; and anorexia
- Adverse effect of medications
- Psychological factors including low mood and anxiety
- Unresolved pain

Management requires active involvement of the multidisciplinary team and best outcomes are gained by using a range of approaches that aim to ameliorate the underlying cause and address symptoms directly. Patients and carers need to be fully involved in decision-making and goal-setting. It is often the carer's job to prepare meals and this sustaining role is of vital importance to them. Before embarking on enteral nutritional support, clear goals and plans need to be thought through and discussed with the patient.

Enteral tube feeding is considered to be a medical treatment in law. Initiation, stopping and withdrawal are a medical decision; however, this needs to be made in concert with the patient (see also Chapter 5). If the patient is not competent to make decisions then it is incumbent on the doctor to make these decisions in the best interest of the patient. In English law relatives or a nominated proxy are not in a position to make decisions on the patient's behalf. However, it is vital to ensure good communication and draw relatives into these decisions in a constructive manner. In children and patients with a persistent vegetative state (PVS), application to the courts is often required with regard to withdrawal of artificial hydration and nutrition. (In England and Wales application to the Courts must be made, however the law differs in Scotland.)

Drugs to increase appetite and weight gain

The following drugs have been shown to have some effect on symptoms in cancer patients [7]. They should initially be used on a trial basis, with treatment being continued if benefit is confirmed. There is no evidence base for their use in non-malignant diseases other than AIDS.

STEROIDS

Dexamethasone 2–4 mg (or equivalent dose of an alternative steroid), is useful for increasing appetite and energy but not weight gain. The side effects of these drugs can limit their use (diabetes, psychological effects, immunosuppression, fluid retention and proximal muscle weakness).

PROGESTERONES

Megestrol acetate 160 mg daily (increased up to 800 mg if required), and medroxyprogesterone acetate 480–960 mg daily, can improve appetite and weight in cancer and AIDS patients. These drugs are usually well tolerated but can cause mild oedema, impotence and vaginal spotting. Unlike steroids their effect is not immediate but may occur within 2 weeks.

OTHER DRUGS WITH POTENTIAL

A number of drugs have been found to have effect on aspects of the pathophysiology of the cachexia anorexia syndrome. Some are in clinical trials to assess their efficacy in patients. These include: Omega-3-fatty acids (fish oils); cannabinoids; melatonin; and thalidomide.

Nutritional support

Nutritional support has benefits for non-terminal patients in terms of quality of life and other outcomes. For example, it increases patient tolerance of chemotherapy and in alcoholic cirrhosis may influence prognosis. Patients with AIDS clearly benefit from nutritional supplements as they recover from acute infections. Patients can find dietary regimes arduous and advice must balance these pros and cons.

Many aspects of nutrition may be deficient but the major one for most patients is the lack of energy substrates. At a basic level, the following advice can be helpful.

- Make food interesting (plan meals)
- Eat a little and often
- Eat what you enjoy (even those ‘bad’ things such as cream and chocolate)

- Prepare food that does not need a lot of chewing
- Encourage fluids
- Use a small plate (it gives the impression of finishing a complete meal)
- Eat when hungry (have food ready)
- Lessen any emotional tension that may surround meal times
- Make use of aperitifs

For some patients, commercially produced supplements are helpful. Unfortunately they are not universally palatable and patients should be encouraged to experiment with different varieties and flavours (e.g. sweet or savoury). They are prescribable in the UK and are therefore free to most patients. They can come in powder form to mix with drinks and yoghurt etc. (e.g. Maxijul LE and Scandishake), liquid to drink (e.g. Fresubin, Ensure and Fortisip) or puddings (e.g. Resource Energy Dessert) and soups (e.g. Vitasavoury). Dieticians provide more detailed advice on nutritional needs of patients and are an excellent source of information on dietary supplementation.

For some patients the normal mechanisms of chewing and swallowing are disturbed and interventional administration of nutrition is required. It is essential that the patient has a functional GI tract.

NASOGASTRIC TUBE FEEDING

Nasogastric feeding is generally only useful for short term intervention (e.g. during chemotherapy or surgery). Various difficulties can be encountered including:

- Accidental displacement of tube (25% of tubes are displaced)
- Aspiration
- Blockage
- Irritation of nasal and pharyngeal tissues
- Narrow bore of tube necessitates prolonged feeding time
- Gastro-oesophageal reflux
- Early satiety
- Diarrhoea
- Patient dislike of tube feeding

A fine bore (5–8F gauge) tube is used which may be useful either for bolus feeds including normal drinks or may be attached to a pump to deliver nutritional supplements over longer time periods. The latter are delivered from the hospital to the patient under the supervision of a dietician.

Sore throat, hoarseness and swallowing difficulties should be addressed proactively. The correct positioning of the tube may be checked by X-ray or aspiration and testing of Ph (should be <5 unless on PPI or H2 antagonist).

PERCUTANEOUS ENDOSCOPIC GASTROSTOMY (PEG) FEEDING

Fixed placement of a tube through the abdominal wall into the stomach is useful for patients who require long-term interventional nutrition (months to years) or those undergoing treatment for head and neck cancer. The procedure is well tolerated even by quite sick patients and is generally done under benzodiazepine sedation (Figure 9.1). It may be placed endoscopically (the majority), radiologically or by a mini laparotomy. It is a day case procedure but patients may remain in hospital whilst learning about the enteral feeding apparatus and techniques. The high 30 day mortality associated with the procedure (up to 40%), reflects patient selection and the underlying poor prognosis of the range of conditions where PEG placement is seen as an option.

Box 9.1 outlines the indications and contraindications and Box 9.2 describes the possible complications of PEG.

PEG tube care

Certain routine measures and guidelines minimise the risks associated with PEG feeding. This includes rinsing the tube before and after each feeding or at least once daily using 30 ml of cooled boiled water or fennel or camomile tea. Any medicine administered via the PEG must be in liquid from or a dissolvable preparation.

Good oral, dental and pharyngeal hygiene is needed and the puncture site should be examined daily.

If late displacement occurs (i.e. once the tract is mature) a urinary Foley catheter can be inserted to maintain the integrity of the tract.

Carbonate drinks and pancreatic enzymes dissolved in water may be useful to unblock tubes. However, the former can cause degradation of the tube. Do not force-flush a tube, seek replacement.

TROUBLE SHOOTING IN TUBE FEEDING

Gastro-oesophageal reflux is common and can be treated with a proton pump inhibitor (PPI). Positional change and avoidance of overnight continuous feeding is also helpful. Aspiration occurs frequently and may present with pneumonia. Patient position, type of feed and

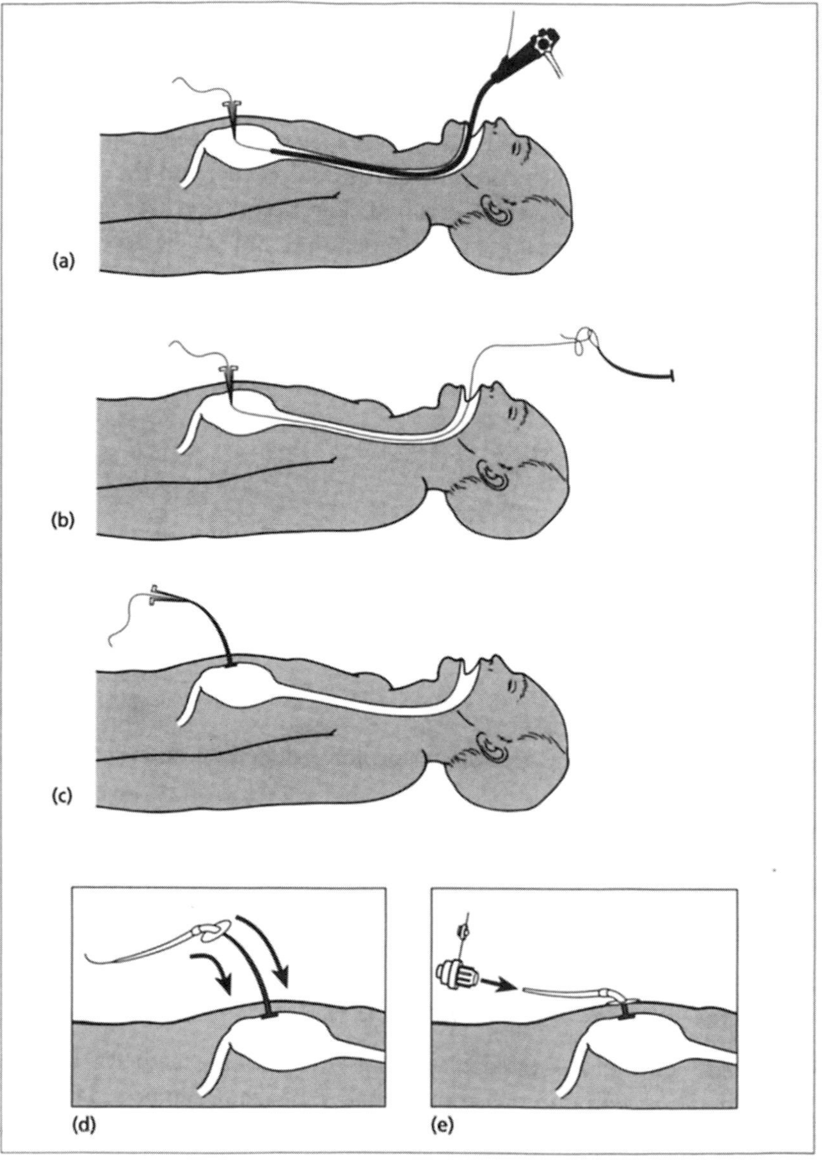

Fig. 9.1 Positioning a PEG tube. (a) Gastric puncture with a sheathed needle and introduction of a string or metal wire through the sheath after removal of the needle. While grasping the string or the metal wire, the endoscope is removed. (b) The loop of the gastrostomy tube is knotted at the string projecting from the mouth and by pulling at the abdominal end of the string the gastrostomy tube passes through the oesophagus and stomach and finally pierces the abdominal wall. (c) The retention disc of the gastrostomy tube is apposed against the gastric wall. (d) The outer retention disc, and (e) the feeding adaptor are put in place. Adapted from [8].

Box 9.1 Factors to assess before PEG insertion

Indications	Contraindications
Tumour cachexia	Lack of diaphanoscopy*
Oropharyngeal disease	Blood coagulation disorder
Inoperable obstruction—upper digestive tract	Poor wound healing
Neurogenic dysphagia without risk of aspiration	Ileus
Major oral surgery	Ascites
Pre-radiotherapy	Sepsis
	Pancreatitis
	Tumour infiltration of stomach

*If it is impossible to site a gastrostomy endoscopically, it may be possible radiologically with ultrasound guidance

Box 9.2 Complications of PEG

Major	Minor
Perforation with peritonitis	Wound infection / stomal leak
Haemorrhage	Regurgitation and aspiration (consider jejunal placement)
Haematoma	Ileus, abdominal bloating, diarrhoea
Death	Tube migration/extubation
	Anorexia

prokinetic medication may be useful. Jejunal feeding may benefit patients with persistent problems (see below).

Nausea, bloating and cramps occur frequently. Diarrhoea occurs in approximately 30% of patients and can present a significant challenge. These problems can be addressed by alteration of feed type and mode of feeding. Close liaison with dieticians and a nutrition support team are essential.

JEJUNAL FEEDING

Some patients have considerable problems with enteral feeding into the stomach with symptoms of: reflux, hiccup, aspiration, nausea and vomiting. If prokinetic agents (e.g. metoclopramide) do not resolve this, then jejunal placement of the NG or PEG tube (usually endoscopically) may alleviate symptoms. However, patients with jejunal feeding tubes will be unlikely to tolerate bolus feeds since there is no longer the gastric reservoir.

PARENTERAL NUTRITION (PN)

If the gut is functional use it! PN is not physiological and fraught with pitfalls. PN is never an emergency. Electrolytes and micronutrients must be corrected to prevent the re-feeding syndrome in malnourished patients.

In the UK most home PN is given for intestinal failure due to the short bowel syndrome. In parts of Europe and the USA however, the bulk of home PN is provided for malignant disease. These practices may in time be more widely adopted. There is, however, no convincing evidence that PN enhances either quality of life or survival. The risks far outweigh the benefits. Patients with advanced cancer who currently receive PN in the UK have usually either been commenced on it prior to diagnosis or before potentially curative treatment and have continued on it; or occasionally it is used in patients who have intestinal failure (complete bowel obstruction) with no other disease spread. For patients with cachexia due to advanced non-malignant disease the place of PN is equally uncertain. This is an area of practice that is likely to challenge us all in the coming years.

Mouth care

A dry mouth (xerostomia) is a common and major problem for many patients with advanced disease. Saliva helps us to chew, talk and swallow. It protects against infection and begins digestion of food. Normally about 1–1.5 litres are produced daily. A reduction in this is most commonly a side effect of drugs (opioids, antihistamines, anticholinergics, diuretics, beta blockers and anticonvulsants) but dehydration, anxiety and mouth breathing also result in a dry mouth. The particular adverse oral effects of radiotherapy and chemotherapy are discussed further in Chapter 11.

Patients may need extra mouth care in order to:

- keep the oral mucosa moist, clean and intact in order to prevent infection;
- keep the lips clean, soft, moist and intact;
- remove food debris/dental plaque without damaging the gingival membrane;
- alleviate pain and discomfort thus enabling greater oral intake;
- prevent halitosis;
- enhance taste and appetite;
- facilitate speech;
- minimise psychological distress.

Key point in mouth care:

The frequency of mouth care is of greater importance than what is used.

Two hourly mouth care was shown to prevent infection more effectively than sporadic mouth care [9].

A sore mouth, from whatever cause, may be helped by sucking anaesthetic lozenges or using local anaesthetic mouthwashes or sprays. A cocaine-based mouthwash may sometimes be helpful in very severe mouth pain.

Management of xerostomia

Table 9.1 outlines the measures that may help patients with dry mouths. A few additional tips: glycerine may make the mouth sticky and chewing gum requires some saliva to be present; moist cotton swabs (e.g. Moistir) or sponge swabs on sticks dipped in water may help very frail patients. Salivary substitutes should be sprayed beneath the tongue and between the buccal mucosa and the teeth (i.e. mimic the pooling of saliva) and not in the back of the throat.

Pilocarpine, a cholinergic agonist, has been shown to increase saliva production post-irradiation. However, it is often poorly tolerated, usually because of sweating or gastrointestinal side-effects. It is contraindicated in obstructive airways disease and asthma.

Table 9.1 A summary of approaches to the management of a dry mouth.

General measures	Cleanliness/ tongue coating	Salivary substitutes	Increased salivary secretion
Sips of water	Pineapple	Carboxymethycellulose	Pilocarpine 5 mg t.d.s. with or after food
Ice poles	Effervescent Vitamin C	Mucin	
Glycerine			
Chewing gum			
Moistened sponges on stick			

Prevention and management of oral infections

THRUSH

Attention to the care of the oral cavity, teeth and dentures will help minimise infection. Patients on steroids, antibiotics or those who have diabetes are at particular risk. Thrush is the commonest infection. Candida prefers an acid environment and sodium bicarbonate mouthwashes (one teaspoon per large cup of water) repeated regularly (2-hourly) coupled with gentle brushing of the teeth (or cleaning dentures) twice per day is effective prevention [10].

Established thrush is treated with nystatin or amphotericin topically. Patients should be instructed to keep the lozenge or suspension in contact with as much of the oral mucosa as possible, for as long as possible. Ice lollipops made with diluted nystatin are soothing and engender a long duration of mucosal contact. Miconazole acts both topically and systemically. If the patient is severely affected, has symptoms suggestive of oesophageal infection, or is taking antibiotics and/or steroids a systemic antifungal is indicated; for example, fluconazole 50 mg o.d. for 7–14 days, or itraconazole 100 mg o.d for 10–15 days. To avoid reinfection dentures must be cleaned in Sterident or Milton with or without nystatin.

HERPES SIMPLEX

Herpes simplex infections present as very painful, vesicular and ulcerating lesions. Oral acyclovir 200 mg five times daily, or valaciclovir 500 mg b.d for 5 days is indicated.

Oesophageal problems

Swallowing may be difficult for patients with oesophageal cancer for several common reasons:

- oesophageal compressive and/or obstructive lesions;
- functional dysphagia;
- odynophagia (painful swallowing);
- oro-oesophageal thrush.

In addition, patients may experience copious thick, tenacious mucus, which may cause coughing.

Treatment options include surgery (not for disease with metastatic spread), external beam and endoluminal radiotherapy, chemotherapy, endoscopic recanalisation and expanding metal stents. Endoscopic interventions are discussed below. General symptom control is vital whatever the cause of obstruction or possibility of intervention.

Mucaine, an antacid containing the local anaesthetic agent oxetacaine and used as often as necessary, may be useful for pain when swallowing. Standard titration through the analgesic ladder should be adopted. Strong (non-oral) opioids, such as subcutaneous diamorphine or transdermal fentanyl, may be required to control background pain. Sucralfate will coat ulcerated tumour and may reduce bleeding and pain.

In total obstruction of the oesophagus, coping with saliva and secretions can be distressing for the patient. The following may be helpful:

- hyoscine hydrobromide (Kwells), 1–2, tablets sublingually q.d.s.;
- hyoscine hydrobromide s.c. 1.2–3.6 mg/24 h;
- hyoscine butylbromide s.c. 40–80 mg/24 h (less sedating than hydrobromide).

Nebulised water or saline may help reduce the tenacity of mucus secreted by the cancer and nebulised local anaesthetic (5 ml of 0.25% bupivacaine) may be helpful in very advanced disease if the pharynx is dysfunctional and swallowing of saliva or mucus results in aspiration with distressing bouts of coughing.

Endoluminal recanalisation

Exophytic growth of tumours into a lumen will lead to obstruction. Endoscopic procedures that recanalise the oesophagus may offer alternatives or additional options to endolimunial stenting (see below) for dysphagia.

- Argon plasma coagulator (APC): This is a safe and effective method. APC provides predictable penetration of normal and abnormal mucosa. The equipment is relatively cheap and has multiple other applications. The main drawback is that it may take a number of sessions to achieve the desired outcome.
- Laser (YAG): Not widely available and has statutory restriction on its use. Very 'powerful' with limited room for error.
- Injection of absolute alcohol: Cheap with good results if injected into exophytic tumour. It usually requires multiple sessions and can give rise to mediastinal discomfort at the time of injection. Will cause ulceration of the normal mucosa if injected into it.

- Dilitation: Useful for constrictive rather than exophytic tumours. Dilitation can be done with bougies over a guide wire or balloons under direct vision. Balloon dilation of the oesophagus, pylorus, duodenum and colon can be undertaken. The perforation rate is 1–5%.

A combination of the above modalities focused on the nature of the individual clinical problem should be employed.

Nausea and vomiting

Nausea and/or vomiting occurs in 40–70% of patients with advanced cancer [11, 12] and can be a major cause of poor quality of life in patients with both malignant and non-malignant diseases. The symptoms may be harder to bear than pain.

Five components are the key to management:

- Careful assessment of the patient to try and identify possible aetiologies
- Knowledge of common syndromes
- Reversal of the reversible (where appropriate)
- An understanding of the mechanism of action of antiemetic drugs (Figure 9.2).
- Consideration of the route of administration of antiemetic and other drugs. Since nausea can cause gastric stasis the subcutaneous or rectal routes may be needed even when there is no vomiting.

Figure 9.3 outlines the management. If the aetiology is really not clear cyclizine is a good first line antiemetic to try. Control of symptoms using one antiemetic is possible in 60% of patients. However, about one-third of patients require concurrent administration of a second antiemetic. In these patients antiemetics of different mechanisms of action should be combined (e.g. cyclizine and haloperidol). This is discussed further below under the section 'Persistent nausea and vomiting'.

Acupuncture and ginger are two commonly used complementary techniques (see Chapter 23). Other approaches such as relaxation therapy, hypnotherapy or neurolinguistic programming are invaluable for patients with a high degree of anxiety or to combat the anticipatory nausea induced by chemotherapy treatments.

Table 9.2 provides a quick view of the range of antiemetics and gives prescription guidance.

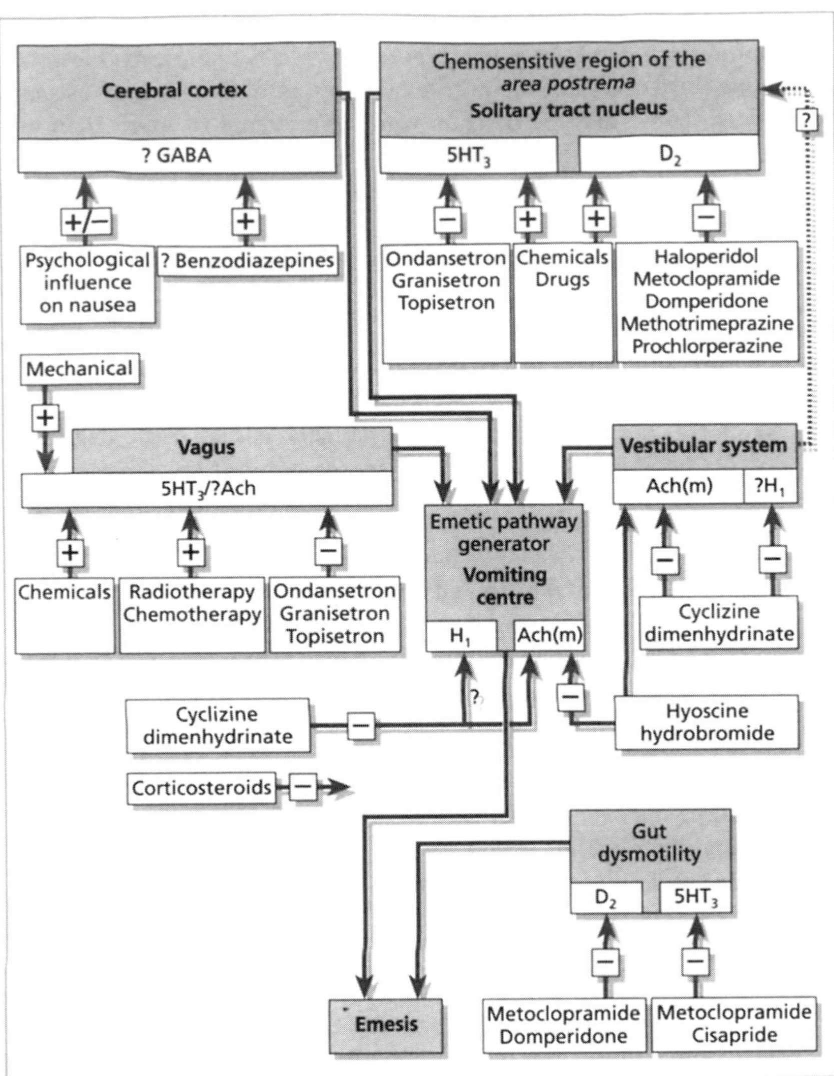

Fig. 9.2 A schema of the pathways of emesis (nausea and vomiting), important neurotransmitters, and site of antiemetics. Receptor types—GABA: gamma-amino-butyric acid, H: histamine, D: dopamine, Ach(m): acetylcholine muscarinic, 5HT: serotonin (5-hydroxytryptophan). Subscript denotes receptor subtype: + denotes agonist or enhancing stimulus—denotes antagonist or blocking stimulus.

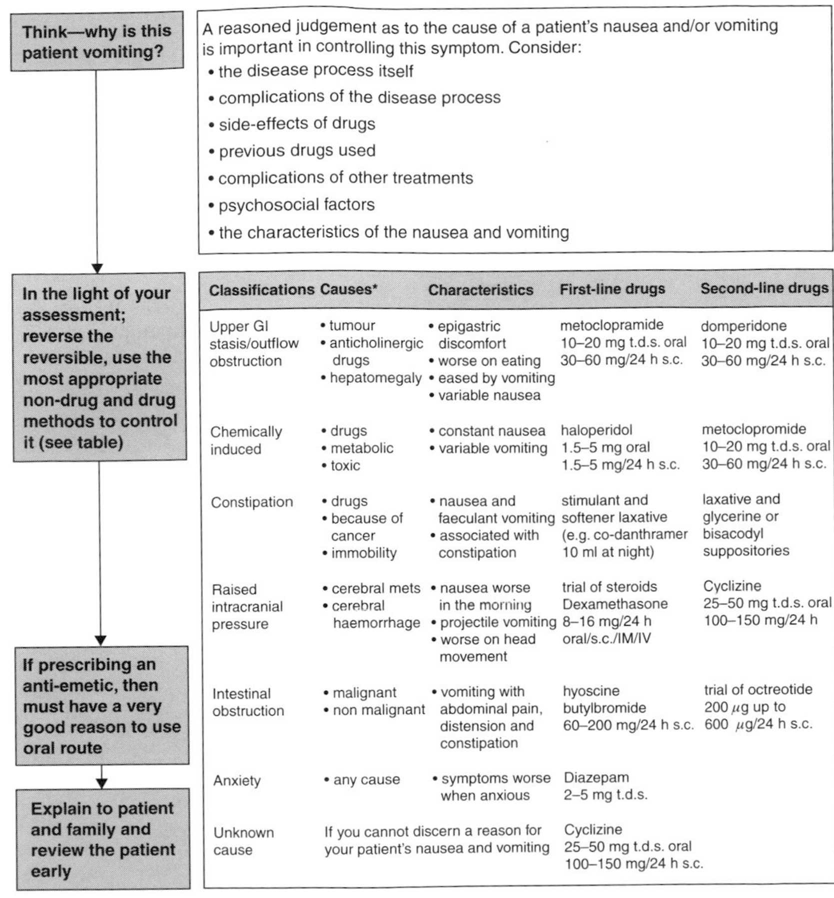

Classifications	Causes*	Characteristics	First-line drugs	Second-line drugs
Upper GI stasis/outflow obstruction	• tumour • anticholinergic drugs • hepatomegaly	• epigastric discomfort • worse on eating • eased by vomiting • variable nausea	metoclopramide 10–20 mg t.d.s. oral 30–60 mg/24 h s.c.	domperidone 10–20 mg t.d.s. oral 30–60 mg/24 h s.c.
Chemically induced	• drugs • metabolic • toxic	• constant nausea • variable vomiting	haloperidol 1.5–5 mg oral 1.5–5 mg/24 h s.c.	metoclopromide 10–20 mg t.d.s. oral 30–60 mg/24 h s.c.
Constipation	• drugs • because of cancer • immobility	• nausea and faeculant vomiting • associated with constipation	stimulant and softener laxative (e.g. co-danthramer 10 ml at night)	laxative and glycerine or bisacodyl suppositories
Raised intracranial pressure	• cerebral mets • cerebral haemorrhage	• nausea worse in the morning • projectile vomiting • worse on head movement	trial of steroids Dexamethasone 8–16 mg/24 h oral/s.c./IM/IV	Cyclizine 25–50 mg t.d.s. oral 100–150 mg/24 h
Intestinal obstruction	• malignant • non malignant	• vomiting with abdominal pain, distension and constipation	hyoscine butylbromide 60–200 mg/24 h s.c.	trial of octreotide 200 μg up to 600 μg/24 h s.c.
Anxiety	• any cause	• symptoms worse when anxious	Diazepam 2–5 mg t.d.s.	
Unknown cause	If you cannot discern a reason for your patient's nausea and vomiting		Cyclizine 25–50 mg t.d.s. oral 100–150 mg/24 h s.c.	

Fig. 9.3 Summary of the approach to the management of nausea and vomiting. (Adapted from Faull C. Woof R 2002: Palliative Care: An Oxford Core Text with permission from the publishers Oxford, University Press)

Common syndromes of nausea and vomiting and their management

GASTRIC STASIS AND OUTFLOW OBSTRUCTION

This is common in patients with GI malignancy because of ascities, liver enlargement and direct effects of tumour on the stomach. It is also common in patients with advanced congestive cardiac failure because of ascites and in diabetics because of autonomic neuropathy. It is a component of the nausea induced by opiates. Nausea is of varying intensity. It may be very transient, just before vomiting and is often relieved by vomiting. The vomitus can be of considerable volume and may contain undigested food. Vomiting may be provoked

Table 9.2 Antiemetic prescription.

Drug	Oral dose	Subcutaneous dose	Rectal dose
Metoclopramide	10–20 mg t.d.s.	40–80 mg/24 h	
Domperidone or	10–20 mg t.d.s.		30 mg t.d.s.
Levomepromazine	5–25 mg o.d.	6.25–25 mg/24 h may be given once daily	
Haloperidol	1.5–5 mg o.d.	1.5–5 mg/24 h may be given once daily	
Ondansetron	8 mg b.d.		16 mg o.d.
Granisetron	1–2 mg o.d.	1–2 mg/24 h	
Tropisetron	5 mg o.d.	5 mg/24 h	
Cyclizine	50 mg t.d.s.	50–150 mg/24 h	
Prochloperazine	3–10 mg t.d.s.	Not suitable	25 mg t.d.s.
Hyoscine hydrobromide	300 μg q.i.d.	0.8–2.4 mg/24 h	

by movement of the torso. A succussion splash and other features of autonomic failure may be present.

Metoclopramide is the drug treatment of choice. Other prokinetics may occasionally be useful: Cisapride 20 mg b.d. p.o may be used on a named patient basis. Erythromycin may need to be given intravenously. Flatulence can be relieved with dimethicone.

In complete obstruction prokinetic drugs should be stopped. Proton pump inhibitors may be helpful in reducing acidity and volume of secretions. A nasogastric tube may help to relieve symptoms and is tolerated well by some patients but many prefer to have intermittent vomiting especially if nausea is controlled. Insertion of a gastrostomy tube (see above) for venting purposes has been found to be effective and acceptable but is not commonly used in the UK [13].

CHEMICALLY INDUCED NAUSEA

A vast array of drugs cause nausea. The initiation of opioids cause nausea in up to 30% of patients It usually settles within 3–4 days but can reappear with an escalation of dose and it persists in a small percentage of patients. Metabolic causes of nausea are common in advanced disease: renal failure, liver failure, hypercalcaemia, hyponatraemia and ketoacidosis. Anti-dopaminergic are the drugs of choice.

$5HT_3$ antagonists are useful for highly emetogenic chemotherapy and perhaps in cases of intractable vomiting of metabolic cause, but their cost-effectiveness in other circumstances is not yet established.

RAISED INTRACRANIAL PRESSURE

Nausea may be worse in the morning, and the vomiting can be projectile in nature. Nausea and vomiting provoked by head movement is associated with vestibular pathway aetiology. There is usually headache, which may be worse in the morning. Neurological signs may be absent. Steroids and cyclizine are the treatments of first choice. If there are signs of vestibular pathway aetiology, hyoscine hydrobromide may be useful.

Persistant nausea and vomiting

Thirty percent of patients require the concurrent use of two antiemetics. These should be selected for different mechanisms of action that are compatible in effects. Haloperidol with cyclizine is a good choice. Both cyclizine and hyoscine hydrobromide will counteract the prokinetic effect of metoclopramide and domperidone but will not counteract the central antiemetic effect of metoclopramide.

Alternatively, low-dose levomepromazine can also be useful. It is a 'broad-spectrum' antiemetic (Achm, D_2 and 5HT antagonist activity) and in low doses does not generally cause troublesome sedation or hypotension.

Corticosteroids are potent antiemetics although their mechanism of action is not fully understood. Dexamethasone at 2–6 mg o.d. is useful to add to an antiemetic regimen for patients with resistant problems.

Hiccup

This is an abnormal respiratory reflex characterised by spasm of one or both sides of the diaphragm, causing sudden inspiration with associated closure of the vocal cords. The phrenic nerve, vagus nerve, thoracic sympathetic fibres brainstem and hypothalamus are all involved in the reflex arc. An inhibitory pathway via the pharyngeal and gloss opharyngeal nerves is present. Disturbance of any of these components may cause hiccup. Identification of cause may sometimes enable a logical and successful approach to treatment.

Management

Stimulation of the pharynx may be successful in reducing hiccup. This can be achieved in various ways, including: holding iced water in the oropharynx, soft palate massage, oropharyngeal or nasopharyngeal catheter placement.

Common empirical treatments are:

- a defoaming antiflatulent before and after meals and at bedtime (e.g. Asilone 10–20 ml);
- domperidone 10–20 mg t.d.s.; or metoclopramide 10 mg t.d.s. half an hour before meals if delayed gastric emptying;
- nifedipine 10–20 mg b.d.-t.d.s.(assess effect on blood pressure);
- baclofen 5–10 mg b.d. (higher doses can be used with caution);
- chlorpromazine—use with care and only if simpler measures fail: 10–25 mg p.o. t.d.s. (it has a diffuse depressant effect on the reticular formation);
- sodium valproate—for hiccup of central origin.

Phrenic nerve stimulation or ablation are only occasionally an appropriate treatment in patients with advanced disease.

Endoluminal stents

Stenting is a widely used therapeutic intervention for palliation of gastrointestinal and hepatobiliary malignant obstruction. Stents are available as an expandable metal systems (covered or uncovered) or in plastic (for biliary obstruction). Stents are usually placed via a guidewire under endoscopic and fluoroscopic guidance, although radiologists do place them under fluoroscopic guidance alone. Uncovered stents embed well in luminal tissues but may become occluded by further tumour growth. Covered stents prevent the ingress of tumour but are more prone to migration and displacement.

Stenting is usually a day case procedure but depends on patient performance status and complications.

Oesophageal stents

Expandable metal stents (EMS) provide relief or improvement of dysphagia in 90% of cases and result in shorter hospital stays and fewer procedures than non-stenting options (see recanalisation above). EMS require less dilation of the oesophagus than previously used plastic stents (Celestin and Atkinson tubes) and have a reduced complication rate of oesophageal perforation, 3% versus 7% respectively.

Stents are most useful in mid to low oesophageal tumours. Tumours of the gastroesophageal junction respond well but stent migration is more common and the function of the lower oesophageal sphincter is lost and can result in problematic gastroesophageal reflux. High tumours can be problematic causing significant and persistent discomfort.

Covered stents are particularly effective in tracheoesophageal fistula.

Complications:

- 0.5–2% mortality as result of stent insertion [14]
- Pain/mediastinal discomfort (NB: surgical emphysema may indicate perforation)
- Bleeding
- Perforation
- Stent migration (more common following chemotherapy and tumour regression)
- Tumour overgrowth
- Food blockage

Trouble shooting

Encourage patient to modify diet: more liquidised/sloppy food; avoid leafy vegetables and chunks of steak etc. Possible acute food blockage may be relieved by carbonated drinks (e.g. coca cola). Total dysphagia with drooling and aspiration requires emergency review.

Tumour overgrowth can be dealt with by laser, alcohol injection or argon (see recanalisation above).

If the stent traverses the gastroesophageal junction, place the patient on a PPI.

Displaced stents can be retrieved endoscopically, but this is challenging.

Gastroduodenal stents

Pancreatic, duodenal and gastric cancers frequently precipitate gastric outflow obstruction and EMS are as effective in relieving this as palliative bypass surgery. Most patients gain significant clinical improvement. Where there is functional gastric-outlet obstruction due to tumour invasion of neural supply or diffuse peritoneal infiltration with bowel encasement and gut failure, improvement will not be seen.

Patients with duodenal involvement frequently develop biliary obstruction and it is advisable that the biliary obstruction is first remedied before stenting of the duodenum takes place as the metal mesh will prevent access to the biliary tract. Biliary stenting in this scenario is best approached via the percutaneous transhepatic route (PTC).

The EMS are best placed using the combined modalities of endoscopic and fluoroscopic guidance, however this can be achieved fluroscopically alone. Gastroduodenal stents can be inserted as an outpatient procedure. Complications are similar to those mentioned above.

Biliary stents

Patients with biliary obstruction experience nausea, anorexia, weight loss, fat malabsorption with steatorrhoea, itch and occasionally cholangitis. Jaundice may be a significant visual reinforcement affirming the disease process. The obstructed biliary tree is decompressed by endoscopic retrograde cholangiopancreatography (ERCP) or PTC. Either metal or plastic stents are used. Plastic stents are cheaper, however they are subject to bacterial and biliary encrustation resulting in occlusion. Stents usually last between 3 and 4 months. Patients may benefit from re-stenting and recurrence of jaundice should not be assumed to be due to tumour progression.

The more expensive EMS have larger diameters and longer patency than plastic stents. If patient survival is greater than 4 to 6 months then metal stents appear more cost effective with fewer endoscopic interventions and hospital admissions required. If EMS block, they can be recanalised by insertion of a plastic stent or a further EMS.

Complications of biliary stenting (ERCP and PTC)

- Pancreatitis
- Bleeding
- Perforation
- Biliary leak and peritonitis
- Malposition
- Cholangitis

COLORECTAL STENTS

Colorectal stents can be used as a bridge to surgery or in patients with extensive disease who are poor surgical candidates. Covered stents are also useful in assisting closure of colo-vesical and colo-vaginal fistulas. Right-sided colonic stents require endoscopic placement. Left sided stents can be placed radiologically.

Complications

- Perforation (devastating as it will cause a florid faecal peritonitis)
- Stent migration
- Stool occlusion

- Bleeding
- Tenesmus*
- Faecal incontinence*

*In stents placed in the lower rectum.

Patients should be advised to consume a low residue diet and take faecal softeners.

Liver disease

Cirrhosis and advanced chronic end-stage liver disease represent a major public health and palliative burden. In 1999 in the the UK 4000 people died from cirrhosis, two thirds of whom were below the age of 65 [15]. Worldwide hepatitis B and C are the most common causes of cirrhosis. In the developed world alcohol is the most common cause, but hepatits C is rapidly increasing.

Prognosis is related to the severity of the underlying disease (see Figure 9.4) and the development of disease related complications. In stable compensated cirrhosis (Childs A) the 5-year survival is excellent, however in decompensated cirrhosis (development of portal hypertension, ascites, portal hypertensive bleeding, encephalopathy)

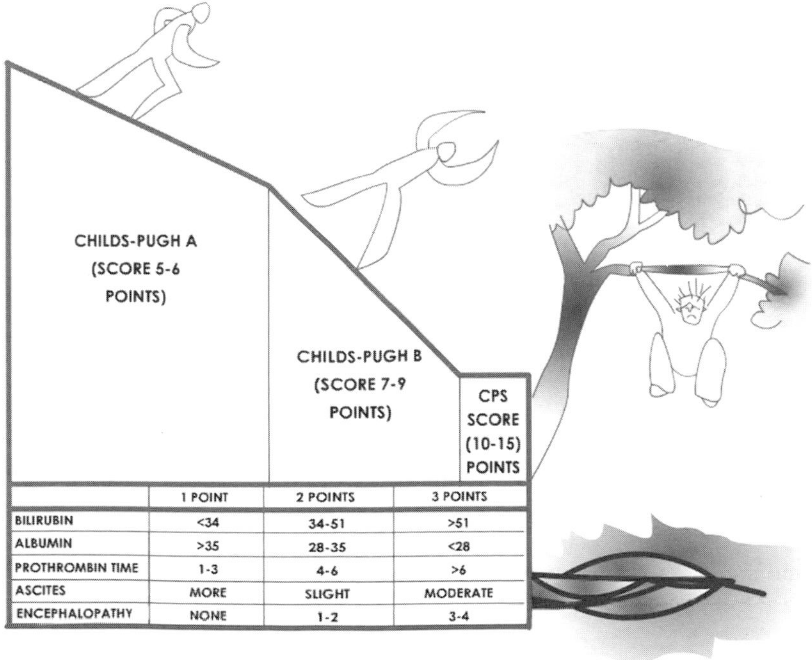

	1 POINT	2 POINTS	3 POINTS
BILIRUBIN	<34	34-51	>51
ALBUMIN	>35	28-35	<28
PROTHROMBIN TIME	1-3	4-6	>6
ASCITES	MORE	SLIGHT	MODERATE
ENCEPHALOPATHY	NONE	1-2	3-4

Fig. 9.4 The Childs-Pugh classification of cirrhosis.

the 5-year survival is 50%. In alcoholic cirrhosis the progression of the disease is directly related to the continued exposure to alcohol.

Complications of cirrhosis

The development of complications associated with decompensated cirrhosis have a marked impact on survival (see Figure 9.5).

- Refractory Ascites (RA)
- Spontaneous Bacterial Peritonitis (SBP)
- Hepatorenal Syndrome (HRS)
- Variceal Bleeding (VB)
- Hepatocellular Carcinoma (HCC)
- Portosystemic Encephalopathy (PSE)

ASCITES AND REFRACTORY ASCITES (RA)

Whilst response to the use of diuretics in malignant ascities is variable and unpredictable, they are highly effective in ascites of decompensated liver disease. Response may be seen using spironolactone up to

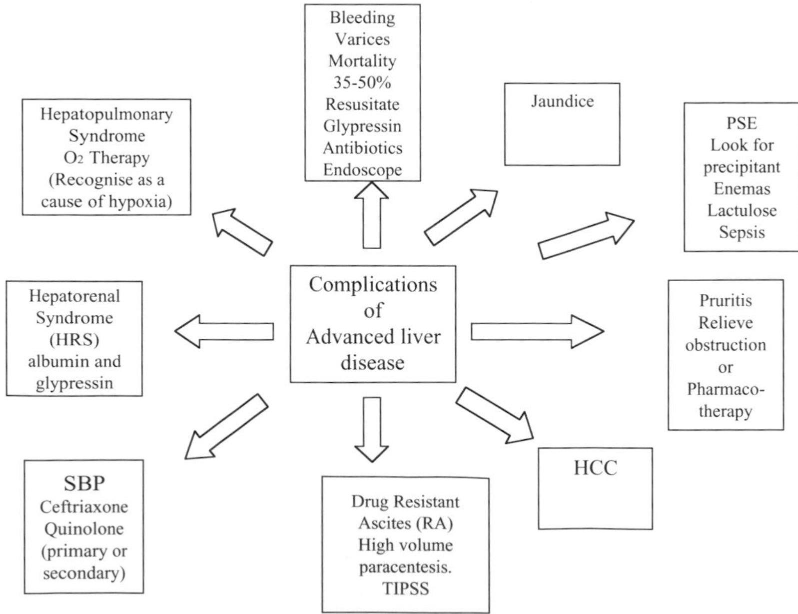

Fig. 9.5 Summary of the complications that may occur in advanced liver disease (HCC: Hepatocellular carcinoma; TIPSS: transjugular intrahepatic portosystemic shunt; SBP: spontaneous bacterial peritonitis; PSE: portosystemic encephalopathy).

400 mg/o.d. and frusemide up to 160 mg/o.d. Diuretics should be titrated to effect whilst monitoring electrolyte balance and renal function.

RA occurs in 5–10% associated with a high frequency of complications (PSE and infections). The one-year survival is approximately 35%. Patients should have the patency of the portal vein checked (ultrasound) and development of a Hepatoma excluded (serum alpha feto protein).

Treatment of RA includes:

- Transplantation: By far the best treatment but not all patients will be suitable.
- Paracentesis (see Box 9.3): The treatment of choice for most patients.
- TIPSS Transjugular intrahepatic portosytemic shunt: Reduces the rate of ascites recurrence and the development of HRS, has no effect on survival and is associated with a 20% incidence of encephalopathy. The ongoing management of patients with TIPSS is hospital intensive.

Box 9.3 High volume paracentesis

- If patient on diuretics, withhold
- Under local anaesthetic insert suprapubic catheter into peritoneal cavity (Banano Catheter ideal)
- Give albumin 1g/kg in total i.v.*
- Drain to dryness
- Remove catheter after 24 hours to reduce chances of infection and peritonitis.
- Place stoma bag over site if ascites leakage.

*As a rule of thumb, give 100 ml of human albumin solution 20% for every 3 litres of fluid removed. Start albumin infusion before or at same time as starting paracentesis.

SPONTANEOUS BACTERIAL PERITONITIS (SBP)

SBP carries a 10–30% mortality with a one-year survival of 38% after the first episode. It may lead to circulatory dysfunction and HRS which has a very poor survival rate. Administration of albumin with antibiotic therapy prevents HRS and improves prognosis.

There is good evidence for the administration of prophylactic quinolone antibiotics in patients with ascites due to cirrhosis for the prevention of SBP, however concerns exist over the emergence of quinolone resistant species of bacteria. The suggested schedule is ciprofloxacin 250 mg o.d.

HEPATORENAL SYNDROME (HRS)

In patients whose renal function deteriorates, HRS should be considered and urgent specialist advice sought. HRS occurs in 5–10% of cirrhotic patients with ascites and is a very sinister development with greater than 90% mortality.

PORTOSYSTEMIC ENCEPHALOPATHY (PSE)

This is common and if mild is easily controlled. There are multiple causes, however the most common are sepsis, dehydration, GI bleed and the co-administration of sedating drugs.

Treatment includes:

- Correction of the reversible (sepsis, SBP, dehydration, hypokalaemia, underlying bleeding)
- Enemas to achieve bowel clearance
- Lactulose to acidify the stool, aiming to achieve two loose stools daily. There is no advantage of giving neomycin with lactulose.

VARICEAL BLEEDING

Varicies are related to elevated portal pressure and the development of a portosystemic shunt through collateral vessels, allowing portal blood to be diverted to the systemic circulation. The size of the varix and the severity of the underlying liver disease are risk factors for bleeding. Propanolol (40 mg b.d.) reduces the incidence of first variceal bleeds by 50%. Alcohol causes marked increase in portal hypertension and every effort should be made to get patients to cease drinking. Banding of varicies has a role in preventing further bleeds, and if practical, should be carried out on a regular basis until the varicies are obliterated.

The average mortality of a first variceal bleed is approximately 50%, however this is closely related to the underlying severity of liver disease. Bleeding may result in severe decompensation and fatal liver injury. Variceal bleeding is always a frightening and dramatic occurrence.

PAIN MANAGEMENT IN ADVANCED LIVER DISEASE

Paracetamol is safe in normal doses in patients with liver disease. NSAIDs should be avoided since their salt retention and other renal effects may lead to decompensation in patients with cirrhosis.

All opiates require liver metabolism and may accumulate in liver impairment. There is no evidence base to inform prescribing advice and we suggest:

- use reduced doses
- avoid drugs with long half lives
- titrate against effect
- re-evaluate daily

Liver transplantation issues

Liver transplant is a highly effective therapy for dealing with all the complications of advanced liver disease; however, for a variety of reasons not all patients will be eligible for transplantation and there is a limited pool of donor grafts available. From July 2002 to August 2003, 766 patients were on the active waiting list for liver replacement in the UK. The median time spent on the active waiting list was 73 days (data from August 2001 to September 2002). In 1999 11% of patients on the active waiting list died from their disease.

For those who are not suitable for transplantation (e.g. those with alcoholic cirrhosis who cannot cease drinking) palliative care is the key focus of care. One in ten patients who are suitable for transplant will not attain this and for all those on the waiting list there is a need to consider quality of life and symptom management issues alongside preparation for transplant. This will include support of their families and consideration of place of death when patients are removed from the transplant list because of deterioration.

Cholestatic liver disease

The key symptoms resulting from stasis of bile are pruritis and jaundice.

PRURITIS

The pruritic effect is mediated through a central mechanisim, a response to a rise in endogenous opioid levels. Large variations in individual response are seen and there is no correlation between plasma bilirubin concentration and intensity of pruritus. Some people get no pruritus at all (see also Chapter 11).

There is no standard or generally accepted regimen for treatment [16]. In 1979 naloxone was observed to have a significant effect on intractable pruritis and the oral derivative naltrexone has been demonstrated to be of value in controlled trials. The use of this requires specialist guidance since opioid withdrawal syndrome may be provoked even in patients not taking opioids.

The most effective treatment is to achieve biliary drainage, although this is not always possible.

Other drugs for pruritis include:

- Antihistamine: Sedating antihistamine have no effect on the itch but may assist in promoting sleep through their sedating effect, best avoided during the daytime.
- Exchange resins: Colestyramine is a bile salt binder, give 4 g b.d. Best taken on an empty stomach first thing in the morning and before the evening meal (can add to orange juice to improve palatability).
- Choleuretic agents: Ursodeoxcholic acid 250 mg t.d.s.
- Enzyme inducers: Rifampacin 150 mg daily or phenobarbital. Moderate to low efficacy with variable response.
- $5HT_3$ antagonists: Anecdotal reports of therapeutic response to i.v. ondansetron.

JAUNDICE

In cholestatic or obstructive jaundice patients frequently feel unwell, anorexic and nauseated. Bile is essential for digestion and absorption of fat, an essential fuel source. They may develop symptoms of malabsorption. Active palliation through decompression of the biliary system (see endoluminal stents above) is the only effective treatment, if at all practical. The approach can be via an ERCP or PTC, either as a day case or a short stay in hospital.

Malignant bowel obstruction

Malignant gastrointestinal obstruction occurs most commonly in patients with advanced abdominal or pelvic cancers: in 25% of patients with a primary bowel cancer; in 6% of patients with a primary ovarian cancer; and in about 40% of advanced ovarian cancer patients.

Where surgery is technically not possible, is inappropriate, or is not acceptable to the patient, medical management of malignant gastrointestinal obstruction can offer good symptom control. Patients may live for surprisingly long periods of time (sometimes months) and be able to take small quantities of food and fluids as desired, usually without the need for a nasogastric tube or parenteral fluids. Most patients can be cared for at home.

The clinical scenario may only have some of the classic features of complete bowel obstruction outlined in Box 9.4. Malignant

Box 9.4 Classical features of complete intestinal obstruction

- Large-volume vomits
- Nausea worse before vomiting
- Nausea relieved by vomiting
- Nil per rectum or per stoma
- Abdominal distension
- Visible peristalsis
- Increased bowel sounds, classically tinkling, but may be absent
- Background abdominal pain
- Colicky abdominal pain

obstruction may present acutely but more commonly is gradual in onset, intermittent, and variable in severity. Gross distension is often absent, even in lower bowel obstruction since the bowel may be constricted at several points. Patients with lower bowel obstruction will often have infrequent, faeculent vomiting, while those with high bowel obstruction may vomit undigested food. It is always useful to determine whether colic is present or absent since this will affect the management strategy (see below).

Non-malignant causes of obstruction must be considered, which may be amenable to surgical or other appropriate intervention. These include: adhesions; constipation; drugs; and unrelated benign conditions.

Investigations can be helpful and may include a biochemical profile (hypokalaemia may cause ileus, hypercalcaemia may cause pseudo-obstruction due to constipation). A plain abdominal X-ray will demonstrate constipation, but can be misleading when multiple levels of obstruction are present. A CT/MRI scan can be indicated if surgery is to be considered.

Chemotherapy may offer a palliative option for some patients with ovarian carcinoma. Any surgical or oncological intervention should run in parallel with more immediate symptomatic treatment. Expanding stents placed endoscopically or radiologically are occasionally helpful and are discussed above.

Surgical intervention

Surgery should always be considered in malignant gastrointestinal obstruction. However, it will often be inappropriate or technically impossible. Surgical intervention is unlikely to be successful in the following situations:

- radiological or previous surgical evidence indicating that a surgical procedure will not be technically possible;
- a stiff, doughy abdomen with little abdominal distension [17];
- diffuse intra-abdominal carcinomatosis;
- massive ascites which re-accumulates rapidly after paracentesis;
- poor general physical status [18];
- previous radiotherapy to the abdomen or pelvis, in combination with any of the above.

Medical management

A nasogastric tube and intravenous fluids are rarely necessary if the following strategy is used.

PAIN

Analgesia for background pain is obtained by using a continuous s.c. infusion of diamorphine (dose: 1/3 total daily morphine dose ± 30–50% increment as dictated by the pain). If opioid naive, start on a diamorphine dose of 10 mg/24 h. Not all patients require opioid analgesia if no background pain is present and colic can be relieved by more appropriate drugs (see below).

COLIC AND GUT MOTILITY

If colic is present avoid all drugs that could worsen this (i.e. metoclopramide, bulk-forming, osmotic and stimulant laxatives). If colic persists, add hyoscine butylbromide s.c., starting at 60 mg/24 h (up to 200 mg/24 h as needed).

If colic is absent a trial of metoclopramide s.c. 40–80 mg/24 h, with or without dexamethasone s.c./i.m./i.v. 6–16 mg daily, may allow resolution of partial obstruction or pseudo-obstruction due to dysfunction of the nerve supply to the gut. In the absence of colic, incomplete obstruction in the large bowel may be helped by a stool-softening laxative, such as docusate sodium 200 mg b.d.-q.d.s.

NAUSEA

The choice of antiemetic depends on whether the patient is experiencing colic. If colic is not a feature, metoclopramide is administered s.c.

40–80 mg/24h (see above). If colic is present, give haloperidol (s.c. 5–20 mg/ 24 h) or cyclizine (s.c. 100–150 mg/24 h). A combination of haloperidol and cyclizine is sometimes necessary.

$5HT_3$ antagonist antiemetics may have a role in relief of the nausea induced by bowel distension and stimulation of the vomiting centre through vagal afferents (see above) but this is unclear. They can be given rectally or subcutaneously.

VOMITING

Reduction in the volume of gastrointestinal secretions will reduce colic, nausea, pain and the need to vomit. This can usually be adequately achieved with hyoscine butylbromide (s.c. 60–200 mg/24 h [19]) with or without an H_2 antagonist or proton pump inhibitor.

If large-volume vomiting persists despite hyoscine butylbromide, the somatostatin analogue, octreotide, will further decrease the volume of intestinal secretions in the gut lumen [20]. A trial of octreotide, given at a rate of 300 μg/24 h by s.c. infusion, should be performed. The dose can be titrated over 2–3 days to 600 μg/24 h; If there is no benefit at 600 μg/24 h it should be stopped. The dose should be reduced daily by 100 μg/24 h to the lowest effective dose (mean dose 300 μg/24 h) [21].

In some cases, particularly in high obstructions such as gastric outlet obstruction, these strategies are not effective. It may then be helpful to use a nasogastric tube or consider a venting gastrostomy to allow the patient to continue to drink and eat as desired without the fear of provoking immediate vomiting. Venting gastrostomy can be performed under local anaesthetic either endoscopically or radiologically and may facilitate discharge and dying at home. In one series of 51 patients median survival was 17 days with a range of 1–190 days; 92% of patients gaining symptomatic improvement of nausea and vomiting with some restoration of diet. [13]

Contraindications to the use of a venting gastrostomy are:

- The presence of significant ascites as it would precipitate peritonitis.
- Tumour infiltration of the stomach.

In an obstructed abdomen with malignant infiltration the risk of perforating the bowel with resultant peritonitis is significant and the patient should be clear about this risk.

It is important that at least a 16–20 F bore gastrostomy tube should be used to facilitate adequate decompression.

SUBCUTANEOUS DRUG DELIVERY

Patients may require the use of more than two drugs to obtain symptom control and not infrequently two subcutaneous infusions are required. Studies of the compatibility of multiple drug combinations are not available (see Chapter 22) but clinical observation suggests the following drugs are compatible and maintain efficacy:

- diamorphine, haloperidol and cyclizine;
- diamorphine, haloperidol and hyoscine butylbromide;
- diamorphine, cyclizine and hyoscine butylbromide;
- diamorphine and octreotide;
- diamorphine, haloperidol and octreotide.

DIET AND HYDRATION

Sensitive, pre-emptive discussion of the situation is a vital part of care for the patient and family. Many patients with obstruction can eat and drink in modest amounts when symptoms are controlled. A liquid, low-residue diet may be the least problematic.

Hydration should be considered on an individual basis. Oral discomfort and dryness can largely be relieved by frequent, attentive mouth care, ice to suck and drinks as desired and tolerated. Profound thirst is not common but some patients may benefit from parenteral fluids, for example s.c. infusion of 1–2 l 0.9% saline/24 h or i.v. fluids.

Constipation

Constipation is a big problem for patients with advanced disease. For instance more than 50% of patients admitted to hospices in the UK complain of constipation [22]. Physical illness, immobility, poor oral intake, opioids and many other drugs are risk factors for constipation. Constipation can be prevented in the majority of patients by prescription of appropriate laxatives and careful review.

All patients prescribed a weak or strong opioid should be advised to also take a stimulant laxative unless a contraindication exists. The dose of laxative will usually need to be increased as the dose of opioid is increased. It is not appropriate to wait until (predictable) constipation occurs before commencing laxative treatment. The vicious cycle of inappropriately treated abdominal pain and constipation should be anticipated in all patients with cancer, or others taking opioid analgesics.

Management

Management will involve removing any underlying causes if possible, prescribing an appropriate oral laxative and considering the use of per rectal/stomal measures (see Table 9.3). It should be remembered that one of the commonest reasons for failure of therapy is prescription of a laxative which the patient dislikes.

Table 9.4 shows the various types of laxative that are available. Movicol and sodium picosulfate are probably best used as second line laxatives for patients with established constipation resistant to other laxatives. Lactulose may cause substantial gaseous distension, especially in resistant constipation.

Rectal laxatives may be needed and include:

- Suppositories: glycerine (softening and mild stimulant); bisacodyl (stimulant);
- Enemas: arachis oil (130 ml) (softening); phosphate, sodium citrate (stimulant).

If the rectum is empty and stool is high in the colon, enemas should be administered through a rubber Foley catheter. Oil enemas should be warmed before use.

Bulk-forming laxatives have a very limited place in the management of constipation in patients with advanced disease, since they are

Table 9.3 Treatment of constipation.

Examination finding	Treatment
Rectum full of hard faeces	Soften with glycerine suppositories +/− arachis oil enema. Commence combined stimulant and softening oral laxative
Rectum full of soft faeces	Stimulate evacuation with bisacodyl suppository +/− stimulant enema. Commence stimulant oral laxative
Empty distended rectum	Exclude obstruction. Stimulant suppository or enema will enhance colonic contraction. Commence oral laxative

Table 9.4 Laxatives and their characteristics.

Laxative TCH type	Drugs	Starting dose	Latency of action
Stimulant	Bisacodyl	10 mg nocte	6–12 h
	Senna	15 mg nocte	
	Movicol	1 sachets daily in 125 ml water	
	Sodium picosulfate	5 ml nocte	
Softening	Docusate sodium	10 mg t.d.s.	1–2 days
	Lactulose	15 ml b.d.	
Combined softening and stimulant	Co-danthramer	Two capsules or 20 ml nocte	6–12 h
	Co-danthrusate	One capsule or 10 ml nocte	

generally troublesome to take, rely on a high oral fluid intake, and are not appropriate for the management of opioid-induced constipation.

All laxative doses should be titrated according to response.

Rectal problems of advanced cancer

The presence of tumour in the rectum may lead to bleeding, faecal incontinence and offensive discharge, in addition to pain. The quality of life may be severely impaired. Such problems occur in patients with primary rectal cancers but also in patients with other pelvic cancers: cervix, vagina, uterus and bladder. Treatment options include:

- radiotherapy;
- palliative surgery with stoma formation;
- endoscopic injection of absolute alcohol;
- laser therapy and diathermy;
- metal stent alone or in combination with laser or alcohol;
- pharmacological palliation.

The stool should be kept very soft to pass through the obstructive lesion. Docusate sodium is given at a dose of 200 mg at least q.d.s. but titrated to stool consistency; it can be combined with a stimulant laxative, such as Co-danthrusate. Careful insertion of softening enemas may be useful.

PAIN AND TENESMUS

Pain from rectal cancer may be troublesome in a number of ways; constant nociceptive, visceral and bone, which may be worsened by movement. In some cases sitting may be impossible. The pain may be present only on, or worsened by, either standing or defecation. Neuropathic pains can result from infiltration of the lumbosacral plexus. Some patients experience tenesmus: a painful sensation of rectal fullness and an urge to defecate.

The WHO ladder (see Chapter 8) will be helpful for all of these pain syndromes. Pain will be additionally helped by keeping the faeces soft. For some patients a palliative colostomy will be the best form of pain relief.

Neuropathic pain, of which tenesmus is one type, may be helped by opioids but will probably require adjuvant analgesics such as amitriptyline 10–150 mg nocte. Tenesmus may also be helped by:

- steroids—dexamethasone 4–16 mg daily;
- calcium channel antagonists—nifedipine 10–20 mg b.d.-t.d.s (smooth muscle relaxant);
- radiotherapy;
- bupivacaine enema;
- sacral epidural injection of steroid and local anaesthetic;
- bilateral lumbar sympathectomy;
- intrathecal 5% phenol to posterior sacral nerve roots.

Occasionally epidural delivery of opioids and local anaesthetic may be appropriate for relief of pain at rest and on defecation, particularly if the obstructive lesion is very low in the bowel. In the ill, dying patient, the most appropriate option is to achieve complete constipation with opioids and hyoscine butylbromide.

Rectal bleeding and discharge

While radiotherapy, alcohol injection, diathermy, or laser therapy is being planned, or if these are not possible or helpful, other measures may be needed to reduce the distress and discomfort from rectal bleeding. Enemas may be performed using various active ingredients, including: tranexamic acid (2–4 g/day made up in KY jelly) [23]; and aluminium coating via an enema (1% alum or sucralfate g in KY jelly) [24]. Distress or discomfort due to rectal discharge may be alleviated by steroid enemas and metronidazole suppositories.

Stoma care

Patients with stomas require both physical and psychological support. Good preparation before stoma formation and adequate time spent with the patient after stoma formation by a specialist (stoma care) nurse help in the transition and continued successful management. Patients vary in the time needed to adapt to and manage their stoma.

The most common physical difficulties are:

- when a bowel stoma becomes overactive, often with a more fluid faecal output;
- when constipation occurs;
- when patients are less able to manage their own stoma care because of the effects of their treatment or their disease.

Evaluation and management of these problems will involve examination of the stoma and effluent, including a digital examination of the stoma. There must also be a review of skin protectives/adhesives and bag size, together with a review of laxatives and antidiarrhoeal agents along with all other drugs.

If a stoma is impacted, suppositories and enemas can be given as for rectal impaction; however, a stoma has no sphincter. Suppositories should be gently pushed through the stoma as far as possible and gauze held over the stoma for a few minutes. If an enema, either oil or phosphate, is used it should be administered via a medium-size Foley catheter. This should be passed well into the stoma (identify direction of the bowel by digital examination beforehand). Inflate the balloon to 5 ml for 10 minutes while instilling the enema.

Control of fluid loss from an overactive ileostomy can be troublesome and specialist advice may need to be sought. Various treatments are available. The administration of opioids can reduce bowel motility; for example loperamide 4–8 mg b.d. or codeine phosphate 30–60 mg q.d.s. If the patient is already taking morphine for pain relief an increase in this may reduce bowel motility further but will also increase sedation and other central effects, and is not the preferred option unless it is also useful to improve pain control. A reduction of bowel motility and secretions may be achieved by use of anticholinergics, for example hyoscine butylbromide s.c. 60–180 mg/24 h, while H_2 antagonists or proton pump inhibitors can reduce gastric secretion.

Ispaghula (1–2 sachets t.d.s.) aids thickening of the motions, as does the use of isotonic and avoidance of hypotonic oral fluids. A subcutaneous infusion of octreotide can reduce small bowel secretions (see above). However, doses required can be much greater than in treating obstruction.

The principles of management of a stoma and stoma-care equipment can also be used to contain the output from faecal fistulae and protect the skin. Subcutaneous octreotide has been used to decrease the volume of fistula effluent and in some cases has aided healing.

Acknowledgement

We would like to acknowledge the work of Marie Fallon and John Walsh for the first edition of this chapter.

References

1 Roth K, Lynn J, Zhong Z, et al. Dying with end stage liver disease with cirrhosis: insights from SUPPORT. Study to Understand Prognoses and Preferences for Outcomes and Risks of Treatment. *J Am Geriatr Soc* 2000; 48(5 Suppl): S122–S130.

2 Dewys WD, Begg D, Lavin PT, et al. Prognostic effect of weight loss prior to chemotherapy in cancer patients. *Am J Med* 1980; 69: 491–496.

3 Wouters EF, Creutzberg EC, Schols AM. Systemic effects in COPD. *Chest* 2002; 121(Suppl): 127S–130S.

4 Anker SD, Negassa A, Coats AJ, et al. Prognostic importance of weight loss in chronic heart failure and the effect of treatment with angiotensin-converting-enzyme inhibitors: an observational study. *Lancet* 2003; 361: 1077–1083.

5 Plauth M, Schutz ET. Cachexia in liver cirrhosis. *Int J Cardiol* 2002; 85: 83–87.

6 Grunfield C. What causes wasting in AIDS? *NEJM* 1995; 333: 123–124.

7 Bruera E, Sweeney C 2003. Pharmacological interventions in cachexia and anorexia. In: Doyle D, Hanks, Cherney N, Calman K, eds. *Oxford Textbook of Palliative Medicine*. 3rd edition. Oxford: Oxford University Press, 2003: 552–560.

8 Mathus-Vliegen EMH. Feeding tubes and gastrostomy. In: Tygat GNJ, Classen M, Waye JD, Nkazawa S, eds. *Practice of Therapeutic Endoscopy*. Philadelphia, PA: Saunders, 2000.

9 Jobbins J, Bogg J, Finlay I, Addy M, Newcombe RG. Oral and dental disease in terminally ill cancer patients. *BMJ* 1992; 304: 1612.

10 DeConno F, Sbanotto A, Ripamonti C, Ventafridda V. Mouthcare. In: Doyle D, Hanks, Cherny N, Calman K, eds. *Oxford Textbook of Palliative Medicine*. Oxford: Oxford University Press, 2003: 673–687.

11 Grond S, Zech D, Diefenbach C, Bishcoff A. Prevalence and pattern of symptoms in patients with cancer pain: a prospective evaluation of 1635 patients referred to a pain clinic. *J Pain Symptom Manage* 1994; 9: 372–382.

12 Dunlop GM. A study of the relative frequency and importance of gastrointestinal symptoms, and weakness in patients with far advanced cancer. *Palliat Med* 1989; 4: 37–43.

13 Brooksbank MA, Game PA, Ashby MA. Palliative venting gastrostomy in malignant intestinal obstruction. *Palliat Med* 2002;16: 520–526.
14 Ramirez FC, Dennert B, Zierer ST, Sanowski RA. Esophageal self-expandable metallic stents-Indications, practice, techniques and complications, results of a national survey. *Gastro Intest Endosc* 1997; 45: 360–364.
15 www.doh.gov.uk/cmo/annualreport2001/livercirrhosis.htm
16 Bergasa NV, Jones EA. Management of the pruritis of cholestasis. Potential role of opiate antagonist. *Am J Gastroenterol* 1991; 86: 1404–1412.
17 Taylor RH. Laparotomy for obstruction with recurrent tumour. *Br J Surg* 1985; 72: 327.
18 Krebs H, Goplerud DR. Surgical management of bowel obstruction in advanced ovarian cancer. *Obstet Gynaecol* 1983; 61: 327–330.
19 DeConno F, Caraceni A, Zecca E, Spondi E, Ventafridda V. Continuous subcutaneous infusion of hyoscine butylbromide reduces secretions in patients with gastrointestinal obstruction. *J Pain Symptom Manage* 1991; 6: 484–486.
20 Fallon MT. The physiology of somatostatin and its synthetic analogue, octreotide. *Eur J Palliat Care* 1994; 1: 20–22.
21 Riley J, Fallon MT. Octreotide in terminal malignant obstruction of the gastrointestinal tract. *Eur J Palliat Care* 1994; 1: 23–25.
22 Sykes NP. Constipation and diarrhoea. In: Doyle D, Hanks, Cherney N, Calman K, eds. *Oxford Textbook of Palliative Medicine*. 3rd edition. Oxford: Oxford University Press, 2003: 483–496.
23 McElligot E, Quigley C, Hanks GW Tranexamic acic and rectal bleeding. *Lancet* 1991; 29: 37–39.
24 Regnard CFB. Control of bleeding in advanced cancer *Lancet* 1991; 337: 974.

Further reading

Nutrition, tube feeding and PEG
Stroud M, Duncan H, Nightingale J. Guidelines for entral feeding in adult hospital patients. *Gut* 2003; 52(suppl VII): vii1-vii12.
Cirrhosis and its complications
Menon KV, Kamath PS. Managing the complications of cirrhosis. *Mayo Clinic Proceedings* 2000; 75(5): 501–509.

10: The Management of Respiratory Symptoms

ROSEMARY WADE, SARA BOOTH
AND ANDREW WILCOCK

Introduction

Respiratory symptoms are a common problem for patients with advanced cancer, cardio-respiratory and neurological disease. In their last year of life as many as 94% patients with chronic lung disease, 78% of those with lung cancer [1] and 50% of patients with heart disease will experience breathlessness [2]. This chapter will discuss the management of the three commonest respiratory symptoms: cough, breathlessness and haemoptysis.

Historically, the evidence base for the symptomatic management of respiratory symptoms in both malignant and non-malignant diseases has been limited, but this is changing. Palliative care is becoming available for patients earlier in the course of their disease, but particular caution, and close, objective evaluation should be used when extrapolating from experience in patients with cancer to manage the needs of patients with chronic, non-malignant disease. Palliative care techniques first used in the management of malignant disease may, however, offer the only ways of maintaining and improving quality of life for patients with non-malignant disease once maximum medical therapy has been used.

Cough

Cough is a physiological reflex and an important defence mechanism that clears the central airways of foreign material and secretions. The central control of cough is in the brain stem (close to the respiratory centre): there is some voluntary control. Cough receptors are few or absent in smaller bronchioles and the lung periphery and cough has a stronger association with mediastinal tumours such as squamous and small cell types. Cough becomes pathological when excessive, ineffective, or persistent.

Patients complain both of the cough itself, and also of its consequences including: exhaustion, self-consciousness, insomnia, musculoskeletal pain and urinary incontinence [3]. In patients with cancer the prevalence of cough varies between 50% and 90% during the course of the disease; it is highest in patients with lung cancer.

In the general population the commonest cause of acute cough is infection of the respiratory tract: the main causes of chronic cough are gastro-oesophageal reflux, asthma and postnasal drip [3]. In the palliative care setting chronic obstructive pulmonary disease (COPD) and cancers, primary and secondary, predominate. (see Table 10.1).

In clinical trials of drugs used to treat the cough of respiratory tract infections, a placebo response of 85% has been demonstrated [4]. This compares to a placebo response of 30–40% in trials in a variety of other conditions making the response to medications alone difficult to assess.

Chronic cough is often a poorly managed symptom with implications for patient, family and carers. Intractable cough interrupts conversation, isolates the patient socially and may affect sleeping arrangements.

Management of the cough

The cause can be established in the majority of patients by a careful history alone. Investigations appropriate to the clinical condition of the patient may include chest X-ray, sputum culture, spirometry (pre- and post-bronchodilator), sinus X-rays or barium swallow. Stimuli that exacerbate coughing such as smoke, cold air and exercise should be established for the individual patient and avoidance measures taken.

It is useful to divide cough into 'wet' or 'dry' [5]. A wet cough serves a physiological purpose and expectoration should be encouraged and facilitated. Conversely, a dry cough serves no purpose and should be suppressed. A wet cough that is distressing a dying patient, who is too weak to expectorate, should also be suppressed.

There are three basic strategies for managing cough (see Figure 10.1):

- Treat the underlying cause of the cough.
- Suppress a 'dry' cough (using demulcents and antitussives).
- Encourage a more productive 'wet' cough (using cough enhancers or protussives).

Table 10.1 Causes of chronic cough and specific treatments.

Cause	Mechanism	Specific treatments
Cancer related		
Primary or secondary cancer causing airway obstruction	Infiltration, compression, distortion, obstruction, leading to collapse +/− infection.	Radiotherapy, chemotherapy
	Tracheo-oesophageal fistula	Stent
Ineffective cough due to:	Generalised weakness	
	Vocal cord palsy	Teflon injection
	Pain on coughing	Analgesics
Treatment related		
Cancer treatment:	Pulmonary infiltration/fibrosis related to chemotherapy and radiotherapy	Corticosteroids
Non-cancer treatment:	ACE inhibitors—increase cough reflex	Stop
	Beta-blockers—induce bronchoconstriction	
Other causes		
Infection	Lung abscess, bronchiectasis Post-infection increased cough reflex	Antibiotics
COPD, asthma		Anti-inflammatory drugs, bronchodilators
Gastro-oesophageal reflux		Antacids, proton pump inhibitor
Post nasal drip syndrome		Decongestants, corticosteroids, antibiotics
Pulmonary oedema		Diuretics
Smoker's cough		
Pulmonary infarction,		

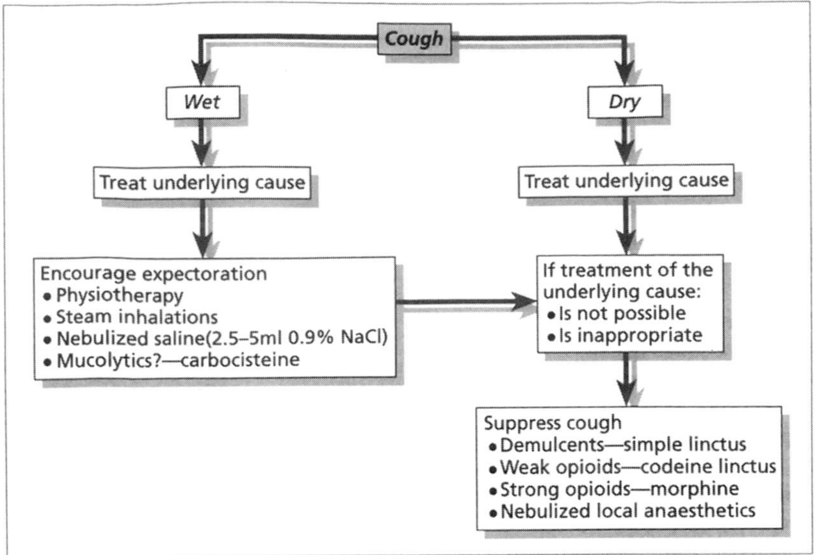

Fig. 10.1 The management of cough in patients with cancer.

Treat underlying cause

Even in patients with cancer, cough often has more than one cause, but it is easy to attribute *all* symptoms to the cancer alone without recognising that other non-cancer-related causes may be important. These may potentially be ameliorated by instigation of appropriate treatment or maximising existing therapies (e.g. for asthma/COPD). If there is any doubt then consult appropriate colleagues for advice.

Active palliative treatments for tumours include radiotherapy, chemotherapy, hormone therapy, surgery, the insertion of a stent and the drainage of pleural effusions. To obtain advice on these treatments contact your local oncology and respiratory medicine teams.

BRONCHODILATORS

Patients known to have asthma and COPD should have their treatment optimised. Standard bronchodilator treatment should be tried in patients where bronchospasm is suspected. Sodium cromoglicate (10 mg inhaled q.i.d.) has been shown to reduce cough in patients with non-small cell lung cancer with no change in lung function [6].

Cough suppression

DEMULCENTS

Demulcents contain soothing substances such as syrup or glycerol. The high sugar content may coat sensory nerve endings and stimulate both saliva production and swallowing and so inhibit the cough reflex. Lemon flavourings promote salivation and may also promote secretion of airways mucus. Herbal antitussives, many including menthol from peppermint, have been shown to reduce cough induced by citric acid in healthy volunteers [7]. Any effect is short lived and there is no evidence to suggest that compound preparations offer any advantage over simple linctus (5 ml t.-q.d.s.) although individual patients often have a preference.

ANTITUSSIVES

Opioids

Opioids primarily work by suppressing the cough reflex centre in the brainstem. Patients will often require concomitant prescription for a stimulant laxative.

Codeine. Codeine, pholcodine and dextromethorphan are common ingredients in compound cough preparations. Evidence supports the use of codeine, dihydrocodeine and dextromethorphan, but not pholcodine [3]. However, the effective dose of codeine or dextromethorphan is greater than that usually delivered by compound preparations, where the sugar content may in fact be the main effective ingredient. Therefore, codeine linctus 5–10 ml (15–30 mg t.-q.d.s.) should be used.

The antitussive effect of codeine, similar to its analgesic effect, may rely partly on its conversion to morphine, an enzymatic process deficient in 5–10% of the population, who may fail to benefit from its use [8].

If codeine is ineffective a strong opioid such as morphine should be used. If a patient is already receiving a strong opioid for pain relief there is no logic in adding codeine or another opioid as a separate cough suppressant. In this situation, check with the patient if an 'as needed/prn' dose helps relieve the cough. If so, use as required, or consider increasing the regular dose. If not, there is little point in further dose increments or addition of another strong opioid.

Morphine. The prescription of morphine is 2.5–10 mg every 4 hours. The dose can be titrated upwards as allowed by side-effects and then converted to a modified-release preparation.

Methadone. Methadone has no clear advantage over morphine for the treatment of cough. There is a wide variation in its pharmacokinetics between individuals, and a risk of accumulation with repeated use.

Nebulised local anaesthetics

Local anaesthetics inhibit afferent nerve endings and clearly reduce cough during bronchoscopy when administered locally. Their use in patients with cough due to cancer or other disease has not been fully evaluated and cannot be routinely recommended. They should be considered only when other measures have failed. Their use is limited by their unpleasant taste, oropharyngeal numbness, risk of aspiration and bronchoconstriction and short duration of action (10–30 minutes). Patients need to abstain from food or drink for 1–2 hours after their use.

Suggested doses are 2% lidocaine (5 ml) or 0.25% bupivacaine (5 ml) t.ds-q.d.s. [5]. A test dose should always be given under close observation to ensure bronchospasm or other adverse effects are rapidly treated. Tachyphylaxis (rapid development of resistance to the effect) is common.

Cough enhancers and protussives

There are occasions when cough is useful and needs to be encouraged. Hypertonic saline, amiloride and terbutaline following chest physiotherapy increase cough clearance in trials but the clinical usefulness of these has yet to be determined. It is consistent to stop drugs that reduce mucus clearance such as anticholinergics, aspirin and benzodiazepines.

CHEST PHYSIOTHERAPY (BRONCHOPULMONARY HYGIENE)

Chest physiotherapy is often prescribed in patients with copious secretions such as those with cystic fibrosis. Although there are no large trials, postural drainage is regarded as effective but time consuming: there is less evidence for the use of vibration and percussion. In a Cochrane review of bronchopulmonary hygiene in COPD and bronchiectasis there was not enough evidence to support or refute its use [9].

MUCOLYTICS

In chronic bronchitis there is good evidence that N-acetylcysteine (400–600 mg a day in 2–3 oral doses) benefits patients, without causing harm, by reducing the number of exacerbations and days of disability [10]. With other diagnoses, a therapeutic trial could be considered e.g. carbocisteine 750 mg t.d.s. Nebulised acetylcysteine sometimes appears to be more effective than nebulised 0.9% saline [11]. However, it has an unpleasant sulphurous odour, is expensive and can cause bronchoconstriction, nausea or vomiting. It is inactivated by oxygen and the nebuliser must be driven by compressed air.

Nebulised isotonic saline 2.5–5 ml t.d.s to q.d.s. is often used in specialist palliative care settings to aid mucolysis.

Breathlessness

Breathlessness is the most common symptom of cardio-respiratory disease. It is a complex experience of the mind and the body and like pain has physical and emotional components. There is no single definition of breathlessness and no unitary theory of causation. The American Thoracic Society, in a consensus statement has defined dyspnoea as "a subjective experience of breathing discomfort ... " : the statement goes on to emphasise that breathlessness is made up of "qualitatively distinct sensations that vary in intensity... " and is derived from the interaction of many factors physiological, psychological, social and environmental [12]. The experience of breathlessness includes the perception of *difficulty* in breathing and the physical, behavioural and emotional responses to it. It should not be confused with an increase in respiratory rate (tachypnoea) or in depth of ventilation (hyperpnoea). Dyspnoea is always unpleasant and often frightening. The terms breathlessness and dyspnoea are often used interchangeably; there is still some debate about this as breathlessness is also a normal accompaniment of enjoyable, strenuous activity and some experts feel that only the term dyspnoea should be used to describe pathological breathlessness. However, most patients will not understand the term dyspnoea: in this chapter they are used interchangeably.

Patients find breathlessness frightening, disabling and restricting. Patients' spouses also suffer significantly, experiencing anxiety and helplessness as they witness their partners suffering and feel powerless to reduce it [13]. Breathlessness imposes many restrictions on patients' lives and the most common adaptive strategies include reducing functional performance, obtaining assistance with activities of daily living, and altering, reducing or discontinuing work [14]. The psychological responses may include anxiety, fear, panic and depression.

The number of people affected by breathlessness is reaching epidemic proportions across the world as the number of people with cardiorespiratory disease increases—in England alone 24 000 patients with COPD and 10 750 patients with chronic heart failure (CHF) died in 2002 [15]. Most of these patients probably suffered breathlessness for some years before their death. Intractable breathlessness in cancer patients is a poor prognostic sign and patients deteriorate and die more rapidly than most patients with non-malignant disease. Both the prevalence and the severity of breathlessness increase as death approaches.

A study of 923 patients (only 4% of whom had lung cancer) to determine the prevalence of dyspnoea in the cancer population found that 46% had some breathlessness. Over 50% of patients with lymphoma, breast, head and neck and gynaecological cancers complained of breathlessness [16].

Pathophysiology

The neurophysiological mechanism that underlies the generation of the sensation of breathlessness remains unclear but it appears related to the degree of activation of brainstem structures concerned with the automatic control of breathing. Inputs from cortical and other higher centres are important and help explain why the threshold and tolerance to breathlessness appears to vary between individuals and is influenced by mood, anxiety [17] and the degree of encouragement and support available to the individual patient [18].

Assessment of breathless patients

Chronic breathlessness is difficult to treat hence it is vital to identify any of the causes that may be partially or fully reversible (Table 10.2). Diagnosing the cause of breathlessness requires a thorough history and examination combined with appropriate investigation (see Box 10.1). A chest X-ray is often valuable as an initial investigation as clinical examination of the chest may reveal few signs even in the presence of significant disease.

Table 10.2 Causes of breathlessness and specific treatments.

Causes	Mechanisms	Specific treatments
Cancer related		
Primary and secondary lung cancer causing:	Airway obstruction (+/− collapse), mass effect, lung infiltration	Chemotherapy, radiotherapy, hormone therapy, stent, cryotherapy, laser treatment
	Lymphangitis carcinomatosis	Corticosteroids, diuretics, bronchodilators
Generalised weakness causing:	Loss of 'fitness', respiratory muscle weakness	Encouragement and support to keep active
Pleural effusion		Pleural drain, pleurodesis
Superior vena cava obstruction		Radiotherapy, corticosteroids; intravascular stents
Anaemia; – of chronic disease – due to marrow infiltration		Transfusion, erythropoietin
Pericardial effusion		Drainage
Phrenic nerve palsy		
Splinting of the diaphragm	Ascites	Paracentesis, diuretics
	Hepatomegaly	
	Chest wall infiltration	
	Chest wall pain	Analgesics
Treatment related		
Cancer treatments	Surgery: lobectomy, pneumonectomy	
	Radiotherapy: pneumonitis/fibrosis	Corticosteroids
	Chemotherapy	
Non-cancer treatments	Drugs precipitating fluid retention, e.g. corticosteroids	Stop
	Drugs precipitating bronchospasm, e.g. beta-blockers	Stop

Continued

Table 10.2 *Continued*

Causes	Mechanisms	Specific treatments
Other causes		
Infection	Bacterial, viral, fungal	Antibiotics/fungal
Chronic respiratory disease	For example, COPD, asthma	Bronchodilators, steroids
Chronic cardiac disease	For example, ischaemic heart disease, CHF	Diuretics, ACE inhibitors, βblockers
Pulmonary oedema		Diuretics
Pulmonary embolism		Anti-coagulation
Pneumothorax		Aspiration
Psychological factors	For example, anxiety, fear, anger, frustration, isolation, depression	Increased support for patients and family; antidepressants, anxiolytics

Box 10.1 The assessment of the breathless patient with cancer.

Aspect of assessment	Detail
Important aspects of the history	Speed of onset Associated symptoms: • pain • cough • haemoptysis • sputum • stridor • wheeze Exacerbating and relieving factors Symptoms suggestive of hyperventilation: • poor relationship of dyspnoea to exertion • presence of hyperventilation attacks • breathlessness at rest • rapid fluctuations in breathlessness within minutes

Continued

Box 10.1 *Continued*

Aspect of assessment	Detail
	• fear of sudden death during an attack • breathlessness varying with social situations. Past medical history: e.g. history of cardiovascular disease and respiratory Drug history: e.g. drugs precipitating fluid retention or bronchospasm Symptoms of anxiety or depression Social circumstances-support networks Level of independence: • ability to care for themselves • identify coping strategies What the breathlessness means to the patient How do they feel when they are breathless
Examination	Very useful to observe the patient walking a set distance or carrying out a specific task Does hyperventilation reproduce symptoms?
Investigations	Commonly performed: • Chest X-ray • Haemoglobin Less commonly performed: • Ultrasound scan—helpful for differentiating between pleural effusion and solid tumour • Oxygen saturation at rest and on exercise: may be useful if assessing value of oxygen • CT Scan and spiral CT scan • Peak flow/simple spirometry: useful for assessing response to bronchodilators or corticosteroids • Electrocardiogram • Echocardiography • Ventilation/perfusion scan

Assessment should also identify any symptoms of anxiety and depression, the impact of the breathlessness on the patient's lifestyle, the patient's (and family's) coping strategies, and the meaning and implications of the symptom for the patient.

Hyperventilation is a common accompaniment of breathlessness and causes a number of physical symptoms such as a feeling of abdominal bloating and circumoral tingling. If hyperventilation is suspected then ask the patient to take up to 20 deep breaths and monitor if this reproduces the patient's symptoms. This is also therapeutic as it helps to demonstrate the cause of the symptoms and allows the introduction of breathing control/relaxation exercises that aim to give the patient a greater feeling of control over their breathing.

The impact of breathlessness on the patient can be observed by asking the patient to carry out a set, everyday task. This may reveal hyperventilation, which can be highlighted to the patient. Alternatively, beneficial coping strategies that the patient uses can be reinforced. The exercise assessment also provides a baseline against which to monitor progress.

It is important to explore what the patient and their carers understand about breathlessness. It is a common erroneous belief that the heart or lungs are being further damaged when the patient becomes breathless and many people fear that they might die suddenly during an episode of breathlessness, which is very rare. Activities are subsequently curtailed or avoided and many become socially isolated. It is important to stress that becoming breathless is in itself not dangerous and patients must be encouraged to remain as active as possible as this prevents deconditioning which exacerbates the symptom. An exploration of the patient's emotional reactions to breathlessness is also important for successful management.

Management of breathlessness

It is essential to find out the patient's aims for treatment and the sort of therapies and investigations that they can, or will, undergo. In the very frail patient or one who has a very poor prognosis it may be inappropriate to investigate aggressively or use treatments that will detain the patient in hospital with only a small prospect of improving the symptom. Although CT scanning is often helpful, some patients are unable to lie flat or dislike the claustrophobia they feel during the investigation. In a patient with cancer other symptoms may be of more importance to the patient and may need immediate attention.

There may be many causes of breathlessness in one individual, which may each require a separate management strategy. A survey of patients with lung cancer attending a chest clinic found that half of them had airflow obstruction which was associated with severe breathlessness. Of these, only 14% were taking bronchodilator therapy. A trial of bronchodilator therapy improved breathlessness in 60% of the previously untreated patients [19]. Such patients should receive appropriate treatment or have any existing treatment optimised.

In patients with cancer, radiotherapy, chemotherapy, hormone therapy and surgery sometimes have a place in palliating breathlessness. Palliative procedures for the secondary effects of cancer should be considered. This may involve the drainage of pleural and pericardial effusions or ascites and the insertion of endobronchial or superior vena caval stents. Corticosteroids are used for their anti-inflammatory effect (thereby reducing peri tumour oedema) to treat the symptoms of superior vena cava obstruction, tracheal compression/stridor or carcinomatosis lymphangitis. As there is little evidence to support their use, corticosteroids should not be a substitute for, or delay the use of, more effective therapies where these are appropriate.

AN OVERALL STRATEGY FOR THE TREATMENT OF BREATHLESSNESS

All chronically breathless patients and their families, whatever the illness, need medical assessment to ensure that the treatment of the underlying illness is as good as it can be and that they are receiving appropriate palliative pharmacological treatments.

Pharmacological and non-pharmacological treatments are both important but the relative contributions made by these two approaches vary according to the patient's prognosis. Pharmacological treatments predominate in the terminal phase and non-pharmacological methods in patients who are breathless on exertion only. It is useful to consider the treatment of breathlessness in the clinical settings that relate to the prognosis of the patient: remember that patients with cancer who are breathless have a very different prognosis from those, for example, with COPD:

- breathlessness on some exertion only—prognosis of months to years;

- breathlessness on minimal exertion (speaking or eating for example)—prognosis weeks to months;
- breathlessness at rest—prognosis of days to weeks;
- terminal breathlessness (with other signs of advanced disease and fall in level of consciousness)—prognosis of hours to a few days.

Breathlessness on exertion is common in patients with COPD, congestive cardiac failure and cancer (especially those with co-existing cardiac disease). A specialist opinion may be necessary to ensure that all possible treatment is being given: this should be considered in patients who have had stable disease for many years and suffer deterioration. All patients with, or in whom breathlessness is predicted in the near future should be instructed in the use of a fan, breathing exercises and positioning strategies. An introduction to physiotherapy and occupational therapy services is often very beneficial. Support for the spouse or other caring family members is also needed, including careful explanation of what is happening and what may happen. It is often reassuring to discuss what a relative or friend can do when the patient has an exacerbation of breathlessness: even such simple things as fetching a fan and a chair, offering any oxygen or prescribed 'as needed' medicines or giving a simple shoulder massage can be helpful for both patient and the relative, who may otherwise feel helpless.

NON-PHARMACOLOGICAL APPROACHES

Pulmonary rehabilitation

Pulmonary rehabilitation is an established therapy for patients with COPD and other respiratory diseases to reduce breathlessness and improve exercise capacity. Patients must be motivated to benefit and it may not help those with significant cardiac disease, musculoskeletal problems or cognitive impairment. Supervised aerobic exercise sessions of 20–30 minutes three times a week have shown reduction in breathlessness and fatigue components of the Chronic Respiratory Questionnaire [20] and can enhance the patient's sense of control. The role of purse-lipped breathing, diaphragmatic-breathing and respiratory-muscle training is controversial [21].

A trial of an 8-week rehabilitation programme in patients with COPD and moderate dyspnoea showed benefits over the non-exercise group, which were maintained at 6 months but lost by 1 year [22].

There is also growing evidence that physical exercise programmes, tailored to the individual, can reduce cancer related fatigue [23].

Palliative care breathlessness clinics

These multidisciplinary clinics have been set up to improve the care of patients with cancer-related breathlessness and use the same approach as pulmonary rehabilitation services within specialist palliative care. The principles that underpin them are outlined in Box 10.2 [24]. The clinics are usually held in cancer centres or hospices and patients and spouses attend the clinic weekly over a 4–6 week period. Patients attending these clinics have been shown to notice a reduction in their breathlessness (which is still present after four weeks) and an improvement in quality of life [25]. Unfortunately, many of the patients referred to breathlessness clinics are not able to attend their first appointment (as they have deteriorated rapidly) and often the reported improvements in breathlessness are small and not sustained as the illness progresses.

Box 10.2 Non-pharmacological approaches to breathlessness

Exploring the perception of the patient and carers
- Exploration of anxieties—especially fear of sudden death when breathless
- Explanation of symptoms and meaning
- Informing patient and carers that breathlessness in itself is not dangerous
- What is/is not likely to happen—'you won't choke or suffocate to death'
- Help come to terms with deteriorating condition
- Help to cope with and adjust to 'losses' (of role, abilities, etc.)

Maximising the feeling of control over breathlessness
- Use of an electric or hand-held fan
- Breathing control advice
- Relaxation techniques
- Plan of action for acute episodes: simple written instructions-step-by-step plan increase confidence in coping with acute episodes
- Complementary therapies may benefit some patients

Continued on p. 200

Box 10.2 *Continued*

Maximising functional ability and support

- Encourage exertion to breathlessness to increase tolerance to breathlessness and maintain fitness
- Assessment by the district nurse, occupational therapist, physiotherapist and social worker may all be necessary to identify where additional support is required

Reduce feelings of personal and social isolation

- Meet others in similar situation
- Attendance at a day centre
- Respite admissions

Oxygen

Supplemental oxygen has been shown to improve exercise tolerance and prolong life [26] in patients with COPD who are severely hypoxic ($Pa\text{O}_2$ < 9kPa). The role of oxygen in less hypoxic and normoxic patients is more difficult to determine as there is great variability between individuals in subjective response to oxygen. In addition, the oxygen saturation level does not predict benefit from oxygen or degree of breathlessness.

Oxygen is expensive to prescribe and the patient and family can incur great cost in terms of quality of life. Activities are restricted and communication can be impaired between patient and family. Patients become psychologically dependent on oxygen and become anxious when oxygen supplies are perceived to be low. Some patients feel stigmatised by using oxygen in public.

The cooling flow of oxygen against the face or through the nose may reduce breathlessness [27] (as does a stream of air) by stimulating facial and nasal receptors of the trigeminal nerve. This finding also supports the use of an electric fan to help relieve breathlessness. In patients with cancer the benefit of oxygen is also variable [28, 29]. An 'N of 1' trial of compressed air compared to oxygen, with breathlessness being formally measured, is recommended to establish the benefit for each individual patient before prescribing oxygen [30].

Oxygen therapy should be available to severely hypoxic patients. In those less hypoxic, a trial of oxygen therapy can be given via nasal prongs for an agreed fixed period of time. If on review the patient has found it useful it can be continued. If the patient has any doubts concerning its efficacy then it should be discontinued.

Oxygen can be delivered at home via cylinders or an oxygen concentrator. All patients suffering from breathlessness should be encouraged to use an electric or hand-held fan.

Non-invasive ventilation

Non-invasive positive pressure ventilation (NIV) is being increasingly used in patients with acute and chronic respiratory failure. NIV uses a tight-fitting mask and small, relatively portable ventilator, to produce a positive pressure, improve ventilation and oxygenation, reduce the severity of breathlessness and reduce CO_2 retention. It can be used in the community for patients with severe COPD and for some patients with neurological disease associated with hypoventilation. Use in the community always needs support from the specialist centre. NIV may be used in the future to help patients with cancer and severe breathlessness.

PHARMACOLOGICAL APPROACHES

Opioids

Morphine and other opioids can reduce the severity of breathlessness probably through three mechanisms: they act centrally to reduce ventilatory drive stimulated by hypercapnia and hypoxia, reduce oxygen consumption at rest and on exercise and alter the central perception of breathlessness.

A Cochrane review of the use of opioids for the palliation of breathlessness in terminal illness was published in 2001 [31]. This included 14 studies were in patients with COPD predominating, two in cancer, one in heart disease and one interstitial lung disease. The opioids used were dihydrocodeine, diamorphine and morphine in parenteral or oral form and nebulised morphine. The review found a strong effect on reduction of breathlessness by oral and parenteral opioids in COPD and cancer patients but this was not seen in the use of nebulised morphine. Since the review was published, two further studies, one involving patients with chronic heart failure and the another in patients with COPD, have also shown a reduction in breathlessness with morphine [32, 33].

For opioid-naive patients use small doses initially (e.g. 2.5 mg oral morphine q.d.s. 4 hourly) and titrate the dose and dose interval according to response and side effects. The use of morphine may arouse fears, and time is required to listen, clarify, explain and reassure patients and families about these. Written information is also useful. For patients already receiving opioids, ask them to assess whether there is benefit from an additional dose. If so, increase the regular opioid in steps of 30–50%. If there is no improvement or if adverse effects occur, then reduce the dose. A modified release preparation or a continuous subcutaneous infusion of opioid may be better tolerated and be more effective for some patients.

Benzodiazepines

There is no good evidence for the use of benzodiazepines in the management of breathlessness but they are widely used in cancer-related breathlessness. In the non-malignant diseases associated with breathlessness they are rarely indicated because patients have time to develop a damaging dependence on them. In addition, the use of benzodiazepines in patients with pulmonary disease requires caution as there are reports of ventilatory depression, although this has not been a universal finding. Alprazolam was not helpful in relieving dyspnoea at rest or during exercise in a 24-patient trial in patients with COPD [34]. Any effect they appear to have on relieving breathlessness is probably due to their anxiolytic effect: drowsiness is common and may be disabling. Benzodiazepines should not be prescribed routinely as a treatment for breathlessness in patients without co-existent anxiety.

The oral benzodiazepine most frequently used is diazepam initially at a dose of 2–5 mg t.d.s., reducing over several days as levels of active metabolites rise, to a maintenance dose of 2–5 mg at night. Careful dose titration is necessary to avoid troublesome sedation as the half-life of the drug and its metabolites is very prolonged. Lorazepam is often prescribed for use sublingually (0.5 mg to 1.0 mg t.d.s as needed); the half-life is 16 hours.

There are only anecdotal reports for the use of low doses of midazolam (2.5 to 5 mg of midazolam plus 2.5–5 mg of diamorphine over 24 hours) in patients with severe breathlessness, who are not terminally ill. Patients can remain ambulant and fully awake on these doses.

Phenothiazines

There is more evidence to support the use of phenothiazines in breathlessness but these are not used commonly—probably because of adverse effects. Chlorpromazine has been used for the relief of terminal breathlessness in patients with cancer [35].

Buspirone

Buspirone is an anxiolytic acting predominantly via serotonin receptors ($5HT_{1A}$). It is as effective as diazepam in the relief of anxiety and is free of sedative or respiratory depressant effects. In patients with COPD, buspirone improves anxiety levels along with breathlessness and exercise tolerance [36]. Further evaluation is necessary but buspirone appears to be an useful alternative to diazepam.

Terminal breathlessness

Patients often fear suffocating to death and it is important to have an active, positive approach to the patients, their families and to colleagues about the potential to relieve terminal breathlessness:

- No patient should die with distressing breathlessness.
- Failure to control is a failure to utilise drug therapy correctly.
- Combination of a parenteral opioid with a sedative anxiolytic such as midazolam is effective (Table 10.3).
- If the patient becomes agitated or confused (sometimes aggravated by midazolam), haloperidol or levomepromazine should be added or substituted.

Usually, due to distress, inability to sleep and exhaustion, patients (and their carers) accept the risk of increasing drowsiness in order to be more comfortable. Sedation is not the primary aim of therapy (unless there is overwhelming distress) and some patients often become 'brighter' with the improvement in their symptoms. However, as increasing drowsiness is usually a feature of their deteriorating clinical

Table 10.3 Drugs used in treatment of terminal breathlessness.

Drug	Starting dose	Upper dose	Route
Diamorphine	5–10 mg/24 h (opioid naive)	Titrate according to symptoms	s.c., infusion
Midazolam	5–10 mg/24 h	60 mg/24 h	s.c., infusion
Levomepromazine	12.5 50 mg/24 h	200 mg/24 h	s.c., infusion

condition it is important to explain clearly to the relatives the aims of treatment and the gravity of the situation.

Haemoptysis

Coughing-up blood is frightening and will lead most people to seek medical attention. In the majority of cases the amount of blood expectorated is small but large bleeds can occur with little or no warning. The most common cause is acute infection but other causes include cancer, congestive heart failure, pulmonary infarction or emboli [37]. One-third of patients with bronchogenic carcinoma experience haemoptysis, with an incidence of acute fatal bleeds of 3%. Haemoptysis from bronchogenic carcinoma can occur with any histological type although massive fatal haemoptysis is most likely to be due to squamous cell tumours (83%) that are located centrally. The management of massive haemoptysis is discussed in Chapter 21.

In patients with metastatic lung disease from solid malignancies, haemoptysis is usually due to erosion of small, friable mucosal vessels. Infection (bacterial and fungal), low platelets and abnormal clotting increase the risk of haemoptysis.

Management of haemoptysis

The history of the patient will help determine if the haemoptysis is related to cancer, to its treatment, or to the common differential diagnoses of infection or pulmonary embolism. Investigations appropriate to the clinical condition of the patient depend upon the causes being considered and the severity of the haemoptysis.

RADIOTHERAPY

Radiotherapy is the treatment of choice for haemoptysis due to cancer, leading to prolonged relief in 85% of patients. The dose given is palliative and the treatment can usually be repeated if the symptom recurs. For patients with unrelieved or recurrent haemoptysis, in whom further external beam irradiation is not possible, brachytherapy, laser therapy, bronchial artery embolisation or cryotherapy may be considered depending on local access to specialist services.

ANTICOAGULATION

If the patient is anticoagulated, review the indication and level of anticoagulation required. It may help to discontinue drugs with antiplatelet effects (e.g. aspirin, non-selective cyclo-oxygenase inhibitor (COX)) or change to a selective COX2 inhibitor or paracetamol, which does not interfere with platelet function.

MEDICATION

Tranexamic acid (500 mg—1 g q.d.s.) inhibits plasminogen activation and thus prevents fibrinolysis. It appears effective in reducing blood loss in a number of conditions from case reports as there are no randomised controlled trials.

Summary

Respiratory symptoms are common in patients with advanced cardio respiratory and neurological disease; they are frightening and very disabling for patients and also severely impair the family and social lives of those closely associated with the patient. Specialist advice is often needed to manage them as effectively as possible, although most patients can be investigated from and treated in the community.

References

1 Edmonds P, Karlsen S, Khan S, Addington-Hall J. A comparison of the palliative care needs of patients dying from chronic respiratoy diseases and lung cancer. *Palliat Med* 2001; 15: 287–295.
2 McCarthy M, Lay M, Addington-Hall J. Dying from heart disease. *J Roy Coll Phys Lon* 1996; 30: 325–328.
3 Irwin RS, Boulet LP, Cloutier MM, Fuller R, Gold PM, Hoffstein V et al. Managing cough as a defense mechanism and as a symptom. A consensus panel report of the American College of Chest Physicians. *Chest* 1998; 114(2 Suppl): 133S–181S.
4 Eccles R. The powerful placebo in cough studies? *Pulm Pharmacol Ther* 2002; 15: 303–308.
5 Twycross R, Wilcox A, Charlesworth S, Dickman A. *Palliative Care Formulary*. 2nd edition. Radcliffe: Medical Press, 2002.
6 Moroni M, Porta C, Gualtieri G, Nastasi G, Tinelli C. Inhaled sodium cromoglycate to treat cough in advanced lung cancer patients. *Br J Cancer* 1996; 74: 309–311.
7 Ziment I. Herbal antitussives. *Pulm Pharmacol Ther* 2002; 3: 327–333.
8 Twycross R. Weak opioids. *Pain Relief in Advanced Cancer*. Edinburgh: Churchill Livingstone, 1994: 233–254.
9 Jones A, Rowe B. Bronchopulmonary hygiene physical therapy for chronic obstructive pulmonary disease and bronchiectasis (Cochrane review). The Cochrane Library, Issue 1, 2004. Chichester, UK: John Wiley & Sons, Ltd.
10 Poole PJ, Black PN. Mucolytic agents for chronic bronchitis or chronic pulmonary disease (Cochrane review). The Cochrane Library, Issue 1, 2004. Chichester, UK: John Wiley & Sons, Ltd.

11 Gallan A. Evaluation of nebulised acetylcysteine and normal saline in the treatment of sputum retention following thoracotomy. *Thorax* 1996; 51: 429–432.
12 Dyspnea. Mechanisms, assessment, and management: a consensus statement. American Thoracic Society. *Am J Resp Crit Care Med* 1999; 159: 321–340.
13 Booth S, Silvester S, Todd C. Breathlessness in cancer and chronic obstructive pulmonary disease: Using a qualitative approach to describe the experience of patients and carers. *J Palliat Supp Care* 2003; 1:337–344.
14 Carrieri V, Janson-Bjerklie S. Strategies patients use to manage the sensation of dyspnoea. *West J Nurs Res* 1986; 8: 284–305.
15 www.statistics.gov.uk. Accessed 15-11-2003.
16 Dudgeon DJ, Kristjanson L, Sloan JA, Lertzman M, Clement K. Dyspnea in cancer patients: prevalence and associated factors. *J Pain Symp Manage* 2001; 21: 95–102.
17 Morgan A, Peck D, Buchanan D, McHardy G. Effects of attitudes and beliefs on exercise tolerance in chronic bronchitis. *BMJ* 1983; 286: 171–173.
18 Guyatt GH, Pugsley S, Sullivan M, et al. Effect of encouragement on walking test performance. *Thorax* 1984; 39: 818–822.
19 Congleton J, Muers MF. The incidence of airflow obstruction in bronchial carcinoma, its relation to breathlessness, and response to bronchodilator therapy. *Respir Med* 1995; 89: 291–296.
20 Lacasse Y, Brosseau L, Milne S, Martin S, Wong E, Guyatt GH, et al. Pulmonary rehabilitation for chronic obstructive pulmonary disease. *Cochrane Database Syst Rev* 2002;(3): CD003793.
21 Gigliotti F, Romagnoli I, Scano G. Breathing retraining and exercise conditioning in patients with chronic obstructive pulmonary disease (COPD): a physiological approach. *Respir Med* 2003; 97: 197–204.
22 Bestall JC, Paul EA, Garrod R, Garnham R, Jones RW, Wedzicha AJ. Longitudinal trends in exercise capacity and health status after pulmonary rehabilitation in patients with COPD. *Respir Med* 2003; 97: 173–180.
23 Dimeo FC. Effects of exercise on cancer-related fatigue. *Cancer* 2001; 92 (6 Suppl): 1689–1693.
24 Corner J, Plant H, Warner L. Developing a nursing approach to managing dyspnoea in lung cancer. *Int J Palliat Nurs* 1995; 1: 5–11.
25 Hateley J, Laurence V, Scott A, Baker R, Thomas P. Breathlessness clinics within specialist palliative care settings can improve the quality of life and functional capacity of patients with lung cancer. *Palliat Med* 2003; 17: 410–417.
26 Crockett AJ, Cranston JM, Moss JR, Alpers JH. *Domiciliary Oxygen for Chronic Obstructive Pulmonary Disease (Cochrane review)*. The Cochrane Library, Issue 1, 2004. Chichester, UK: John Wiley & Sons, Ltd.
27 Schwartzstein R, Lahive K, Pope A, Weinberger S, Weiss J. Cold facial stimulation reduces breathlessness induced in normal subjects. *Am Rev Resp Dis* 1987; 136: 58–61.
28 Bruera E, de Stoutz N, Velasco-Leiva A, Schoeller T, Hanson J. Effects of oxygen on dyspnoea in hypoxaemic terminal-cancer patients. *Lancet* 1993; 342: 13–14.
29 Booth S, Kelly MJ, Cox NP, Adams L, Guz A. Does oxygen help dyspnea in patients with cancer? *Am J Resp Crit Care Med* 1996; 153: 1515–1518.
30 Booth S, Wade R, Anderson H, Swannick M, Kite S, Johnson M. The use of oxygen in the palliation of breathlessness. A report of the expert working group

of the scientific committee of the association of palliative medicine. *Respir Med* 2004; 98: 66–77.

31 Jennings AL, Davies AN, Higgins JPT, Broadley K. *Opioids for the Palliation of Breathlessness in Terminal Illness (Cochrane Review)*. The Cochrane Library, Issue 1, 2004. Chichester, UK: John Wiley & Sons, Ltd.

32 Abernethy AP, Currow DC, Frith P, Fazekas BS, McHugh A, Bui C. Randomised, double blind, placebo controlled crossover trial of sustained release morphine for the management of refractory dyspnoea. *BMJ* 2003; 327(7414): 523–528.

33 Johnson MJ, McDonagh TA, Harkness A, McKay SE, Dargie HJ. Morphine for the relief of breathlessness in patients with chronic heart failure–a pilot study. *Eur J Heart Fail* 2002; 4: 753–756.

34 Man GC, Hsu K, Sproule BJ. Effect of alprazolam on exercise and dyspnea in patients with chronic obstructive pulmonary disease. *Chest* 1986; 90: 832–836.

35 McIver B, Walsh D, Nelson K. The use of chlorpromazine for symptom control in dying cancer patients. *J Pain Symp Manage* 1994; 9: 341–345.

36 Argyropoulou P, Patakas D, Koukou A, Vasiliadas P, Georgopoulos D. Buspirone effect on breathlessness and excersise performance in patients with COPD. *Respiration* 1993; 60: 216–220.

37 Eddy J-B. Clinical assessment and management of massive hemoptysis. *Crit Care Med* 2000; 28: 1642–1647.

11: Managing Complications of Cancer

RACHAEL BARTON

Introduction

Metastatic or advanced cancer may cause complications which require intervention to palliate symptoms, restore function or prevent deterioration. Although common, some complications are rarely seen by those working outside the field of oncology. Such complications often have a profound effect on a patient's functional ability and quality of life. It is important to identify early those who may benefit from specific treatment since a prompt referral allows the rapid palliation of symptoms and may prevent loss of function and independence. It is equally important to identify those patients who are in the terminal stage of their disease, and who may be helped more by symptomatic measures alone.

This chapter outlines the clinical problems most frequently encountered and gives management guidelines so the non-specialist may have confidence in dealing with what is often a frightening situation for both the patient and their carer.

Spinal cord compression

This requires early recognition and prompt referral. Restoration of sphincter and motor function is rarely possible for those who have lost it by the time they start treatment. Despite the development of cord compression being a poor prognostic sign, active management is indicated in all but very terminally ill patients.

Epidemiology

Malignant spinal cord compression (MSCC) is common, affecting 5% of all cancer patients and in up to half of these, it is the first presentation of cancer. It is particularly frequent in myeloma, lymphoma and in those cancers which metastasise readily to bone, i.e. breast, prostate, lung and renal carcinomas, affecting up to 10% of all patients with these diseases. Of those with spinal cord compression, 60% have primary tumours of the breast, lung or prostate [1]. In children, MSCC is very rare but may occur with Ewing's sarcoma, neuroblastoma, Hodgkin's disease, germ cell tumours and soft tissue sarcomas [2].

Pathophysiology

Neurological dysfunction is caused by a combination of spinal cord oedema, ischaemia, and direct pressure. Of the total, 85–90% are due to vertebral metastases, while 10% are due to compression from growth of a paraspinal mass (commonly lymphoma). A small proportion is due to meningeal carcinomatosis. Metastatic disease is present in more than one vertebra in >70% of patients.

Site of cord compression by vertebral level:

- thoracic: 70%
- lumbar: 20%
- cervical: 10%
- multiple sites: 20%

Diagnosis and early suspicion

Any patient with cancer is at risk of MSCC, especially those with vertebral metastases. A history of increasing back pain is the presenting symptom in 60–95% of patients. This may be localized pain but often a radicular pain develops. The pain may be worsened by coughing, sneezing, straining, movement, lying supine, percussion over the vertebrae, or neck and hip flexion. The cardinal features of MSCC are:

- pain
- muscle weakness
- sensory loss
- abnormal reflexes
- sphincter dysfunction

Muscle weakness generally occurs symmetrically in the proximal leg groups. Sensory loss may be in any pattern. Sphincter dysfunction occurs late except in compression of the cauda equina, with painless urinary retention, constipation or faecal incontinence. Cauda equina syndrome produces the following:

- sciatic pain
- saddle anaesthesia
- urine retention
- loss of anal tone

Prognostic factors

AMBULATORY STATUS AT PRESENTATION

Of patients with MSCC, 30–40% can walk at presentation (with or without help) and of these, 70% will still be able to walk after treatment. In contrast, 50% of patients with spinal cord compression have complete paraplegia at presentation and few of these will regain function. Early diagnosis is therefore important before irreversible damage occurs.

HISTOLOGY OF THE PRIMARY

Myeloma, lymphoma, small cell lung cancer and germ cell tumours have the most favourable prognosis. Breast and prostate cancer have a better outlook for mobility and survival than non-small cell lung cancer or metastases of unknown primary.

RATE OF NEUROLOGICAL DETERIORATION PRIOR TO PRESENTATION

A slower development of neurological deficit predicts for a better outcome in terms of maintaining mobility. A rapid deterioration over 24–48 hours suggests irreversible cord damage, probably with infarction [3].

Treatment

IMMEDIATE MANAGEMENT

A patient with MSCC should be prescribed dexamethasone 8 mg immediately followed by 16 mg daily in divided doses. The first dose should be given parenterally where there is doubt about absorption. Suitable analgesia is required using NSAIDs, opioids and antispasmodics. Urgent telephone referral to an oncologist or neurosurgeon for further management is vital. The investigation of choice is an MRI scan that shows the location and number of spinal levels affected.

There is no need to keep the patient immobile in bed with log-rolling unless the spinal lesion is considered to be unstable and at risk of progression if the patient bears weight. The patient should be encouraged to sit up, sit out of bed and, if possible, mobilise unless this causes severe pain.

SUBSEQUENT TREATMENT OPTIONS

Surgery. Surgery should be considered when the histology of the primary cancer is unknown. Patients with spinal cord compression without complete paraplegia should also be discussed with the neurosurgical team as a matter of urgency. Spinal decompression and stabilisation followed by radiotherapy improves the outcome in terms of maintenance of mobility and continence compared with radiotherapy alone [4]. Surgery should also be considered when there is spinal instability causing pain or when the tumour is radioresistant. In cases such as these, the multidisciplinary assessment and management of the patient is essential.

Radiotherapy. For many patients, radiotherapy (RT) is the mainstay of treatment. It relieves pain, may prevent deterioration but rarely restores function that has been lost unless the cord remains viable and the tumour responds rapidly enough to relieve pressure. In general, radiotherapy is more effective when cord compression occurs without bony collapse [5]. Five to ten fractions are often given but a single fraction may suffice to relieve pain in the patient with a poor prognosis and complete paraplegia. RT should ideally be started within 24 hours of presentation with a maximum delay of 48 hours [6].

Chemotherapy. Chemotherapy (CT) may be indicated for chemosensitive tumours such as lymphoma, small cell lung cancer, germ cell tumours and myeloma and is usually followed by radiotherapy.

Rehabilitation and discharge planning

Most patients have a dramatic change in both their functional ability and independence. The physiotherapist and occupational therapist play a key role in rehabilitation. Patients and carers may need to adapt not only to loss of mobility but also to catheterisation and faecal incontinence.

Patients and their carers may need:

- special equipment;
- adaptations to home or a new place of care;
- a 'package' of social and health care including respite care;
- support in psychological adaptation to the life change and poor prognosis.

It is vital that the hospital and primary health care teams, social workers and the community occupational therapists, physiotherapists and palliative care services work together to achieve optimal results.

Outcomes

FUNCTION

Overall, 40% of patients with MSCC will walk again. However, 25% of patients relapse at the same site within 6 months and 50% of those living long enough relapse within a year. Of those who do not require a urinary catheter prior to treatment, 80% will remain catheter-free compared to 20% of those who require a catheter at diagnosis.

SURVIVAL

Overall median survival is 7–10 months; 10% die within 1 month and 18–30% live for more than 1 year. Lung cancer carries a particularly poor prognosis, with a median survival of 2–3 months.

PLACE OF CARE

Many people who are paretic or paraplegic will require care in a nursing home. If life expectancy is very short or there are particular physical, psychological or other problems, a palliative care unit may be appropriate.

Follow-up

Patients with MSCC are at increased risk of further spinal cord compression since >70% will have other vertebral sites affected by metastatic disease. To continue to optimise function, pain control and quality of life, regular follow-up in the community is vital.

Superior vena cava obstruction (SVCO)

SVCO describes a syndrome characterised by obstruction to blood flow through the superior vena cava. There is a malignant cause in 88% of cases, lung cancer causing 70%, lymphoma 8% and other malignancies 10%. In 50% of cases with an underlying malignancy, SVCO is the first manifestation of disease and therefore an urgent specialist referral is important to make an accurate diagnosis.

Active treatment of SVCO may give good relief from distressing symptoms and is indicated in all but the frail, terminally ill patient who may be helped more by symptomatic measures alone.

Pathophysiology

Malignant obstruction to blood flow usually results from extrinsic compression by tumour or lymph nodes although intracaval thrombus may also occur. Swelling of the face and arms results from elevation of venous pressure above the obstruction.

Diagnosis and early suspicion

Any patient known to have a primary lung tumour, especially right-sided, is at particular risk. The onset is usually insidious, which allows collaterals to develop, visible as engorged subcutaneous veins. Two-thirds of patients complain of breathlessness and half of facial swelling or a feeling of fullness in the head. All symptoms and signs (see Box 11.1) may be exacerbated by bending forwards or lying down.

Box 11.1 Symptoms and signs of superior vena cava obstruction

Symptoms
- Dyspnoea
- Facial/arm swelling
- Head fullness
- Headache
- Cough
- Chest pain
- Dysphagia

Physical signs
- Neck vein distension
- Facial/arm swelling
- Chest vein distension
- Breathlessness
- Plethora
- Facial +/or conjunctival oedema
- Central +/or peripheral cyanosis

Management

Although the symptoms are often uncomfortable, the syndrome is rarely life-threatening unless oxygenation is severely compromised. Urgent telephone referral should be made to a chest physician if there is no prior diagnosis, or to the oncologist if the patient has known malignant disease.

IMMEDIATE MEASURES

The patient is prescribed bed rest. Elevation of the bed head is helpful. Oxygen should be used only if it gives symptomatic relief. Hypoxia, if present, is usually due to the underlying tumour.

The role of steroids is unproven. Dexamethasone 16 mg daily in divided doses may help but should not be given 'blind' if the underlying diagnosis is not known. Rarely, high-grade mediastinal lymphoma may present as SVCO, in which case steroids may induce tumour lysis, threatening renal function and obscuring a histological diagnosis. Anticoagulants are not indicated routinely.

SUBSEQUENT TREATMENT

The aim of treatment is to relieve symptoms and, if possible, cure the underlying process. Patients with SVCO who are otherwise well can be treated as outpatients.

Both radiotherapy and chemotherapy may be used to treat the underlying cancer, the rates of relief depending on the histology. Approximately 77% of patients with small cell lung cancer and 60% of those with non-small cell lung cancer will have relief of symptoms regardless of whether chemotherapy, radiotherapy or a combination are used [7]. Radiotherapy is usually complete in 1–2 weeks and symptoms usually improve within 2–3 weeks. Lymphoma is usually treated initially with chemotherapy.

Insertion of a stent under radiological control gives rapid and often immediate relief of symptoms, most resolving within 72 hours [7]. Urgent referral for stenting should be considered for severe symptoms or for relapse following treatment with other modalities. Thrombolysis may be indicated for extensive thrombus, although this increases the chances of adverse side effects.

Symptomatic measures alone may provide some relief for terminally ill patients who are too unwell for active treatment. These include steroids, oxygen, raising the head of the bed, analgesia and antitussives.

Outcome

The average survival of a patient diagnosed with a malignant cause of SVCO is 8 months, but the prognosis depends on the underlying histology and stage of their disease.

Relapse occurs following radiotherapy and/or chemotherapy in approximately 17% of patients with lung cancer over a period of 1–16 months following treatment.

Follow-up

During active treatment and until toxicity has settled, care should be centred on the specialist unit providing the treatment. Patients with incurable lung cancer are best followed by infrequent routine hospital visits with an 'SOS' option. The patient, family, palliative care and primary health care teams should all be made aware of the likely symptoms of advanced lung cancer and who to contact should the need arise.

Bone Metastases

Bone metastases are common, especially in cancers of the breast, prostate, lung and kidney and in multiple myeloma which primarily affects the bones. Up to 70% of women dying of breast cancer will have bone metastases, although many of these will have been asymptomatic. The complications of bone metastases include pathological fracture, nerve compression and hypercalcaemia, which are discussed below.

Diagnosis and early suspicion

The cardinal feature of a bone metastasis is pain. This is commonly unrelenting, may be present at rest and may be associated with referred pain, restriction of movement and neurological impairment.

The initial investigation should be an X-ray of the affected area, asking for orthogonal views of long bones (i.e. perpendicular) as some metastases may be obscured from one direction. At this stage it is important to rule out a pathological fracture or a bone at imminent risk of fracture (see below). Prostate cancer classically results in sclerotic metastases although lytic disease may occur, whereas myeloma causes marked lysis of the bone. Breast and lung cancer often give a mixed picture of sclerotic and lytic metastases and renal cancer metastases are often large and vascular. Bone metastases are frequently multiple although many will not cause symptoms.

An isotope bone scan is a more sensitive investigation than an X-ray, assessing the whole skeleton and detecting small areas of increased isotope uptake which may indicate a metastasis. The distinction between metastases and degenerative disease is improved by comparing the bone scan with X-rays. Noticiably, metastases which cause a great deal of bony lysis, e.g. myeloma, may appear 'cold' on a bone scan. In cases of difficulty, an MRI scan of the affected area may be diagnostic.

MANAGEMENT

General measures

The initial priority is analgesia. NSAIDs are often useful although severe pain from bony metastases often requires opiates. Steroids, e.g. dexamethasone, 4–6 mg daily can be helpful as a short term adjunct to other analgesics but if not helpful after a week's trial, should be discontinued. Pain may also be reduced by resting the affected area. Consultation with physiotherapists may be helpful if walking aids are required.

Systemic anticancer treatments

Consideration should be given to systemic treatments, e.g. hormones for breast and prostate cancer or chemotherapy for sensitive cancers, e.g. small-cell lung cancer, breast cancer and myeloma as these will often improve the pain of bony metastases.

Radiotherapy

For most painful bony metastases, local radiotherapy is the treatment of choice. In uncomplicated bone metastases, a single dose of radiotherapy, planned and delivered in one day will achieve pain relief in 60–80% of patients with a complete response in 30%.

The side effects of radiotherapy depend on the site treated and include fatigue, nausea and vomiting and looseness of the bowels. GI side effects are most common when the treatment field includes the abdomen and can be reduced by a $5HT_3$ antagonist plus dexamethasone 2 mg t.d.s. beginning on the day of radiotherapy and continuing for 3 days. Palliative radiotherapy given in this way can be repeated if the pain recurs with a good chance of a second response and little added toxicity.

Widespread bony metastases are impractical to treat with several local fields. One option is 'hemibody radiotherapy' in which a single dose is delivered either to the upper or lower half of the skeleton. Toxicity can be severe, mainly comprising nausea, vomiting and diarrhoea. A $5HT_3$ antagonist plus dexamethasone as above allows outpatient treatment in patients of good performance status but admission for treatment should be considered in frail patients. If necessary, the untreated hemibody can be treated 4–6 weeks later, allowing bone marrow recovery. An alternative is the use of bone-seeking radioactive isotopes, e.g. ^{89}Strontium and ^{153}Samarium which are concentrated in the affected bone and deliver a local dose of radiotherapy. There is little acute toxicity and any bone marrow suppression is usually asymptomatic.

Bisphosphonates

Bisphosphonates have a role in prophylaxis against bone pain, fractures and hypercalcaemia in patients with myeloma and bony metastases from breast cancer. Bisphosphonates can also be used to treat patients with malignant bone pain in myeloma, breast, lung and prostate cancer and are usually delivered as an i.v. infusion every 4 weeks. The response rate in common solid tumours is 40% but up to 80% in myeloma. Oral preparations are being developed which may improve the convenience of treatment.

Radiotherapy is cheaper than bisphosphonates and has a higher response rate for bone pain in common solid tumours but the side effects are greater. Except in myeloma, bisphosphonates are usually reserved for when radiotherapy has failed.

OUTCOME

For bony metastases not complicated by nerve compression, fracture or hypercalcaemia, the outlook is relatively good and many patients will be able to reduce their analgesic requirement and/or improve their mobility. For most common solid tumours, the prognosis is better for patients with metastases in the bones alone than for patients with visceral metastases.

Follow-up

Patients with bony metastases often have several sites of pain and more will usually reveal themselves with time. Close follow-up is therefore required in the community to ensure adequate analgesia and appropriate and prompt referral back to specialist services. Social services, occupational and physiotherapy services may also be needed to allow patients with reduced mobility to return safely and comfortably to their own homes.

Pathological fracture

Pathological fractures are usually associated with lytic bone metastases, particularly in weight bearing bones. The early diagnosis and treatment of impending pathological fractures may prevent unnecessary pain and loss of function.

Impending pathological fracture

DIAGNOSIS AND EARLY SUSPICION

Myeloma, metastatic breast, lung and renal cell cancer are commonly associated with pathological fracture. However, any primary cancer may give rise to a metastatic fracture and all patients with metastases in long bones are at risk. Pain on limb movement (functional pain) especially on bearing weight, raises the possibility of a lesion at high risk of fracture. The diagnosis is usually made on plain X-ray.

MANAGEMENT

Prophylactic fixation of an impending fracture can be carried out with good results in all but the most unfit patient and an orthopaedic team should be consulted in all cases.

There is a well established scoring system to estimate the probability of a given metastatic lesion fracturing [8] (Table 11.1). A score of eight or more indicates a high risk of fracture and such lesions should be considered for surgical treatment.

Those with an impending pathological fracture should take as little weight through the affected region as possible until definitive treatment. Admission may be necessary to achieve this. All patients will require adequate analgesia.

OUTCOME

Functional outcome is usually excellent after surgical treatment of an impending pathological fracture but may be less so if fracture has already occurred.

Table 11.1 Mirels' score for impending pathological fracture.

	Score		
Variable	1	2	3
Site	Upper limb	Lower limb	Peritrochanteric
Pain	Mild	Moderate	Functional
Lesion	Blastic	Mixed	Lytic
Size	<1/3	1/3–2/3	>2/3

Established fracture

DIAGNOSIS

The sudden loss of function or mobility or a sudden increase in pain raises the possibility of a pathological fracture. Spinal cord compression should also be considered and urgent specialist referral for admission is indicated.

MANAGEMENT

Established pathological fracture in weight-bearing long bones are treated surgically in all but the most frail patient. Those of the upper limb may be fixed surgically but in unfit patients, immobilisation, often with radiotherapy, provides pain relief.

Radiotherapy

Following surgical treatment of either an impending or an established fracture, radiotherapy is usually given to prevent local progression. A 5-day course of radiotherapy would typically be given approximately four weeks after the surgery to allow for healing of the soft tissues. A pathological fracture, which is not to be treated surgically, or a painful lesion, which is not at high risk of fracture, is usually managed with radiotherapy alone.

Rehabilitation and discharge planning

As for spinal cord compression, discharge planning may require the coordinated action of several teams.

Brain metastases

Metastases to the brain are a common problem in oncology, affecting 17–25% of the cancer population. They are common in carcinomas of the lung (26% of patients), breast (16%) and kidney (13%), in colorectal carcinomas (5%) and in melanoma (4%). In the majority of patients, the diagnosis carries a poor prognosis.

Diagnosis and early suspicion

Brain metastases frequently masquerade as a stroke or less commonly as seizures in patients not previously known to have a diagnosis of cancer and the correct diagnosis is made on CT scanning. Brain metastases should be considered in all those known to have cancer presenting with any of the symptoms or signs listed in Table 11.2.

Management

In many patients, the presence of cerebral metastases is a component of widely disseminated disease with a poor performance status and prognosis. The focus of management for this group is general symptomatic care and consideration of psychosocial needs. For a selected group of patients with a better prognosis, active treatment may be appropriate.

GENERAL SYMPTOMATIC MEASURES

Cerebral oedema and raised intracranial pressure is treated acutely with steroids giving dexamethasone 8 mg immediately followed by

Table 11.2 Frequencies of symptoms and signs associated with brain metastases.

Symptom	Frequency (%)	Sign	Frequency (%)
Headache	53	Cognitive impairment	7
Focal weakness	40	Hemiparesis	66
Confusion	30	Sensory loss	27
Unsteadiness	20	Papilloedema	26
Seizures	15	Ataxia	24
Visual disturbance	12	Aphasia	19
Speech abnormality	10		

16 mg daily in divided doses. The first dose should be given parenterally if there is any chance that absorption will be poor. Occasionally steroids can induce distressing side effects (e.g. agitation). Intravenous mannitol may rarely be needed to reduce the intracranial pressure in a patient whose condition is worsening rapidly.

Seizures are often controlled once the intracranial pressure is reduced but some patients require anticonvulsant drugs. The terminally ill patient with cerebral metastases and uncontrolled fitting may require rectal or infusional benzodiazepines (see Chapter 21). The nausea and vomiting of raised intracranial pressure respond best to measures which reduce pressure, but antiemetics (e.g. cyclizine 50 mg t.d.s.) may be required and may need to be given parenterally at first.

Headache is very common and may be helped by steroids and analgesics. An NSAID and/or codeine phosphate given regularly is often helpful but stronger analgesia may be required. Confused, agitated or psychotic patients may require sedative medications.

SPECIFIC TREATMENT OPTIONS

Surgery

Surgery may be carried out where there is no known primary cancer and the differential diagnosis lies between a primary brain tumour and a solitary metastasis. There is also a role for surgery followed by radiotherapy to the whole brain in patients with a solitary brain metastasis and a good performance status. In such cases, combined treatment reduces the frequency of local recurrence and extends symptom-free and overall survival compared to radiotherapy alone [9]. Surgery may also be indicated to relieve obstructive hydrocephalus caused by posterior fossa metastases or if symptoms persist from a metastasis which has proved resistant to other treatment. The multidisciplinary team is vital in the management of brain metastases.

Radiotherapy

Radiotherapy to the whole brain has been a common treatment and is usually given over 2–5 days. Steroids are continued throughout the treatment but are tailed off once it is complete, at a rate determined by symptoms. It is often not possible to stop steroids completely. Good response rates have often been quoted but studies using patient rated scales suggest that symptomatic benefit is the exception and benefit is often outweighed by side effects [10, 11]. For the patient with a poor performance status and poor prognosis, treatment with steroids and general supportive measures may be the best option.

Side-effects are frequent following whole brain radiotherapy and include: temporary alopecia; headache which often responds to simple analgesia or an increase in steroid dose; nausea, requiring antiemetics and often an increase in steroid dose.

Precisely targeted stereotactic radiotherapy may be an alternative to resection for up to three brain metastases not amenable to surgery [12]. It may be given as the sole initial treatment or combined with whole brain radiotherapy. It may also be used for retreatment at relapse following prior radiotherapy to the whole brain [13].

Chemotherapy

Chemotherapy is useful for some tumours which are chemosensitive, such as small-cell lung cancer and germ cell tumours and may also be useful in patients with breast cancer. Chemotherapy is usually followed by radiotherapy.

Rehabilitation and discharge planning

Many patients with brain metastases have a dramatic change in their functional ability, independence and personality. Many of their rehabilitation needs are similar to those outlined for patients with MSCC. In addition, some patients need speech therapy and/or nasogastric or gastrostomy feeding. There is a need for psychological support for both patient and carers.

Outcomes

SYMPTOMS AND QUALITY OF LIFE

One month following whole brain radiotherapy, 20% of patients report an improvement or resolution of their neurological symptoms and a similar number are stable. The rest will have progressive symptoms or have died [10]. The majority of patients are likely to have a worse quality of life one month after radiotherapy than before treatment. Disease progression and the side effects of radiotherapy are likely to contribute to this.

SURVIVAL

The survival of patients with cerebral metastases is usually short. Performance status is the strongest predictor of survival although patients with lung cancer have a particularly poor prognosis with a median survival of around 2 months. Box 11.2 summarises the factors influencing survival.

Box 11.2 Factors affecting survival in patients with brain metastases

Factors that improve survival

- Brain as first site of relapse of disease
- Long disease-free interval prior to relapse
- Primary site breast

Factors that reduce survival

- Poor performance status
- Meningeal disease

PLACE OF CARE

Many patients will be unable to be cared for at home because of loss of independence in activities of daily living, nursing care needs and cognitive impairment. Changes in cognitive function in particular make care at home problematic and distressing to relatives.

Follow-up

Relapse of brain metastases is common and close follow-up in the community is essential. Occasionally, further radiotherapy may be useful although there is a risk of necrosis of the treated area.

Surgical management of other metastatic disease

Liver metastases

Liver metastases are common in colorectal cancer affecting 15–25% of patients at presentation and a further 20% at a later stage in their disease. Radical treatment of liver metastases has been shown to result in long term survival and, in some cases, cure [14].

SURGERY

The resectability of liver metastases largely depends on the tumour bulk, the number of metastases and their location within the liver but each case should be considered individually. Patients must have good liver function and be fit enough to undergo major surgery and the success rate is improved if a clear resection margin can be achieved. In selected groups with optimally resectable metastases, 5-year survival rates of 35–40% are reported.

LOCAL ABLATION

Liver metastases may be unresectable because of their number or location. Local ablative techniques such as radiofrequency ablation and cryotherapy may be directed at individual metastases to destroy tumour tissue. As an adjunct to surgery or chemotherapy these techniques may increase survival.

Lung metastases

Lung metastases are common, affecting 25–30% of patients dying of cancer. Rarely, resection will result in long term survival or cure in selected patients [15]. Cures are seen in metastatic teratoma when multiple lung metastases are resected following chemotherapy. Curative resections may also be carried out in patients with colorectal cancer and a solitary pulmonary metastasis.

Bone metastases

Renal cell carcinoma may recur as a solitary bone metastasis. Surgical excision and reconstruction may be curative and early specialist referral is mandatory.

Metabolic emergencies

Hypercalcaemia

Hypercalcaemia is the commonest metabolic emergency associated with cancer and is usually, but not always, associated with widespread bone involvement (80%). The outlook is poor, but prompt active treatment may relieve symptoms rapidly with minimal toxicity. Specific therapy should be offered in all but the very frail, terminally ill patient in whom hypercalcaemia is a terminal event and who may be helped more by simple symptomatic measures.

Hypercalcaemia is common in breast cancer and myeloma, affecting up to 50% of patients with these diseases. It is also common in carcinoma of the kidney, cervix and head and neck and in non-small cell carcinoma of the lung.

PATHOPHYSIOLOGY

Tumour-induced hypercalcaemia results from the action of various factors released by the immune system or from the tumour. The most common is parathyroid hormone-related protein (PTH–RP), which increases the release of calcium from bone and its renal tubular reabsorption. Others include prostaglandins and cytokines.

Hypercalcaemia induces vomiting and an osmotic diuresis leading to polyuria, dehydration, hypovolaemia and compromised renal function, further escalating calcium levels. The action of a raised serum calcium concentration on smooth muscle and the CNS leads to the characteristic symptoms of constipation, confusion and nausea.

DIAGNOSIS AND EARLY SUSPICION

The diagnosis should be considered in any patient with advanced cancer who becomes unwell. Bony metastases are usually, but not always, associated. Onset is often gradual and the symptoms are non-specific, often mimicking the general debility of a patient with advanced cancer (see Box 11.3)

Box 11.3 Clinical features of hypercalcaemia

General

- Thirst
- Polyuria
- Polydipsia
- Dehydration
- Weight loss
- Anorexia
- Lethargy
- Fatigue

Continued on p. 226

Box 11.3 ***Continued***

Neurological
- Confusion
- Psychosis
- Coma

Gastrointestinal
- Nausea/vomiting
- Constipation
- Peptic ulceration
- Pruritus

Cardiac
- Bradycardia
- Arrhythmias

Investigations

Serum calcium, corrected for the serum albumin should be checked along with renal function. Uncontrolled diabetes should be excluded as the clinical features are similar.

MANAGEMENT

For patients at home with mild symptoms suggestive of hypercalcaemia, the results of blood tests should be established within 48 hours.

A patient with cancer who becomes unwell with suspected hypercalcaemia should be admitted urgently under the oncology or medical team for investigation and treatment. Many hospices will have facilities for treatment of patients who have more advanced disease and recurrent hypercalcaemia. The admission should be discussed with palliative care and oncology teams and with the patient to ensure the most appropriate place of treatment.

Immediate treatment

Rehydration is the first requirement. Oral fluids are encouraged and intravenous normal saline is infused at a rate determined by the clinical condition. Drugs that inhibit urinary calcium excretion or decrease renal blood flow are stopped (e.g. thiazide diuretics, NSAIDs). High-dose steroids are no longer recommended.

Symptom control

Rehydration alone may be sufficient to relieve many of the symptoms. Analgesia may be required for the pain of bony metastases or abdominal symptoms. Constipation and nausea are often severe and should be treated vigorously (see Chapter 9).

Specific treatment of hypercalcaemia

Intravenous bisphosphonates are the mainstay of the treatment of malignant hypercalcaemia and several drugs are available in this class. They differ in their potency, the more potent formulations having a shorter duration of infusion which may be more convenient in the outpatient setting [16]. Bisphosphonates are given after rehydration, reducing the risk of inducing a deterioration in renal function. The serum calcium concentration begins to fall rapidly reaching a nadir after 7–10 days. Symptomatic improvement is often rapid.

Maintenance bisphosphonate therapy either as intermittent intravenous infusions (usually 4 weekly) or oral formulations have been shown to reduce the incidence of subsequent skeletal events, including symptomatic bone metastases and episodes of hypercalcaemia.

Specific treatment of the underlying cancer

Unless treatment is directed at the underlying problem, hypercalcaemia will recur. In patients for whom there is a therapeutic option, specific anticancer treatment such as chemotherapy or hormonal therapy should be started as soon as the clinical condition allows. Rarely, the initiation of tamoxifen therapy may induce hypercalcaemia in patients with bony metastases from breast cancer.

OUTCOME

With the exception of myeloma the prognosis for most patients with cancer-induced hypercalcaemia is poor. If an anticancer treatment is available, the median survival is 3 months, otherwise it is only 1 month. Similarly, if the patient becomes normocalcaemic with the administration of bisphosphonates the median survival is 7–8 weeks but if not, it is less than 3 weeks [17].

FOLLOW-UP

Close follow-up at home is vital as hypercalcaemia commonly recurs. Recurrent hypercalcaemia may be a pre-terminal event and the appropriateness of admission to a hospice or hospital oncology unit should always be fully considered.

Obstructive nephropathy

Pelvic malignancies predispose to the development of ureteric obstruction. If left untreated, progressive disease will lead to acute or chronic renal failure, which will ultimately prove fatal. Relief of the ureteric obstruction is a relatively simple procedure with good resolution of symptoms in most patients. However, if renal failure is relieved in the absence of a therapeutic option for the cancer itself, the original disease process will continue to progress, causing suffering and ultimately leading to death. This gives rise to a dilemma commonly encountered in palliative care: *is relief of the obstruction, and therefore prolongation of life, in the patient's best interests?* Discussion with the patient and their informed consent are crucial, but this is often very difficult if this issue is only raised when the need for treatment has become urgent.

Of patients presenting with acute renal failure secondary to bilateral ureteric obstruction, two-thirds have underlying malignant disease. For half of these it will be their first manifestation of disease. This is particularly common in cancers of the cervix, bladder and prostate.

DIAGNOSIS AND EARLY SUSPICION

Obstruction of a single kidney is often not noticed unless imaging of the abdomen takes place. Once the second kidney becomes involved, the clinical features of obstructive nephropathy become evident (see Box 11.4). As with hypercalcaemia, the features are non-specific unless anuria occurs and may mimic the general debility of a patient with advanced cancer.

Box 11.4 Clinical features of obstructive nephropathy

- Anorexia
- Anuria/oliguria

Continued

Box 11.4 ***Continued***

- Bleeding tendency
- Cardiac arrhythmias
- Confusion
- Drug toxicity
- Hypertension
- Myoclonic jerks
- Nausea
- Oedema
- Susceptibility to infection
- Vomiting

Investigations

Both blood urea and creatinine and often potassium are raised. Ultrasound and/or CT scan of the renal tracts and pelvis will usually be able to confirm obstruction to renal outflow with dilation of thc renal pelvis and may be able to demonstrate the cause of the obstruction.

MANAGEMENT

If appropriate, the obstruction needs to be relieved promptly before irreversible damage is caused to the kidneys. This is commonly carried out by nephrostomy or ureteric stenting [18]. Acute management of the associated hyperkalaemia, metabolic acidosis, and fluid overload may be necessary if the deterioration in renal function has been rapid. Bilateral ureteric obstruction in carcinoma of the prostate has been successfully relieved with the administration of high dose dexamethasone, 16 mg daily as an initial dose, tapering rapidly once definitive treatment is underway [19].

Symptomatic measures

Hydration should aim to replace losses and prevent thirst while avoiding fluid overload and the distressing features of pulmonary oedema. All drugs should be used with caution in renal failure (see British National Formulary, Appendix 3). Haloperidol 1.5–5 mg o.d.-t.d.s. orally or 5–20 mg/24 h by subcutaneous infusion will help control nausea, myoclonic jerks, confusion and agitation.

Pain from hydronephrosis may require strong opioids. Many opioids accumulate in renal failure and should be used with longer dosing intervals and daily review. Fentanyl has little renal excretion and accumulates less in renal failure than morphine (see also Chapter 18).

Haemorrhage

There are several reasons why a patient with cancer may haemorrhage including:

- bleeding directly from tumour or metastases;
- invasion of tumour into blood vessels;
- bleeding tendency due to thrombocytopenia, DIC, uraemia or anticoagulants;
- bleeding from post-radiotherapy telangiectasia (especially bladder and GI tract).

The management of massive, terminal haemorrhage is discussed in Chapter 21.

Radiotherapy

Palliative radiotherapy to control bleeding is usually restricted to a short course of treatment with few planning stages. A typical course lasts 1–3 weeks. Radiotherapy is useful for bleeding skin metastases but locally recurrent breast cancer usually occurs in skin which has already received radiotherapy to tolerance doses. Advice should be sought from the treating radiotherapist.

Haemoptysis responds well to radiotherapy (see Chapter 10).

Previous radical radiotherapy to the pelvis usually rules out further treatment to a bleeding central pelvic lesion but this is not always so and the advice of a radiotherapist should be sought in individual cases.

Vascular embolisation

Occasionally, bleeding from a vascular tumour can be reduced by embolisation of its blood supply. Advice should be sought from an interventional radiologist on the suitability of the lesion and the need for further investigation.

SYMPTOMATIC MEASURES

Drugs which decrease the tendency to bleed may be helpful, e.g. tranexamic acid 500 mg q.d.s. or ethamsylate 500 mg q.d.s. Mucosal bleeding may be reduced by using 1% alum as a bladder irrigation or enema. Tranexamic acid enema (5 g in 50 ml water twice daily or 1–2 g mixed with KY jelly) may reduce bleeding from rectal tumours. The application of adrenaline-soaked swabs (1:1000), alginate dressings, and sucralfate paste (in KY jelly) may reduce capillary bleeding [20]. Oral or rectal sucralfate (1 g b.d.-q.d.s.) may stop bleeding from oesophageal, gastric, or rectal tumours, respectively.

Itch

Itching is a sensation that produces a desire to scratch and is a problem for many patients with cancer. It can cause profound debility as it prevents sleep and leads to painful excoriation of skin. It is associated with various conditions.

- Blood disorders: lymphoma (itch may be the presenting feature of Hodgkin's disease); leukaemia; polycythaemia rubra vera
- Iron deficiency
- Cholestatic jaundice (see Chapter 9)
- Uraemia
- Allergens causing eczema and contact dermatitis
- Drugs: opioids (histamine release); chlorpromazine (cholestasis)
- Skin infections and infestations: scabies; fungal infection
- Advanced cancer

Pathophysiology

Irritant substances in the skin stimulate receptors of unmyelinated nerve fibres (C fibres). The chemical irritant may be histamine, tissue proteases, prostaglandins or bile acids.

Management

If possible the underlying cause should be addressed. There are no specific antipruritic drugs.

GENERAL MEASURES

Avoiding the following may be helpful: friction from rough clothing and bed linen; overheating; vasodilators and soap that dries the skin. Scratching exacerbates the itchiness.

Cooling and moistening the skin with moisturizers and emollients is helpful, e.g. menthol 0.25–1% in aqueous cream. Cucumber is soothing but may be impractical if the itch is generalized. Calamine lotion may over-dry the skin.

Oral antihistamine in the form of a sedative preparation may be useful at night (e.g. chlorphenamine 4 mg). A less sedative preparation may be tried in the day (e.g. loratidine 10 mg) but may not prove as effective.

A trial of oral corticosteroids may be of value in some patients, particularly those with lymphoma or bile duct obstruction due to tumour or lymph nodes. NSAIDS are helpful in some patients, presumably where prostaglandins play a role in the pathophysiology. They are particularly helpful for the itch of cutaneous tumour infiltration. A hypnotic may be helpful. Acupuncture may also be helpful in treating itch.

OTHER MEASURES

Various treatments can reduce itch in certain conditions. For instance, cimetidine may be helpful in Hodgkin's disease, whereas erythropoietin is helpful for the itch of chronic uraemia.

$5HT_3$ antagonists such as ondansetron and granisetron have been found to be effective for itch associated with cholestatic jaundice of advanced cancer and of non-malignant origin. Both tricyclic and selective serotonin re-uptake inhibitor antidepressants have been found to have some effect. Other treatments with potential in resistant and very problematic instances require discussion with a specialist. These include disodium cromglycate, thalidomide, parenteral lidocaine, naloxone and propofol.

Fever and sweating

Patients with cancer may experience troublesome fever and sweating. The two are related but sweating may occur without fever. These symptoms are generally distressing to patients and can result in fatigue, drowsiness and confusion. The aetiology can be related directly to the tumour (neoplastic fever) or secondary to co-morbidity (e.g. infective process). Both fever and sweating are more common in patients with Hodgkin's disease, leukaemia and tumours with liver metastases.

Management

Although it is inappropriate within a palliative care setting to exhaustively investigate patients with fever and sweats, it is important to consider the differential diagnoses which may aid appropriate treatment.

- Infection. Look for common foci of infection (e.g. chest, urine, upper respiratory tract, pressure sores, tumour site). Be especially cautious in patients who are susceptible to neutropenia (e.g. chemotherapy, marrow invasion). Fever may not occur if patients are on steroids or have a markedly suppressed white cell count.
- Neoplastic fever.
- Treatment related e.g. some chemotherapy drugs produce fever (e.g. bleomycin), as can blood transfusion.
- Hormonal (e.g. thyrotoxicosis and menopause).
- Anxiety.
- Physiological (secondary to environmental conditions).

In many cases it is necessary to resort to general measures to provide relief. Paramount among these is a high standard of nursing care, including: the provision of a fan, sponging and regular washing and encouraging the intake of oral fluids. The effectiveness of paracetamol may be reduced in neoplastic fever. Other options include aspirin, NSAIDs [21] and thioridazine. High-dose steroids have a role in chronic lymphatic leukaemia.

Side-effects of palliative oncology treatments

Severe side-effects of chemotherapy and radiotherapy weigh heavily in the cost-benefit analysis of palliative interventions. It is important for the patient, the health care teams, and the carers to know what effects are likely, how long they may last and what can be done to alleviate them. Late side-effects of palliative treatments are rarely a concern.

Gastrointestinal system

PROBLEMS OF THE MOUTH, OROPHARYNX AND OESOPHAGUS

Oral mucositis is most common with radiotherapy to head and neck tumours, whereas oesophageal mucositis is seen with radiotherapy to the mediastinum or neck. Reactions begin 1–2 weeks after the start of treatment and continue for the same period after completion [22].

Chemotherapy often temporarily affects taste and may give a mild to moderate mucositis, which may be accompanied by mouth ulcers.

Management

Patients having radiotherapy which includes the mouth and particularly the salivary glands may develop a marked mucositis with lack of normal saliva [23].

The following measures may help:

- avoiding exacerbating agents e.g. smoking, spicy foods and alcohol;
- basic oral hygiene: cleaning the teeth with a soft brush and fluoride toothpaste after each meal and before retiring to bed, rinsing well with 0.9% saline after brushing;
- hourly saline mouthwashes for moisture as the mouth becomes more sore;
- anti-inflammatory mouthwashes eg. benzydamine diluted 1:1 with water.

Commercial mouthwashes containing alcohol cause mucosal irritation and are not recommended. Chlorhexidine mouthwash is useful as an antiseptic but may irritate the mucosa. Moisturising creams should be used for dry lips.

Patients with painful mucositis having chemotherapy may find relief in the use of chlorhexidine, dilute benzydamine or oraldene mouthwashes in addition to scrupulous oral hygiene.

Severe pain on swallowing affects nutrition and a full nutritional assessment is vital prior to treatment, with careful follow-up during radiotherapy. As swallowing becomes more difficult, softer foods are introduced along with supplement drinks. If swallowing is impossible, artificial feeding may be necessary e.g. via a temporary percutaneous gastrostomy.

Analgesia must receive careful attention and patients often require opioids orally. It is worthy of note that many liquid oral opioid preparations contain alcohol, which will cause pain on contact with ulcerated mucosa. Topical medication consists of: dilute benzydamine mouthwash 1–3 hourly; mucaine 10 ml before meals, particularly for oesophagitis; sucralfate suspension 1 g before meals (coats raw mucosa of mouth and oesophagus) or mucilage swilled and swallowed 10 minutes before meals for lubrication. Consider the use of an antifungal, for example nystatin suspension 1 ml q.d.s. or fluconazole 50 mg o.d. Also consider oral acyclovir if the ulcers are very painful as herpes simplex sometimes becomes activated in these cases.

NAUSEA AND VOMITING

Nausea and vomiting are worsened by anxiety about cancer, the treatment and its side-effects, so psychological support is vital throughout treatment (see also Chapter 9).

Highly emetogenic chemotherapy

Nausea and vomiting usually occur in the first 24–72 hours post chemotherapy. They can be managed by administering a $5HT_3$ antagonist plus dexamethasone intravenously pre-chemotherapy, followed by metoclopramide 10 mg p.o. q.d.s. (domperidone if extrapyramidal side-effects) plus dexamethasone 2 mg p.o. t.d.s. for 3 days afterwards.

Less emetogenic chemotherapy

Where chemotherapy is less emetogenic, oral antiemetics usually suffice e.g. cyclizine 50 mg t.d.s. or metoclopramide 10 mg t.d.s. Rarely, $5HT_3$ antagonists are required.

Radiotherapy

Nausea and vomiting can follow radiotherapy, especially if the stomach or liver is in the treatment field. The symptoms usually occur acutely after each treatment and remit once treatment is complete. Oral antiemetics usually suffice, e.g. cyclizine 50 mg t.d.s. or haloperidol 1.5 mg b.d. Vomiting may be a side-effect of radiotherapy to the brain, in which case it will usually respond to an increase in the dose of oral steroids with the addition of cyclizine.

PROBLEMS OF THE LOWER BOWEL

Diarrhoea

Diarrhoea is common with pelvic or abdominal radiotherapy. It often begins in the second week of radiotherapy and lasts 1–2 weeks after completion.

Management includes:

- Dietary assessment
- Loperamide titrated to effect

- Codeine phosphate 30–60 mg 6 or 12 hourly (if the patient is not already receiving a strong opioid)
- Oral rehydration
- Barrier creams to perianal skin

Proctitis

Proctitis is common with pelvic radiotherapy. The timing of its occurrence is the same as for diarrhoea (see above). Rectal bleeding may occur. Management involves the use of steroid foam enemas and appropriate analgesia. Warm baths may help to alleviate symptoms.

Rectal bleeding occurring more than 6 months after radiotherapy is unusual but may require surgery, although this is hazardous as tissue healing is poor.

Skin

Skin reactions are common with high-dose radiotherapy [24]. Reactions occur 1–2 weeks after the start of radiotherapy and take approximately the same time to heal. Table 11.3 details the types of skin reactions.

Table 11.3 Skin reactions to radiotherpy.

Category of skin reaction	Detail of signs and symptoms
Erythema	The area in the radiotherapy field becomes slightly inflamed and may tingle, usually occurring after 1–2 weeks of treatment
Dry desquamation	The skin becomes hot, flaky, very itchy and uncomfortable usually occurring after 2–3 weeks
Moist desquamation	Blisters form on the epidermis which sloughs leaving a denuded, painful area of dermis which may exude serum. Moist regions with opposed skin surfaces, such as the perineum or inframammary fold, are particularly affected

The skin is less commonly affected by chemotherapy although rashes are common. Discoloration, erythema and peeling of the palms and soles are sometimes seen.

Several steps can be taken to improve the comfort of the skin and prevent further damage.

- Protect from friction, by avoiding tight clothing, elastic straps underwired bras, etc.

- Avoid strong sunlight, hot baths, wet shaving, cosmetics, deodorants, adhesive plasters and perfumed creams.
- Wash with warm water and usual soap. Pat dry with a soft towel and air-dry if possible.
- For erythema, apply moisturising cream e.g. aqueous cream twice daily.
- For dry desquamation increase frequency of moisturising cream to 4–5 times daily.
- For worsening irritation from dry desquamation, use hydrocortisone cream 1% avoiding the genital area.
- Intrasite® gel is soothing for dry desquamation and with a non-adherent dressing, lifts debris from the skin.
- For very itchy dry desquamation, a glycerine-based hydrogel sheet e.g. Novogel® is very cooling.

Moist desquamation heals best in a warm, moist environment. Dressings should be conformable, comfortable, non-adherent, must not contain metals or cause further skin damage. Intrasite gel® absorbs exudate and helps lift debris and can be used with mepilex® dressing, which is a low adherence silicone dressing.

Hair loss

Temporary hair loss is a variable feature of many chemotherapy regimes and radiotherapy will also cause temporary alopecia if the scalp is irradiated. The psychological impact should not be underestimated and wigs and camouflage should be discussed pre-treatment.

Marrow suppression

Patients with advanced cancer may have reduced bone marrow reserve and symptomatic anaemia is common. Thrombocytopenia is less common without current chemotherapy although it may occur in the presence of marrow infiltration by tumour. The platelet count may be especially low if there has been prior chemotherapy, wide field radiotherapy or bone seeking isotopes, particularly in prostate cancer. Anaemia and thrombocytopenia may require transfusion.

Clinically significant neutropenia is uncommon without current cytotoxic chemotherapy treatment. It predisposes to overwhelming bacterial sepsis, particularly when the absolute neutrophil count is less than $1 \times 10^9/l$. Neutropenic sepsis requires urgent specialist inpatient treatment with intravenous antibiotics. Urgent admission to the treating oncology unit should be arranged for assessment of any patient on chemotherapy who develops symptoms or signs of sepsis, particularly: sore throat, fever >38°C, rigors, cough productive of purulent sputum or shock.

References

1 Levack P, Graham J, Collie D, et al. Don't wait for a sensory level—listen to the symptoms: a prospective audit of the delays in diagnosis of malignant cord compression. *Clin Oncol* 2002; 14(6): 472–480.
2 Klein SL, Sanford RA, Muhlbauer MS. Pediatric spinal epidural metastases. *J Neurosurg* 1991; 74(1): 70–75.
3 Rades D, Heidenreich F, Karstens JH. Final results of a prospective study of the prognostic value of the time to develop motor deficits before irradiation in metastatic spinal cord compression. *Int J Radiat Oncol Biol Phys* 2002; 53(4): 975–979.
4 Patchell R, Tibbs PA, Regine WF. A randomized trial of direct decompressive surgical resection in the treatment of spinal cord compression caused by metastasis. *Am Soc Clin Oncol*; 2003: 1.
5 Loblaw DA, Laperriere NJ. Emergency treatment of malignant extradural spinal cord compression: an evidence-based guideline. *J Clin Oncol* 1998; 16(4): 1613–1624.
6 Board of the Faculty of Clinical Oncology. *A National Audit of Waiting Times for Radiotherapy*. London: Royal College of Radiologists; 1998. Report No.: BFCO(98)3.
7 Rowell NP, Gleeson FV. Steroids, radiotherapy, chemotherapy and stents for superior vena caval obstruction in carcinoma of the bronchus: a systematic review. *Clin Oncol* 2002; 14(5): 338–351.
8 Mirels H. Metastatic disease in long bones. A proposed scoring system for diagnosing impending pathologic fractures. *Clin Orthop* 1989(249): 256–264.
9 Patchell RA, Tibbs PA, Walsh JW, et al. A randomized trial of surgery in the treatment of single metastases to the brain. *N Engl J Med* 1990; 322(8): 494–500.
10 Bezjak A, Adam J, Barton R, et al. Symptom response after palliative radiotherapy for patients with brain metastases. *Eur J Cancer* 2002; 38(4): 487–496.
11 Gerrard GE, Prestwich RJ, Edwards A, et al. Investigating the palliative efficacy of whole-brain radiotherapy for patients with multiple-brain metastases and poor prognostic features. *Clin Oncol* 2003; 15(7): 422–428.
12 Sneed PK, Suh JH, Goetsch SJ, et al. A multi-institutional review of radiosurgery alone vs. radiosurgery with whole brain radiotherapy as the initial management of brain metastases. *Int J Radiat Oncol Biol Phys* 2002; 53(3): 519–526.
13 Davey P, PF OB, Schwartz ML, Cooper PW. A phase I/II study of salvage radiosurgery in the treatment of recurrent brain metastases. *Br J Neurosurg* 1994; 8(6): 717–723.
14 Ruers T, Bleichrodt RP. Treatment of liver metastases, an update on the possibilities and results. *Eur J Cancer* 2002; 38(7): 1023–1033.

15 Davidson RS, Nwogu CE, Brentjens MJ, Anderson TM. The surgical management of pulmonary metastasis: current concepts. *Surg Oncol* 2001; 10(1–2): 35–42.
16 Major P, Lortholary A, Hon J, et al. Zoledronic acid is superior to pamidronate in the treatment of hypercalcemia of malignancy: a pooled analysis of two randomized, controlled clinical trials. *J Clin Oncol* 2001; 19(2): 558–567.
17 Ling PJ, RP AH, Hardy JR. Analysis of survival following treatment of tumour-induced hypercalcaemia with intravenous pamidronate (APD). *Br J Cancer* 1995; 72(1): 206–209.
18 Watkinson AF, A'Hern RP, Jones A, King DM, Moskovic EC. The role of percutaneous nephrostomy in malignant urinary tract obstruction. *Clin Radiol* 1993; 47(1): 32–35.
19 Hamdy FC, Williams JL. Use of dexamethasone for ureteric obstruction in advanced prostate cancer: percutaneous nephrostomies can be avoided. *Br J Urol* 1995; 75(6): 782–785.
20 Regnard CF. Control of bleeding in advanced cancer. *Lancet* 1991; 337 (8747): 974.
21 Tsavaris N, Zinelis A, Karabelis A, Beldecos D, Bacojanis C, Milonacis N, et al. A randomized trial of the effect of three non-steroid anti-inflammatory agents in ameliorating cancer-induced fever. *J Intern Med* 1990; 228(5): 451–455.
22 Feber T. Mouth Care. In: Head and Neck Oncology: Whurr Ltd.; 1999.
23 Shih A, Miaskowski C, Dodd MJ, Stotts NA, MacPhail L. A research review of the current treatments for radiation-induced oral mucositis in patients with head and neck cancer. *Oncol Nurs Forum* 2002; 29(7): 1063–1080.
24 Porock D, Nikoletti S, Kristjanson L. Management of radiation skin reactions: literature review and clinical application. *Plast Surg Nurs* 1999; 19(4): 185–192.

12: The Management of People with Advanced Head and Neck Cancers

NICKY RUDD AND JANE WORLDING

Introduction

The care of patients with advanced or relapsed head and neck cancer poses a unique challenge to the clinician. This group experiences unpleasant local symptoms: swallowing, speech and breathing difficulties and sometimes disfigurement, which can lead to added psychological distress and social isolation.

Fortunately, head and neck tumours are rare and many are curable, but their rarity may disadvantage the patient, who does not have access to support systems and the self-help groups, which are in place for patients with commoner cancers. Patients for whom heavy drinking and self-neglect have been an aetiological factor, often find themselves socially isolated prior to diagnosis, living alone in poor circumstances with little help or social contact (see case example Box 12.1). The primary health care team may lack confidence in dealing with these patients as they are unlikely to see many in their professional life. To address this some case examples have been included in the text.

Box 12.1 Case example

A 60-year-old unemployed man who drank and smoked heavily presented with a left cheek mass. He underwent extensive surgery and was referred for post-operative radiotherapy. He failed to attend on several occasions and was eventually found in the pub outside the hospital gates. He refused admission to the radiotherapy hostel for his treatment but agreed to a daily visit from the district nurses. With their help, he completed his radiotherapy.

He continued to smoke and drink and although he remained disease-free at his original site, he went on to develop a primary bronchial carcinoma from which he died two years later.

Epidemiology of head and neck cancers

Squamous head and neck cancer accounts for approximately 40 400 new cancer cases worldwide per year [1]. In developing countries cancer of the mouth and pharynx is the third commonest cancer in men and the fourth commonest in women.

The highest rates of oral cancer reported in France, the Indian subcontinent, Brazil and eastern Europe.

Head and neck cancers account for approximately 4% of all solid tumours in the UK. They occur two to three times more commonly in men than in women and there is a higher incidence in immigrants from the Indian subcontinent, who present 10–15 years earlier than the indigenous population [2].

The predominant risk factors are tobacco and alcohol use; however, family studies demonstrate a genetic component possibly related to increased sensitivity to chromosomal damage by carcinogens and reduced ability to repair damage [3]. The major determinants of survival are age, socio-economic status, nutritional factors, intercurrent disease and the continuing presence of risk factors such as smoking [4].

Other risk factors are chewing of betel nut and tobacco and poor dental hygiene. Nasopharyngeal cancer is associated with the Epstein Barr virus. In addition, patients who are cured of their initial carcinoma are at higher risk of a second primary tumour [5].

Challenges of head and neck cancer

The natural history of the disease and the management options depend on the stage at presentation and fitness of the patient [6]. Patients with early stage disease are treated with either surgery or radiotherapy or a combination of both. Some tumours are treated with combined chemotherapy and radiotherapy.

Surgical procedures are major but recent advances in techniques have reduced disfigurement. Patients may be left with residual disability, for example, partial glossectomy may cause speech impediment, while laryngectomy may entail the need for tracheal stoma care and communication aids. Radiotherapy requires careful planning, which may entail an anxious delay for patients before treatment can start. Even palliative treatment may mean daily visits for several days or weeks. Nearly all treatment requires plaster cast moulding and the wearing of a mask. Chemotherapy is increasingly used either in combination with radiation treatment or as a monotherapy for both locally advanced disease and systemic metastasis.

Locally recurrent and advanced primary head and neck tumours can be most unpleasant, causing mainly localised symptoms. These may include:

- pain;
- dysphagia;
- trismus;
- respiratory difficulties;
- dribbling;
- an unpleasant taste;
- facial oedema;
- the disconcerting constant presence of a tumour within the oral cavity;
- fistulae;
- highly visible, fungating offensive-smelling tumours;
- bleeding.

Studies of relapsed patients have shown 85% experience pain, 62% feeding problems and 43% respiratory problems [7].

Effective care of these patients demands a team approach, with different professionals intervening as the situation demands. The full team will comprise doctors, nurses, speech therapists, dieticians, dentists, physiotherapists, occupational therapists, social workers and chaplains (see also Chapter 2).

Body image counsellors and specialist nurses are invaluable in preparing for and supporting patients through their initial treatment and rehabilitation. They may visit patients in their homes, accompany them on clinic visits and make regular contact when they are in hospital. They can help advise the primary health care team and other professionals on specific aspects of care such as the care of tracheostomies. The relationship which is forged is of great benefit if the patient relapses and a good specialist nurse will remain an important psychological support to the patient and their family throughout the illness, acting as a source of professional support and advice to the primary health care team.

Oncological management of advanced disease

Palliative radiotherapy

Radiotherapy is frequently employed for symptom control if the patient has not already received a maximum dose to the area of

Table 12.1 Side effects of radiotherapy to the head and neck

Side effect	Treatment
Loss of taste	None
Xerostomia	Artificial saliva-water sprayer
	Room humidification
	Pilocarpine 5–10 mg t.d.s/q.d.s. (a,b) Bethanechol 25 mg t.d.s, increase to 50 mg t.d.s. if no improvement after 2 weeks
	Orobase gel
Mucositis/stomatitis	Good oral hygiene
	Raspberry mucilage
	NSAID mouthwashes
	Local anaesthetic gel
	Sodium chloride 4.5 g + sodium bicarbonate 9 g in 500 ml water
Furred tongue	Half tablet effervescent vitamin C dissolved on the tongue
Infection	Chlorhexidine gluconate 10mls qds Nystatin 1 ml five times daily
Odynophagia/dysphagia	Mucaine 10 ml q.d.s.
Desquamation (moist)	Keep clean and dry as possible
Desquamation (dry)	Aqueous cream if itching is a problem

Patients who continue to smoke and drink whilst having radiotherapy may potentiate its side effects and compromise the success of treatment.

recurrence. Reduction in tumour size may improve pain and secondary mechanical difficulties. It is also useful for controlling bleeding from a fungating wound and for reducing odour. A young fit patient, with a late recurrence, may be retreated radically.

The aim of palliative radiotherapy is to relieve symptoms whilst keeping side-effects to a minimum. Table 12.1 [8, 9] illustrates some of the typical and less frequently encountered side-effects and their subsequent treatment.

Chemotherapy

The role of chemotherapy as a palliative treatment in head and neck cancer is less well defined but is used when radiotherapy options have been exhausted and for symptomatic systemic metastasis. Combined modality treatment for locally advanced disease [10] and for nasopharyngeal cancer may improve local disease control and symptom relief but has not yet been shown to alter prognosis. Commonly used regimes are: (1) low dose Methotrexate 25–50 mg/m^2 given as a weekly outpatient bolus injection. The most usual side effects are tiredness, mucositis and mild myelosuppression. Mucositis can be treated as per Table 12.1. Contraindications to the use of methotrexate are pleural fluid or ascites, hepatic and renal dysfunction. (2) Cisplatin 50–100 mg/m^2 with infusional 5-Flurouracil 750–1000 mg day 1–5 given as an inpatient. Common side effects are nausea and vomiting requiring a 5HT3 antagonist; mucositis and diarrhoea. Diarrhoea can be treated with Loperamide, Buscopan and/or Codeine. Cisplatin requires good hydration throughout the treatment and reasonable glomerular filtration rate (GFR).

Dysphagia, nutrition and feeding

Patients with advanced head and neck cancer will usually have altered anatomy as a consequence of previous surgery as well as their recurrent tumour. Neurological dysfunction and the side effects of radiotherapy (e.g. mucositis or xerostomia) may further exacerbate dysphagia and interfere with the complex action of swallowing. Many patients are nutritionally disadvantaged prior to presentation as a result of high alcohol intake combined with a poor diet. Finally, malignancy itself causes cachexia via cytokines.

The consequences of malnutrition are impairment of immune function and hence increased susceptibility to infection; decreased tolerance of chemotherapy or radiotherapy; reduced skin integrity leading to pressure sores and poor wound healing; and increased morbidity and mortality. The enormous psychological distress to both patient and carers should never be underestimated. Continued weight loss, alteration of eating habits, and inability to participate in communal eating are all significant factors.

Criteria for identifying the nutritionally high-risk patient

Various criteria can be used to help identify the patient who is at high risk of malnutrition. These include:

- recent loss >12% of body weight;
- alcoholism;

- no oral intake >10 days (on i.v. fluids only);
- protracted nutrient loss-fistula, fungating wounds;
- hypercatabolic state-infection, rapidly advancing tumour, protracted fever;
- drugs with antinutrient or catabolic properties, e.g. steroids, chemotherapy;
- severe mucositis secondary to radiotherapy.

Nutritional support

Nutritional support should be provided in consultation with a dietician and considered *before* the at-risk patient starts to lose a large amount of weight. High-calorie and high-protein drinks, liquidised food and eating and drinking little and often are helpful steps in maintaining an adequate daily intake. Helping to reduce family stress around meal times is also important (see also Chapter 9).

More invasive support is appropriate in some patients but requires very careful consideration and fully informed consent (see case example Box 12.2). Many professionals will consider nasogastric or percutaneous endoscopic gastrostomy (PEG) feeding unnecessarily invasive. However, the patient may find contemplation of 'starving to death' worse than that of a protracted illness with worsening local symptoms. It is debatable whether supplementary feeding does prolong life. However, it does seem to improve quality of life, particularly

Box 12.2 Case example

A frail 87-year-old smoker attended the GP's surgery with her daughter. She had presented initially three years ago with a squamous carcinoma of the floor of mouth and was treated with surgery and radiotherapy. A further recurrence was excised eighteen months later, after which she experienced some difficulty eating solids. She now has a further inoperable squamous cancer extending the length of her upper lip within the previous radiation field.

Her family is worried as she is reluctant to take much in the way of nutrition, and declined further outpatient follow-up. When seen by her GP, she said that she did not think that any further procedures, antibiotics or artificial feeding was in her best interest. Her GP agreed with her and reassured her that good mouth care and the use of ice cubes could give relief if she felt thirsty. Her family accepted her decision. She died of pneumonia six weeks later, still managing small amounts of water.

if the procedure is carried out as dysphagia is developing. The timing of enteral feeding can be arranged to suit the patient's needs; it is usually done for 12–16 hours but can be interrupted. Overnight feeding is usually preferred but bottles may need to be changed during this period. Equipment is arranged via the community or hospital dietetic service. Biochemical monitoring of electrolytes, calcium and magnesium is desirable whilst feeding is on-going.

Parenteral nutrition is seldom appropriate or necessary if the gut is functional and can be accessed [11].

Airway patency and tracheostomies

A tracheostomy may be necessary to maintain airway patency and allow expectoration of secretions. The indications for tracheostomy include: bilateral vocal cord paralysis, laryngectomy and a tumour occluding the airway.

A tracheostomy tube used in the palliative setting is usually a plastic single-lumen uncuffed tube suitable for long-term use. These tubes are lightweight and soften at body temperature, which reduces tracheal abrasion. They have an inner cannula, which can be removed for cleaning or to allow suctioning and can be periodically replaced. The outer housing and neck plate should not be replaced unless blocked, as resiting in the presence of tumour may be difficult. Some inner cannulae are designed to allow speech, but more frequently (if the vocal cords are intact) the patient is taught to vocalise by temporary occlusion of the stoma with a finger. Occasionally a patient will have an 'electronic voice-box' or communicate by writing. This is often very frustrating and tiring for both patients and carers—patience is required!

Complications of tracheostomies

The complications arising from a tracheostomy can be considered under three categories: immediate, early and late.

- Immediate (0–24 h): anaesthetic complications; primary haemorrhage; damage to local structures, e.g. recurrent laryngeal nerve.
- Early (1–14 days): accidental decannulation; surgical emphysema; pneumothorax; tube obstruction; infection-wound, perichondritis, secondary haemorrhage; necrosis of the trachea leading to stenosis or fistulae; swallowing difficulty.
- Late (14+ days): subglottic or tracheal stenosis; fistulae-oesophageal, blood vessels, cutaneous; stomal recurrence tumour.

Care of a tracheostomy

Many patients manage effective self-care and will wish to do so even in very advanced disease. They should be counselled to avoid polluted atmospheres, for example smoke or dust, and to avoid freezing temperatures. They should also wear a lint-free scarf or bib over the stoma to warm inspired air and trap foreign bodies. There are three basic aspects of care [12, 13]: humidification of inspired air; mobilisation of secretions; and suctioning.

HUMIDIFICATION

Due to the loss of air passing through the moist mouth and oropharynx, extra humidity is essential to keep secretions thin and easily removable in patients with tracheostomies. This can be provided by dampening the covering bib (not all varieties require this), by installing a room or bedside humidifier, or by using an ultrasonic nebuliser with a specialised mask.

MOBILISATION AND REDUCTION OF SERCRETIONS

Regular deep-breathing exercises and chest physiotherapy will help move secretions and reduce pulmonary complications. If the patient is bed-bound, regular turning will aid drainage. Even a low level of activity, such as transferring from a bed to a chair, should be encouraged to help prevent basal atelectasis. Some patients will have coexistent chronic obstructive pulmonary disease: ipratropium bromide nebulisers, administered via the tracheostomy, may be useful in reducing secretions.

SUCTIONING

This is required if viscid secretions or mucous plugs develop and/or the cough reflex is ineffective. The catheter used for suctioning should be half the internal diameter of the tracheostomy tube. A sterile technique should be observed and the procedure explained to the patient.

Some patients may need preoxygenation. The catheter should be inserted 15 cm into the trachea. Suction should be applied as the tube is withdrawn, whilst being slowly rotated. Suctioning should not last longer than 15 seconds to enable the patient to breathe.

FOR PATIENTS WITH A LOT OF SECRETIONS

Special measures are required for patients who produce very high volumes of secretions. Cuffed tubes will prevent blood and secretions entering the airway. Inner tubes should be changed and cleaned (in sodium bicarbonate) frequently (2–6 times daily). Outer tubes may need specialist help in changing (1–2 times weekly).

EMERGENCY CARE OF ACUTE TRACHEOSTOMY OBSTRUCTION

Tracheostomy tubes may become blocked acutely by bleeding from tracheostomal recurrence or severe crusting of secretions, often associated with tumour recurrence and poor humidification of inspired air. When this happens follow the steps in Box 12.3.

Box 12.3 The management of acute tracheostomy obstruction

- Remove the inner tube
- Suction through the outer tube (catheter < half diameter of the tube)
- Tilley's forceps (long fine prongs) may be introduced in the tube to relieve obstruction
- If necessary instil 5 ml 0.9% saline into the tube and resuction, repeat as necessary
- If the obstruction persists remove and clean the outer tube holding the stoma open by tracheal dilators or immediate placement of a new tube

Tracheal dilators and a spare tube set must always be available in case both inner and outer tubes are displaced and the stoma is closed.

Prosthesis

Some patients with advanced head and neck cancer may have facial prostheses to restore functional and cosmetic anatomy. For example, a maxillary bridge to facilitate swallowing and improve speech, or a false nose to support glasses and restore facial integrity. However, the process of facial reconstruction is time-consuming, requiring several long outpatient visits to a prostho-orthodontist as well as extensive laboratory work. Hence, many patients who have advanced disease would not be suitable for referral. Some patients who have relapsed following initial radical treatment and reconstruction may have a facial or dental prosthesis which requires revision.

Symptom control and terminal care

The management of the last phase of life for patients with locally advanced disease may present some challenges. Many patients will become very weak and malnourished, while those with PEG feeding may remain systemically well, but may experience particular complications specific to local tumour growth. These complications may include:

- pain;
- local infections;
- respiratory infections;
- tracheal obstruction/stridor;
- oesophageal obstruction;
- tracheo-oesophageal fistulae;
- pathological, compound fracture of mandible;
- arterial bleeds.

Pain

Pain may be a feature of early disease and those who present with advanced disease may have considerable problems. A small number of disease-free patients experience chronic post-operative pain, particularly those who have undergone radical neck dissection followed by radiotherapy, but more commonly pain will be the first clue to relapsing disease [14]. It is important to exclude intraoral infections and abscesses as a cause for a new pain or worsening of pre-existing pain and a trial of antibiotics is justified.

The principles of pain control, discussed in Chapter 8 should be followed in all patients. The head and face have a rich nerve supply and many patients will experience neuropathic pain. The following is a guide to the management of patients with pain:

- Elicit the cause and type of pain. Consider infections and abscesses.
- If recurrence, follow the WHO analgesic ladder [15].
- Non-steroidal anti-inflammatory drugs are often very effective because of bone involvement and general inflammation.
- Tricyclic antidepressants or anticonvulsants should be introduced early for neuropathic pain, which is unresponsive to moderate doses of opioid analgesics.
- Ketamine or other drugs for neuropathic pain may be appropriate but specialist advice should usually be sought.
- Nerve blocks may be helpful, but if permanent the associated anaesthesia or paralysis needs to be discussed with the patient.

- Steroids may be a useful adjuvant treatment (e.g. Dexamethasone 4–12 mg daily)

It is important to consider routes of drug administration in this group of patients as treatment is commenced, bearing in mind that swallowing difficulties may develop as the tumour progresses. Most medicines can be given as liquids, but may taste unpleasant and be in large volumes. A gastrostomy or jejunostomy tube may be helpful. Transdermal, subcutaneous and rectal routes are useful if acceptable to the patient (see case example Box 12.4).

Box 12.4 Case example

A 70-year-old presented three years after treatment for a tonsillar carcinoma with deep aching pain in his jaw, radiating across his face. A nasendoscopy confirmed recurrence. He was started on a NSAID and titrated onto morphine. In view of trismus he was given fentanyl and diclofenac suppositories with good initial effect. A few months later, amitriptyline via his PEG was effective for lancing facial pains.

Local infections

A large proportion of fungating and recurrent tumours may become locally infected. It is usually worthwhile treating these aggressively with antibiotics as they ease unpleasant additional symptoms including pain, foul-smelling discharge and a constant distressing unpleasant taste in the mouth. Superadded infection may rapidly worsen swallowing in the dysphagic patient.

Treatment involves culturing the organism and commencing appropriate antibiotics, including cover for anaerobic organisms.

Intra-oral infections

Candida and herpes simplex infections are the commonest infections and require prompt treatment to avoid needless distress. *Candida* usually produces white plaques but also may be present in the sore, red mouth. Herpes may cause ulcers, mucositis and plaques. A diagnosis of herpes should be suspected in the presence of any painful oral lesions and should be rapidly treated.

Rhinorrhea

This is a rare problem but can be treated with ipatropium nasal spray (0.03–0.06%) b.d.

Hypersalivation

Saliva is not usually over-produced but the patient is unable to swallow or clear secretions from the mouth normally. This often results in drooling, which is embarrassing for the patient and can exacerbate stomatitis. Anticholinergics can be helpful, as can anti-depressants such as amitriptyline, especially if agitated depression or neuropathic pain is a co-existent problem. Initial dose for hypersalivation alone should be amitriptyline 10 mg nocte.

Respiratory infections

Respiratory infections are the predominate infections in this group, often precipitated by fistulae and aspiration. Treatment decisions depend on the individual case, but antibiotics may alleviate cough and sputum production.

Large airway compression: stridor

The onset of tracheal compression may be slow, due to tumour growth, or rapid, precipitated by haemorrhage or infection (it may occur earlier in the disease and then requires urgent management by referral to the ear, nose and throat (ENT) or other relevant specialist team). Most patients will have previously received radical radiotherapy and treatment is therefore supportive.

- High-dose Dexamethasone: start at 16 mg daily, either orally dissolved or subcutaneously.
- Benzodiazepines may reduce the sensation of panic: e.g. Lorazepam 1 mg sublingually, Diazepam 5 mg orally or titrated i.v., or Midazolam 2.5–5 mg titrated s.c. or i.v.
- Nebulised 0.9% saline + 2% Lidocaine (5 ml volume).
- Oxygen: high flow (28% or more if possible).
- If there is no response to Dexamethasone it may be appropriate to offer sedation. This may be via the PEG tube or subcutaneous infusion via a syringe driver.

Arterial bleeding

The possibility of arterial bleeding causes great anxiety to patients, carers, and health professionals. Many patients will have fungating, eroding tumours close to their carotid arteries but despite this arterial bleeding is a rare occurrence. Patients at risk may have a small warning bleed (see also Chapter 21).

Patients who are told about the possibility of bleeding may be fearful and loathe to leave the hospital. This should be considered when balancing the need for information with the likely ensuing anxiety. If a patient asks or is reported to be (or appears to be) worrying about such an event, facilitating discussion may allow a more realistic scenario to be portrayed, with the opportunity to reassure the patient and the carer that suffering would be transitory as unconsciousness develops quickly. It is also an opportunity to inform many patients that such events are, in fact, very rare. Following this, a plan of care can be formulated together with the patient and carer.

Although unconsciousness and death usually occurs very rapidly following an arterial bleed, it may be helpful to have sedation, such as Midazolam or sublingual Lorazepam, available in the house in case of emergencies. Dark coloured towels or blankets and advanced planning for what to do in such an event are also useful for relatives and staff.

Psychological problems

Contemporary society places great importance on physical attractiveness and the ability to communicate. It is therefore not surprising that head and neck cancer poses unique and distressing psychological problems. For example, when loss of speech is compounded by loss of facial expression, the powers of communication are doubly diminished. Facial deformity or functional changes, for example dysarthria, may draw unwanted attention to a patient already struggling to cope with loss of self-confidence, self-esteem and sexuality (see case example Box 12.5).

Box 12.5 Case example

A 48-year-old Gujarati mother-of-four was initially seen with a T1 carcinoma of the tongue. She was well for five years after surgery but then required further surgery and radiotherapy for a local recurrence. She represented with a large left-sided mass which was thought to be an abscess. An MRI showed a left parapharyngeal soft tissue mass which compressed the pharynx. She was very distressed at the news of recurrence and this was exacerbated by her youngest child who would not approach her bed.

When seen in clinic she had not left the house for five weeks and spent most of the day in bed. She admitted to a low mood and wished that she could go to sleep and not wake up. Other problems were facial pain and

Continued on p. 254

Box 12.5 ***Continued***

distress over her daughter. She was treated with amitriptyline, both for pain and depression and agreed for the clinical nurse specialist to visit home to talk to her daughter. She started attending hospice day care; and although her daughter was still reluctant to have physical contact, she spent much more time with her mother.

Rapport et al. [16] suggest that patients with congenital abnormality cope better than those with acquired abnormality, as do longer-term survivors of facial injury who presumably have longer to come to terms with psychological problems. Another study of patients with facial disfigurement from a variety of causes, including cancer, found that a large proportion had psychosocial problems but this was not related to the degree of disfigurement. Those patients at risk are those already socially isolated, single and those who have pre-existing poor coping strategies [17, 18]. Clearly, when the cause of the acquired abnormality is malignancy, there is a two-fold problem: the cancer itself as well as change in body image and self-concept.

Health professionals should be sensitive to the problems of depression and the social withdrawal which may arise. Consideration must also be given to the reaction of relatives and friends when faced with the altered appearance of someone they are close to. The patient and family may have a constant visual or audible reminder of their disease. Daily activities such as shaving, cleaning teeth, eating and simply talking may become an ordeal. Each time the patient looks into a mirror, they may be confronted by their cancer or consequences of the treatment, such as surgical scarring or radiation damage to the skin. Most cancer patients are able to assume a relatively 'normal' lifestyle in between symptomatic episodes, but this may not be the case for a patient with head and neck disease [19, 20].

There have been several small studies looking at psychosocial interventions for this group, the results of which have been contradictory with some demonstrating benefit from interventions such as support groups, whilst others have not shown benefit [21–26].

Cultural difficulties in dealing with cancer may also pose challenging difficulties in patient care. Disease may be viewed as a 'shame' or punishment, which has been visited on an individual and/or his or her family. Frequent reassurance and clear communication must aim to dispel such beliefs and minimise social isolation and guilt.

References

1 Papadimitrakopoulou VA. Carcinogenesis of head and neck cancer and the role of chemoprevention in its reversal. *Curr Opin Oncol* 2000; 12(3):240–245.

2 Bhurgri Y, Bhurgri A, Hassan SH, Zaidi SH, Rahim A, Sankaranarayanan R, Parkin DM. Cancer incidence in Karachi, Pakistan: first results from Karachi Cancer Registry. *Int J Cancer* 2000; 85 (3):325–329.

3 Sturgis EM, Wei Q. Genetic susceptibility—molecular epidemiology of head and neck cancer. *Curr Opin Oncol* 2002; 14 (3):310–317.

4 Hall SF, Groome PA, Rothwell D. The impact of comorbidity on the survival of patients with squamous cell carcinoma of the head and neck. *Head Neck* 2000; 22 (4):317–322.

5 Larson JT, Adams GL, Fattah HA. Survival statistics for multiple primaries in head and neck cancer. *Otolaryngol Head Neck Surg* 1990; 103 (1):14–24.

6 Jones AS, Fenton JE, Husband DJ. Performance data and survival in head and neck cancer. *Clin Otolaryngol* 2000; 25 (5):396–403.

7 Shedd DP, Carl A, Shedd C. Problems of terminal head and neck cancer patients. *Head Neck Surg* 1980; 2 (6):476–482.

8 Jacobs, van de Pas M. A multicentre maintenance study of oral Pilocarpine tablets for radiation-induced xerostomia. *Oncology* 1996; 10(3 supp):16–20.

9 Johnson JT et al. Oral Pilocarpine for post-irradiation xerostomia in patients with head and neck cancer. *N Engl J Med* 1993; 329 (6):390–395.

10 Department of Veterans Affairs Laryngeal Cancer Study Group. Induction chemotherapy plus radiation compared with surgery plus radiation in patients with advanced laryngeal cancer. *N Engl J Med* 1991; 324:1685–1690.

11 Koretz RL. Parenteral nutrition: is it oncologically based? *J Clin Oncol* 1984; 2 (5):534–539.

12 Leicester Royal Infirmary. *Tracheostomy—ENT Ward Guidelines*. Leicester: Leicester Royal Infirmary.

13 Shiley-Europe. *Tracheostomy Care*. Shiley instruction booklet. Staines: Shiley-Europe.

14 Talmi YP, Bercovici M, Waller A, Horowitz Z, Adunski A, Kronenberg J. Home and inpatient hospice care of terminal head and neck cancer patients. *J Palliat Care* 1997; 13 (1):9–14.

15 World Health Organisation. *Cancer Pain Relief*. Geneva: WHO 1986.

16 Rapport Y, Kreider S, Chaitchik S, Algor R, Weissler K. Psychosocial problems in head and neck cancer patients and their change with time since diagnosis. *Ann Oncol* 1993; 4:69–73.

17 de Leeuw JR, de Graeff A, Ros WJ, Blijham GH, Hordijk GJ, Winnubst JA. Prediction of depressive symptomatology after treatment of head and neck cancer: the influence of pre-treatment physical and depressive symptoms, coping and social support. *Head Neck* 2000; 22 (8):799–807.

18 Katz MR, Irish JC, Devins GM, Rodin GM, Gullane PJ. Psychosocial adjustment in head and neck cancer: the impact of disfigurement, gender and social support. *Head Neck* 2003; 25(2):103–112.

19 McEleney M. The psychological effects of head and neck surgery. *J Wound Care* 1993; 2(4):205–208.

20 Kelly R. Nursing patients with oral cancer. *Nurs Stand* 1994; 8 (32):25–29.
21 Burgess L. Facing the reality of head and neck cancer. *Nurs Stand* 1994; 8(32): 30–34.
22 de Leeuw JR, de Graeff A, Ros WJ, Bblijham GH, Hordijk GJ, Winnubst JA. Negative and positive influences of social support on depression in patients with head and neck cancer: a prospective study. *Psychooncology*; 2000; 9 (1):20–28.
23 Rumsey N, Clarke A, White P. Exploring the psychosocial concerns of outpatients with disfiguring conditions. *J Wound Care* 2003; 12(7):247–252.
24 Hutton JM, Williams M. An investigation of psychological distress in patients who have been treated for head and neck cancer. *Br J Oral Maxillofac Surg* 2001; 39 (5):333–339.
25 Kugaya A, Akechi T, Okamura H, Mikami I, Uchitomi Y. Correlates of depressed mood in ambulatory head and neck cancer patients. *Psychooncology* 1999; 8 (6):494–499.
26 Hammerlid E, Persson LO, Sullivan M, Westin T. Quality of life effects of psychosocial intervention in patients with head and neck cancer. *Otolaryngol Head Neck Surg* 1999; 120(4):507–516.

Further reading

Diamond J. *C: Because Cowards Get Cancer Too*. London: Vermillion 1998.

13: Palliative Care for People with Progressive Neurological Disorders

FIONA HICKS AND HAZEL PEARSE

Introduction

There are a number of different progressive neurological disorders including motor neurone disease (MND), multiple sclerosis (MS), muscular dystrophies, prion disease and Huntington's disease, for which treatment is largely palliative. Whilst these illnesses have many differences, there are principles of care that are common to them all. Good palliative care can help to maximise patient function and comfort within the confines of the disease.

Caring for such patients will be a rare experience for the primary health care team. This chapter will help the team to understand the issues facing patients and their carers, and to feel confident in the management of specific problems.

Background

Motor neurone disease (MND)

In MND there is a progressive loss of motor neurones. Muscles are not directly affected, but show denervation atrophy and irritability, leading to cramps and fasciculation. Some people with MND may have episodes of paroxysmal laughing or crying which do not represent true emotion; this can be difficult for both patients and carers. The mechanism behind this is not clear. The main features of MND depend on the areas affected.

Unlike other progressive neurological conditions such as multiple sclerosis, there are no occasions in MND where function improves. However, periods of stabilisation of the disease may occur but are of unpredictable duration.

MND is a relatively rare condition. It has an incidence of approximately two per 100 000. A general practitioner with an average list size might expect to see one new patient with MND every 25 years. Affected individuals have a median survival of 3 years, leading to an overall prevalence of about 6 per 100 000. In a primary care trust of 250 000 there will be 15 patients at any one time with MND, with three new patients and three deaths a year.

MND is largely a disease of middle to late life. Males are more commonly affected than females. A rare, hereditary form may have an onset in childhood or adolescence.

Three clinical variants of MND have been described (Table 13.1). These may present differently in their early stages but there is inevitably some overlap between them as the disease progresses.

In the 1990s, riluzole was discovered. This is the first compound shown to have efficacy against the course of MND. In practice, riluzole should be given early in the course of the disease where possible, as it appears to slow the rate of loss of motor neurones but does not restore function. It is unclear how well riluzole preserves functional ability, although it certainly does appear to have a modest effect on survival. Riluzole 50 mg b.d. is well tolerated by patients but should only be initiated by specialist physicians with experience in the management of MND.

Multiple sclerosis (MS)

MS is characterised by demyelination affecting the central nervous system. Symptoms depend on the areas affected, as with MND, and

Table 13.1 Summary of the variants of MND.

Variant of MND	Clinical findings	Prognosis
Amyotrophic lateral sclerosis (ALS); 66% of patients	Lesions of lower motor neurones, combined with involvement of the corticospinal tracts	Median survival in this group is around 3 years
Progressive muscular atrophy (PMA); 8% of patients	Largely affects lower motor neurones in the first instance	The most favourable prognosis, with some patients surviving more than 15 years
Progressive bulbar palsy (PBP); 26% of patients	Involvement of the brainstem motor nuclei predominates	The most sinister prognosis with death often occurring within a year

Table 13.2 Summary of the variants of MS.

Variant of MS	Clinical features
Primary progressive	Gradual worsening of illness without clear exacerbations
Relapsing remitting	Characterised by acute exacerbations with remissions in between
Secondary progressive	The gradually worsening state of someone who initially had relapsing remitting disease
Progressive relapsing	Those patients who initially have progressive disease but then go on to develop exacerbations

include hemiparesis or hemisensory loss, internuclear opthalmoplegia and optic neuritis, ataxia and tremor. Bladder and bowel function can be affected and cognitive impairment may be a feature.

MS can be divided into groups depending on the course of the illness as shown in Table 13.2. Patients may experience progressive symptoms or intermittent exacerbations, which are often precipitated by infection.

MS is more common than MND with a life-time risk in the UK of about 1:1000. More women than men are affected. There may be hereditary factors involved in the aetiology. Most patients develop the disease between 20 and 50 years of age.

Treatments may be purely palliative with the aim to reduce symptoms, or aimed at reducing inflammation and demyelination. Pulse methylprednisolone or ACTH can be used for acute exacerbations but their use to reduce long-term disability is unclear [1]. Other options include interferon [2], cyclophosphamide [3], immunoglobulins [4, 5], and aminopyridines [6], all of which need specialist instigation and monitoring.

Muscular dystrophies

These are a group of inherited disorders characterised by degeneration of different muscle groups. Although not strictly neurological disorders, they exhibit similar symptomatology. There are distinct variants of muscular dystrophies (Table 13.3). Duchenne muscular dystrophy (DMD) is the commonest seen in adult palliative care and is the variant that will be referred to in the remainder of this chapter.

Table 13.3 Summary of three variants of the muscular dystrophies.

Variant of muscular dystrophy	Inheritance	Clinical Features
Duchenne	X linked recessive	Proximal muscle weakness, cardiomyopathy, pseudohypertrophy of the calves and (sometimes) low IQ
Beckers	Autosomal recessive	Milder than Duchenne and has a longer life expectancy but shares many common features
Facioscapulohumeral	Autosomal dominant	Weakness of the facial and shoulder muscles. Winging of the scapulae. Normal life expectancy

DMD is an X-linked recessive disorder, which means it is carried by females and is expressed in males. Thirty percent are due to spontaneous mutations.

It is due primarily to a reduction in muscle cell membrane dystrophin, which causes progressive muscle weakness. Proximal muscles are affected initially with patients having increasing difficulty walking and standing. The typically occurs between 4 and 5 years of age. This progresses to being wheelchair bound, usually in the teenage years. With artificial ventilatory support patients are now living longer into adulthood.

Due to its genetic nature, genetic counselling can be important for parents when making decisions about future family planning.

Treatments for DMD are aimed at prevention and treatment of complications and include physiotherapy, surgery for scoliosis and artificial ventilation for respiratory failure.

Huntington's chorea

Huntington's disease is thought to be due to reduced GABAnergic and cholinergic neurones in the corpus striatum.

It presents usually in the fourth decade although patients can present at a younger age with a more aggressive form of the illness. Its estimated prevalence is 1:20 000.

The disease is characterised by early personality changes such as irritability, in association with chorea, increased muscle tone, bradykinesia and slowness of speech. Dysphagia may also occur. In young patients fits can be a feature. Depression and dementia are common.

This is an autosomal dominant disease with implications for the children of an affected parent. Predictive testing is possible but careful pre and post-test counselling is essential.

Currently there is no treatment to alter the course of Huntington's disease.

Creutzfeldt–Jakob disease (CJD)

CJD remains thankfully rare with an incidence of one in a million. This may, however, be an underestimate as cases may be misdiagnosed.

There are four main variants of CJD. Table 13.4 compares some of the features of sporadic and new variant CJD. There is a genetic form of the illness, which is rare, and features depend on the site of the genetic mutation. Iatrogenic CJD can occur, such as from corneal transplants and makes up a minority of the cases seen each year.

There are a number of theories about transmission of CJD. The prion theory postulates the accumulation of prion protein within the CNS. This protein may be transmitted, or be a result of a mutation or a spontaneous change.

There is no link with sporadic CJD and diet but there is often confusion amongst patients and carers. Infection control issues must also be addressed.

Although different treatments have been tried e.g. quinacrine, there are no treatments of proven benefit in altering the underlying disease process.

Table 13.4 Comparison of sporadic and variant CJD.

CJD subtype	Age of onset	Prognosis	Features
Sporadic (most common)	Middle age/ elderly	Weeks to months	Neurological impairment, impaired cognition, ataxia
Variant	Late 20s	Months to years	Behavioural and psychiatric presentations, neurological features and dementia are presented later in the disease. Possible link with BSE

Organisation and co-ordination of care

Efficient organisation of care is mandatory for patients with progressive neurological disorders and contributes to a sense of control, maintaining quality of life for patients and families wherever possible. As these conditions are comparatively rare, the primary health care team may have little experience of the diseases. However, the majority of the work will fall to them. Neurological disorders are complex requiring the skills of many professionals at different times. The number of people involved can be bewildering for patients and professionals alike and may lead to a breakdown in communication. It is essential that each patient is nominated a key worker from the time of diagnosis, whose name and contact number is known to both the patient and the caring team.

The key worker may be drawn from any discipline and should have an interest in the disease, a good relationship with the patient, and the ability to communicate well with all those involved in the patient's care.

Occupational therapists, speech and language therapists, and physiotherapists can be of great help to patients facing progressive disability.

Common physical symptoms in people with progressive neurological disorders

Whilst these illnesses are very different in many ways, they share many of the same physical and psychological symptoms. The remainder of the chapter tries to address some symptoms common to the diseases mentioned above.

As outlined in Chapter 1, good symptom control requires:

- a thorough history of each symptom;
- a careful physical examination;
- conducting relevant investigations;
- discussing the problem with the patient (and carers where appropriate) including the therapeutic options and their potential advantages and disadvantages.

Constipation

Constipation is the most common symptom found among MND patients and is frequently troublesome in the other conditions. Possible causes include a low-residue diet, immobility, drug side-effects (e.g. anticholinergics, opioids) and reduced power of the abdominal muscles used to aid evacuation.

MANAGEMENT

Remove the cause of the constipation if possible, especially if drug-related. It is possible to give dietary advice even in patients with swallowing difficulties. If aperients are needed, they must be easy to swallow by patients with dysphagia. Oral aperients are usually preferable to suppositories. A combination of a stimulant laxative and a softener is usually required, for example:

- Co-danthramer, initially 5–10 ml b.d. (dose maybe increased or given as Co-danthramer forte as necessary);
- Movicol sachets, 1–2 per day, which can be increased, as needed, up to eight sachets a day;
- Senna syrup 5 ml b.d. with lactulose 5–10 ml b.d. (dose titrated as required). Flatulence may limit the dose of lactose that can be tolerated.

Pain

MUSCULOSKELETAL PAIN

There are two main factors that contribute to the development of musculoskeletal pain: (i) restricted movement leading to stiff joints; and (ii) reduced muscle tone around joints leading to loss of the normal positioning (shoulder joints are most commonly affected).

Pain should be prevented wherever possible by careful positioning. Physiotherapy, including passive movements, helps to maintain joint mobility. Once musculoskeletal pain has become established, joint positioning and exercise remain critical but pharmacological treatment will also be necessary.

- Non-steroidal anti-inflammatory drugs (NSAIDs) in tablet, suspension or suppository form as required.
- NSAID gel applied to the affected areas may be of benefit.
- Intra-articular injections of local anaesthetic and steroid are worth considering, especially for shoulder pain.
- Acupuncture may be of benefit.

MUSCLE CRAMPS

Muscle cramps can be a very troublesome problem and may respond to simple stretching exercises. However, if drugs are required, various muscle relaxants may be tried, for example: baclofen 5–20 mg t.d.s. (larger doses may be necessary for some patients); tizanidine 2 mg daily increasing in increments of 2 mg usually up to a maximum of 24 mg daily in 3–4 divided doses; dantrolene 25–100 mg q.d.s.; diazepam 5 mg nocte increased as necessary to 10 mg q.d.s. or more, depending on side-effects; or quinine sulphate 200 mg nocte, increased to 300 mg as necessary. Other options include botulinum toxin and cannabinoids.

These drugs should be titrated against the response of the patient until cramps are controlled or side effects become troublesome. Some authors would advocate higher maximum doses than described here [7]. A combination of drugs may be used if necessary, although drowsiness is a common problem with higher doses. All these drugs may also be used for troublesome spasticity (e.g. adductor spasm) but it is important to remember that in ambulatory patients, some spasticity may be necessary to keep the patient mobile.

SKIN PRESSURE

Skin pressure causes pain in patients with advanced disease who are unable to move and change position. Attention to the care of pressure areas is very important both for patients in wheelchairs and for bed-bound patients (see also Chapter 20). Unfortunately some patients with established pressure sores often need a period of admission to a hospital or hospice unit for intensive nursing support. Pain may be relieved with NSAIDs as before, but analgesics may well have to be increased according to the WHO analgesic ladder (see Chapter 8).

Topical opioids for pressure sores can be helpful [8].

Breathlessness (dyspnoea)

Breathlessness in these patients can have several possible causes.

- Lower respiratory tract infection, often caused or compounded by aspiration pneumonia.
- Weakness of the muscles of ventilation, particularly the diaphragm and intercostal muscles, sometimes aggravated by poor nutrition. This commonly occurs in MND and DMD.
- Coexistent cardiac or lung pathology (e.g. left ventricular failure, chronic obstructive pulmonary disease). Patients with DMD have an associated cardiomyopathy. Particular care needs to be taken with

diuretics in this group of patients as a low potassium contributes to muscle weakness and arrythmias.

MANAGEMENT

Infection

Management of infective causes should comprise appropriate antibiotics, physiotherapy and consideration of alternative methods of feeding if aspiration is a problem.

Weakness of ventilatory muscles

Nocturnal ventilatory failure may precede daytime breathlessness. Precarious ventilatory reserve is exhausted by lying supine at night. Raising the head of the bed or sleeping in a reclining chair may be of benefit. In many patients breathlessness is a poor prognostic sign, and ventilatory failure sufficient to cause daytime breathlessness usually heralds the terminal phase of MND and DMD.

In patients with MND or DMD who may be otherwise fit, non-invasive nocturnal ventilation may be considered and is possible in the home. For patients with muscular dystrophy it is increasingly used successfully. It is important to have a full and frank discussion with patients before embarking on such treatment, as increasing dependence on the ventilator is likely and the limits of such treatment should be made clear [9]. Life can be prolonged indefinitely in this way, which raises many ethical issues.

For most patients treatment is purely symptomatic (see Chapter 10). Sitting upright with a stream of air passing across the face is helpful. Calm reassurance, company, relaxation and breathing exercises have important therapeutic roles. Pharmacological treatment is aimed at reducing anxiety and decreasing the subjective experience of breathlessness. This may be done using diazepam 2–5 mg t.d.s. Lorazepam 0.5–1 mg may be given sub-lingually for acute attacks, as it is shorter acting. Another option is morphine sulphate 2.5–5 mg every four hours. These drugs can be given together as required, but must be titrated carefully as these patients have poor respiratory reserve and are often sensitive to small doses of respiratory sedatives.

Salivary drooling

Bulbar palsies make it difficult for patients to manipulate saliva in the mouth and then swallow it. This may be compounded by weakness of facial and neck muscles, causing parting of the lips and a tendency for the head to fall forwards. This then leads to salivary drooling which is often a distressing symptom for patients, who may isolate themselves from company due to embarrassment.

MANAGEMENT

Explanation to the patient and carer and attention to posture may be all that is needed. Drug treatment may be used to dry up saliva, and in this case a compromise must be reached between drooling and a dry mouth. Anticholinergic drugs are the mainstay of treatment:

- hyoscine hydrobromide patches (1 mg over 72 h); 1 to 3 patches may be needed, titrated according to response; or
- hyoscine hydrobromide 300–600 μg sublingually q.d.s.; or
- glycopyrronium bromide 1.2 mg s.c. over 24 h.

If a patient is also suffering from depression, amitriptyline may be used for both problems. Beta blockers may be useful, for example propranolol 10 mg t.d.s.

A few patients may tolerate having a dry mouth but dislike taking medication in the longer term. Radiotherapy to the salivary glands may then be considered. This is usually done unilaterally in the first instance to assess its acceptability to the patient.

Cough

A weak, ineffectual cough may be a troublesome symptom. This is often compounded by a lower respiratory tract infection.

MANAGEMENT

If aspiration is a problem, consider alternative methods of feeding. Treat infection appropriately and consider physiotherapy and suction. If mucus is tenacious, this may compound the difficulties of a weak cough. Consider mucolytics such as: nebulised saline 5 ml prn, or carbocisteine 500–750 mg t.d.s. A distressing cough, particularly at night, may be helped by nebulised local anaesthetic.

Insomnia

Insomnia may have various causes, including: pain/discomfort, anxiety and depression. The patient's sleep may be disturbed by a troublesome nocturnal cough due to increased secretions. Moreover, nocturnal ventilatory failure causes hypoxia resulting in frequent night-time wakening, morning headache (CO_2 retention) and daytime somnolence.

The management should be directed at the underlying causes of the insomnia, which have been discussed elsewhere in this chapter.

Weakness and the need for aids and appliances

The introduction of new aids and appliances requires sensitive handling. The necessity for new equipment serves to remind patients of their deterioration. Equipment may be rejected or simply not used if it is introduced too early or with inadequate explanation. However, there is nothing more demoralising than waiting so long for a much-needed piece of equipment that by the time it arrives, the disability has progressed too far for it to be of any use. For example, an electric wheelchair is of no use to a patient who has lost the function of their hands.

There is a large variety of equipment available for most conceivable needs. Equipment should be loaned wherever possible, as its usefulness may be short-lived if disability progresses rapidly. Various agencies may be of help:

- Disablement Resettlement Officers.
- Disablement Living Centres.
- The Disablement Living Foundation.
- REMAP (Rehabilitation Engineering Movement Advisory Panels).

Enhancing communication

Many patients will develop difficulties with speech, ranging from quiet speech, to dysarthria and anarthria. Speech problems are rare in DMD. It is vital that wherever possible, the caring team builds up a good relationship with the patient while speech is still preserved. This may entail visiting the patient more often than is strictly necessary during the early part of their illness. During this time, attitudes to illness and treatment can be explored along with other issues and fears that are important to the patient. This will aid communication in the later phases of the disease when speech may be difficult or absent, although the patient's attitudes and fears may change. When a patient becomes anarthric, it is important to remember that their hearing and intellect may be preserved, although patients with CJD or Huntingdon's disease will exhibit an associated dementia.

A speech and language therapist is an important team member. He/she will establish the cause of speech problems and give advice on maintaining intelligible speech where possible. Advice on the choice and use of communication aids will be given. These range from amplifiers for those with a weak voice to a keyboard operated by hand or by eye movements. Communication Aid Centres have been set up around the country, where aids can be tried out.

Feeding problems

Feeding difficulties may be due to upper limb weakness or difficulty in swallowing. These are often of great embarrassment to patients as feeding is often a social event. A speech and language therapist will help diagnose causes of swallowing problems and advise on how a patient may optimize their swallowing. Oral or oesophageal candidiasis should not be overlooked in patients with dysphagia; this can be treated with fluconazole 50 mg for 5 days. Food of uniform, semisolid consistency is the easiest to swallow in patients with bulbar palsies. Dieticians can advise on palatable, nutritious recipes.

If oral feeding becomes untenable, usually due to recurrent aspiration into the trachea, alternative methods of feeding may be considered with the patient. This may remove the stress of needing to maintain nutrition and will probably prolong survival. It should be remembered, however, that the risk of aspiration remains even when the patient only has the occasional cup of tea. The reason for considering alternative feeding methods should be weighed up carefully.

Nasogastric feeding has little place now for these patients. Percutaneous endoscopic gastrostomy (PEG) feeding is a much more satisfactory alternative (see Chapter 9).

Psychosocial problems commonly affecting people with progressive neurological diseases

Anxiety

Anxiety affects many patients, often becoming more manifest as the illness progresses. It is often most disabling at night. Management may include reassurance and cognitive or behavioural techniques. A good therapeutic relationship and efficient management of coexisting symptoms are of great benefit. If medication is needed, a short-acting benzodiazepine, such as temazepam 10–20 mg at night is often sufficient.

If daytime anxiety is also a problem, a longer acting preparation such as diazepam 5–10 mg at night is preferable, although some people prefer to take 2–10 mg t.d.s.

Depression

A low mood may be expected in patients suffering from progressive, ultimately fatal, disorders such as these, but a treatable, clinical depression should not be overlooked. The diagnosis of depression poses a particular challenge in those with severe speech difficulties alongside a severe physical illness, and in those with an associated dementia. An all-pervading sense of hopelessness and loss of self-worth may point to the diagnosis. Treatment is with conventional antidepressants. If insomnia is a problem, amitriptyline 25 mg at night, increased as necessary to 150 mg, is the drug of choice. Care must be taken in patients with coexistent cardiac disease e.g. cardiomyopathy of DMD. Alternatively a selective serotonin reuptake inhibitor (SSRI) such as citalopram 20 mg o.d. may be used.

RESTLESSNESS AND AGITATION

The environment is very important if a patient is restless or agitated. Nursing a patient in a calm quiet and constant setting may be all that is needed. It is important to exclude reversible causes of agitation such as constipation and infection. Severe ventilatory difficulties causing hypoxia can also present with agitation. If drug treatment is needed risperidone or olanzepine could be tried. These can be used in combination with benzodiazepines, particularly if anxiety is a component of the agitation.

Fear about the manner of death

With many of these illnesses the media play a role in the portrayal of death, and choking is often mentioned. The fear of choking combined with impending loss of speech and function in the arms and legs leads some patients to make advance directives requesting assisted suicide or euthanasia. Requests like this must be handled with great sensitivity and the underlying fears explored. An explanation about the likely mode of death, including signs that the terminal phase is approaching, can be of great benefit to some people. Reassurance about the drugs that are available to manage symptoms in the terminal phase can be helpful.

Difficulties for lay carers

The physical and emotional demands on the families and friends of people with severe neurological diseases can be enormous. These demands are compounded where speech problems hinder normal communication and in inherited conditions where more than one family member may be affected. The possibility of respite care should be explored. Options include day care, a home sitting service, or periods of inpatient care in hospital, hospice or nursing home.

Difficulties for professional carers

Caring for patients with progressive neurological diseases and their families can be difficult. Managing patients with a disabling condition with no cure may elicit feelings of hopelessness and despondency among the caring team. Reactions may vary; typical ones include:

- keeping a distance, not getting too involved;
- referring the patient to someone else;
- being over-optimistic about the prognosis;
- being nihilistic about any interventions;
- being drawn towards physician-assisted suicide or euthanasia.

However, there is no substitute for getting involved, being honest and sensitive with the patient and family, and striving to address each problem as it arises. This will maximise physical function and comfort within the limits of the disease.

Professionals should ensure that their own coping strategies are optimised when caring for patients who may cause these predictable impacts on the team.

Terminal care

Terminal care for patients follows the same principles as for other conditions (see Chapter 21). Ideally, a decision about the place of death will have been made in advance by the patient and their carers. Every effort should be made to achieve those wishes wherever possible.

Management

Medications given for symptomatic benefit should be continued in a convenient form during the terminal phase. This may be via a gastrostomy tube where present, or a subcutaneous syringe driver. Common drugs used subcutaneously in terminal care include:

- diamorphine for pain or breathlessness;

- midazolam 10–30 mg/24 h for sedation or anxiety. An alternative is levomepromazine 12.5–150 mg/24 h;
- hyoscine hydrobromide 1.2–2.4 mg/24 h for distressing secretions. Glycopyrronium or hyoscine butylbromide can be used as an alternative in this instance.

Supportive organisations

MND

The Motor Neurone Disease Association (MNDA) is a national, voluntary organisation and registered charity. It has regional care advisors who have direct contact with patients and families and also play an educational role to health care professionals. The MNDA also runs an information service, with a wide range of publications written for both the lay public and professionals involved in the care of people with MND. A comprehensive list of useful addresses and telephone numbers is provided in the MNDA booklets.

MS

There are a number of MS support groups two of which are listed below. They offer help and support with all aspects of care and treatment as well as enabling patients and their families to contact other people in similar situations for advice and friendship. The Multiple Sclerosis Society of Great Britain and Northern Ireland can be contacted on 0808 800 8000 and sited at www.mssociety.org.uk Alternatively the Multiple Sclerosis Trust is at www.mstrust.org.uk or 01462 476700.

Muscular dystrophies

The Muscular Dystrophy Campaign is a charitable organisation that supports all forms of muscular dystrophy. It provides useful information about current treatments, grants and equipment and offers a good support network. The contact number is 020-7720-8055 and web address is www.muscular-dystrophy.org

Huntington's disease

The Huntington's Disease Association can be contacted on 020-7223-7000. Its website is www.hda.org.uk. It offers news updates, information and support for families, patients and professionals.

CJD

The National CJD care team can provide help and support to patients, families and professionals regarding all aspects of the illness. They are based within the National CJD Surveillance Unit and can be contacted on 013-1537-3073 or at their website mail to: cjd.ed.ac.uk. They help coordinate care and provide education. A neurologist can be available for advice if required. They can also help access care packages when, all too often, current services fall short. Support continues after a patient has died.

Conclusions

This chapter outlines various aspects of a strategy designed to help professionals work successfully with patients and their carers in order to achieve good palliative care.

- Get involved early, while the patient can still communicate.
- Nominate a key worker to educate the team, provide a focus for care and ensure that appropriate actions are taken at appropriate times.
- Remember to pay attention to details, especially with aids, appliances and symptom control.
- Remember the psychosocial impact of these illnesses, particularly for patients with communication difficulties and in inherited disorders.
- Be mindful of experts/agencies that can help.

References

1 Flippini G et al. *Corticosteroids or ACTH for Acute Exacerbations in Multiple Sclerosis (Cochrane Review)*. The Cochrane Library, Issue 4. Chichester, UK: Wiley, 2003.
2 Rice G PA. et al. *Interferon in Relapsing-Remitting Multiple Sclerosis (Cochrane Review)*. The Cochrane Library, Issue 4. Chichester, UK: Wiley, 2003.
3 La Mantia L. et al. *Cyclophosphamide for Multiple Sclerosis (Cochrane Review)*. The Cochrane Library, Issue 4. Chichester, UK: Wiley, 2003.
4 Gray OM. et al. *Intravenous Immunoglobulins for Multiple Sclerosis (Cochrane Review)*. The Cochrane Library, Issue 4. Chichester, UK: Wiley, 2003.
5 Sorensen PS. Treatment of multiple sclerosis with intravenous immunoglobulin: review of clinical trials. *Neurol Sci*.2003; 24(Suppl 4): S227–S230.
6 Solari A et al. *Aminopyridines for Symptomatic Treatment in Multiple Sclerosis (Cochrane Review)*. The Cochrane Library, Issue 4. Chichester, UK: Wiley, 2003.

7 Norris F, Smith R, Denys E. Motor neurone disease: towards better care. *BMJ* 1985; 291: 259–262.
8 Flock P. Pilot study to determine the effectiveness of diamorphine gel to control pressure ulcer pain. *J Pain Symptom Manage*. 2003 Jun; 25: 547–549.
9 Shneerson J. Motor neurone disease, some hope at last for respiratory complications. *BMJ* 1996; 313: 244.

14: Palliative Care for People with HIV Infection and AIDS

SURINDER SINGH AND NICK THEOBALD

Introduction and scene-setting

HIV infection and AIDS continue to cause high levels of morbidity and mortality throughout the world. In developing countries as many as one in three deaths can be HIV-related. Most of this chapter will describe palliative care practice in the United Kingdom. We will also bring readers up-to-date with some of the changes that are occurring as a result of the success of antiretroviral therapy.

One illustration of the success of antiretroviral therapies is that HIV-related deaths in the UK have diminished to very small numbers as a result of which, in London for example, one of the two major residential units catering for those with terminal care needs closed all beds and the other one has had to diversify to include respite care for those infected with HIV and their families. How long these successes continue is a major question and a source of uncertainty for patients and doctors alike.

This chapter will not cover the more specialist area of paediatric palliative care, except to say that as time goes on, the number of children born in the UK with HIV will diminish—as records already show—not least because of the success of the antenatal HIV-testing programme [1]. Please also see www.bhiva.org/chiva/index (see Useful Addresses).

Issues about safety and control of infection—including the use of universal precautions are included in the appendix to this chapter.

Global epidemiology

According to UNAIDS the continuing AIDS epidemic claimed more than three million lives in 2002. This occurred in a world where an estimated five million people acquired HIV infection—the virus that ultimately causes AIDS—bringing the number of people living with the infection to forty-two million [2]. Almost two thirds of this vast figure lives in sub-Saharan Africa. HIV is also spreading in areas of large populations, such as India and China, which until recently have experienced lower levels of transmission.

The HIV epidemic in the UK is similar to other Northern European countries (Germany, Holland), while in contrast, Southern European countries (Spain, Portugal) have experienced larger numbers, especially among injecting drug users. Russia and several Baltic States have seen a meteoric rise in numbers, mostly fuelled by injecting drug use.

Recent work in palliative care and HIV/AIDS in resource-poor African countries [3, 4] indicated that, for those dying from a terminal disease, the following factors were critical in a 'good death':

- the relief of pain and other distressing symptoms;
- the avoidance of stigma;
- being cared for by family or members of the local community;
- financial security, if only to not feel totally dependent on direct care-givers.

The World Health Organisation (WHO) has attempted to use these findings to launch palliative care initiatives in some of these same countries concentrating on pain-relief, including the judicious use of opioids, and importantly, financial support at such times of distress [3, 4]. Several Western studies have highlighted very similar features in patients with late stage HIV infection or AIDS.

HIV and AIDS in the UK

HIV continues to be one of the most important communicable diseases in the UK. In 2002 over 5500 individuals were diagnosed with HIV for the first time [5]. It is estimated there are about 49 500 HIV infected people alive in the UK. This means that the estimated prevalence of HIV infection in adults increased by 20% over the previous year. Anti-retroviral therapy (ART) has resulted in a sustained decline in HIV-associated deaths, which, with a rise in the number of new diagnoses has resulted in a steep increase in the number of people requiring long term treatment. London, Brighton and Manchester are the cities in England and Edinburgh in Scotland, with the largest HIV-infected populations. In 2002, 31% of all adults with HIV infection were unaware of their status [5].

Who is Affected?

MALE HOMO/BISEXUAL TRANSMISSION

The majority of infections reported to the Communicable Disease Surveillance Centre have occurred through sex between men. Over 1500 new diagnoses of HIV occur in this group per year with no evidence of any decline in these figures. Despite general levels of awareness, 24% of HIV infected men who have sex with men have not had their infection diagnosed. Almost 60% of those infected through sex between men live in London.

HETEROSEXUAL TRANSMISSION

The number of heterosexually acquired HIV infections diagnosed in the UK has risen enormously since 1985. As a result, since 1999 there have been more diagnoses of heterosexually acquired infection than of infections acquired through sex between men. Three-quarters of heterosexually acquired HIV infection diagnosed in the UK in 2002 were in people from Africa, or were associated with exposure there. Of the 'heterosexuals' 38% of are unaware of their infection and this is the group with the highest proportion not yet diagnosed. Lastly, around 7% of this group have been infected through a blood transfusion or blood factor treatment.

WOMEN WITH HIV

With the rise in heterosexual transmissions, there has been an increase in the number of women diagnosed. The male to female ratio of all new infections diagnosed in the mid 1980s was approximately 14:1 whereas in 2000–2001 it was 1.7:1. At least one ramification of this is in pregnancy—although the number of births to HIV-infected women has risen, the estimated proportion of infants born with HIV declined from about 19% in 1997 to about 9% in 2001.

UNDIAGNOSED HIV

There are over 15 000 people who remain undiagnosed in the UK. This is the group most likely to experience declining health and a subsequent diagnosis of AIDS. HIV-related morbidity and mortality are increasingly concentrated among those who remain undiagnosed until late into their disease, by which time ART may not be as effective.

Many heterosexuals remain undiagnosed until prompted by HIV-related symptoms late in the course of the illness. Around two thirds of those with heterosexually acquired infection are diagnosed at a late stage of progression of the disease.

Issues relating to palliative care

Prognosis and the transition to palliative care

Life expectancy for patients with HIV infection in the developed world has improved significantly following the introduction of combination antiretroviral therapy (ART). The clinical course for any individual patient can be variable and is dependant upon factors such as tolerance of drugs, adherence to complex regimes and the development of drug resistance. For the majority of people, HIV infection can now be regarded as a chronic, manageable disease.

It is therefore even more difficult than ever to determine when the emphasis of care should turn towards palliating symptoms rather than pursuing investigations and curative treatment regimens. In the majority of cases, the processes may run in parallel—with the expertise of palliative care controlling adverse symptoms while the HIV physician works to control the virus and consequences of impaired immunity.

Many patients with HIV and AIDS choose to receive much of their care from hospitals, often for reasons of familiarity, relative anonymity and continuity of care. The availability of 'walk-in' clinics also means that patients can be treated almost exclusively by hospitals. Unfortunately this sometimes means that the primary care team may have very little involvement with the patient until the end of their illness, which is not ideal for all parties concerned. It is therefore important to remind patients that the general practitioner ought to be involved at all stages of their illness. There are of course many resources within primary care that can provide a great deal of help and support to those living with HIV; several GPs have advocated a much greater involvement of the primary care team in their day-to-day management [6].

The average age of the patient with HIV/AIDS is much younger than for most malignant conditions. Some will have battled through numerous opportunistic infections, each potentially life threatening, but then turn the corner, to remain well for many years and stay out of hospital. Others may be diagnosed with a serious HIV related malignancy after years of good health and face a situation with relatively poor prognosis.

A small number of conditions are associated with a particularly poor prognosis and the likelihood of death in less than six months. This should prompt a change in focus with more consideration of quality of life, palliating symptoms and anticipating the terminal care needs of both the individual and their families or partners. Death is predicted by baseline functional status rather than traditional HIV disease markers such as lymphocyte count [7].

Patients with advanced disease often have multiple physical and psychosocial issues and comprehensive care for late-stage HIV disease commonly involves an increasingly complex mixture of therapies—both disease-specific and palliative. This requires co-ordination and collaboration between acute HIV treatment centres, palliative care services and primary care. Recently a set of standards covering twelve clinical areas, palliative care included, has been introduced in the UK which is designed to provide guidance on service networks and best practice (see Medfash website in section on useful addresses). Below are characteristics which render the care of patients with advanced HIV/AIDS as a particular challenge to health care workers:

Characteristics of patients with HIV infection/AIDS [8]

- Predominantly younger age group;
- Multi-system disease;
- Polysymptomatic;
- Polypharmacy/interactions;
- Concurrent active/palliative;
- Changes in prognosis following treatment advances;
- Patient involvement/knowledge/empowerment;
- Social issues of isolation, stigma, confidentiality, housing problems, language, cultural issues, religious issues, housing problems, lack of family and/or support.

Psychosocial issues specific to HIV and AIDS

STIGMA AND CONFIDENTIALITY

In a global, regional or local context HIV and AIDS continue to be stigmatised. So huge is this problem that the 2002–2003 World AIDS Campaign was aimed at spurring worldwide efforts to remove the barriers of stigma and discrimination. The reason for this was simple,

HIV/AIDS-related stigma and discrimination rank among the biggest and most pervasive barriers to effective responses to the AIDS epidemic. Stigma and discrimination target and harm those who are least able to enjoy their human rights: the poorest, the least educated and the most marginalised. In fact stigma, discrimination and human rights violations form a vicious circle generating, reinforcing and perpetuating each other [1].

Stigma affects people in many ways and the issues of confidentiality, anonymity and disclosure are closely linked. The fear of disclosure may extend even to close family members. Professional staff should enquire who has been informed of the diagnosis and make no assumptions. Written and verbal communications with the patient, family, friends and other professionals should always be sensitive and discreet. For some patients there is additional concern that their family should not be aware of their sexuality.

Furthermore, some of those infected earlier in the epidemic may have often cared for friends and/or partners who have died and may be socially isolated as a result of this multiple bereavement. Some people from Africa may have experienced family and community decimation from AIDS and may suffer further isolation, worsened by stigma, as a result of these major life-changes.

In the context of HIV/AIDS confidentiality is crucial. It is an integral part of patient care, as it should be in all conditions. Since HIV and AIDS remain stigmatised conditions it is all the more important that here all services, including those in palliative care, need to guard against complacency, ensure awareness and provide training when necessary. Confidentiality is a team issue. A lapse by one member of staff means that the patient and family or caregiver is compromised. A breach of confidentiality cannot be easily rectified for an individual or family. Some patients perceive negative attitudes towards them from doctors—and perhaps general practitioners are perceived to be worse than most in this regard (though there is no evidence that they are). Many patients crave anonymity and confidentiality, which is one of the reasons why people with HIV infection would commonly move home to be within a major conurbation like London, Manchester or Brighton.

Several studies involving general practice have shown that a practice declaration (often in the form of a visible practice statement) can be important in allaying the fears of adults regarding confidentiality—and the more prominently these are displayed the better. Other features of an HIV-friendly practice include:

1 All members of the team are non-judgmental and empathic to different lifestyles.
2 Development and implementation of a non-discrimination policy.
3 Development and implementation of an appropriate confidentiality policy.

The association of HIV/AIDS with illegal drug use has inevitably led to many patients with HIV spending time in prison and clearly this has implications for confidentiality. Whilst release on compassionate grounds may be considered appropriate for some terminally ill patients, others will be transferred to hospital/hospice under custodial supervision in the final stages of their illness. This can lead to additional stress for all involved and demands careful and considerate organisation to preserve patient dignity (as well as confidentiality) yet fulfil Home Office supervision requirements.

In the specific context of palliative care it must be remembered that the duty for confidentiality continues 'beyond the grave' [9]. This may present dilemmas later, for example third parties needing information about a particular client. This often requires formal legal advice as well as advice and support to the clinician from medical defence bodies.

ELIGIBILITY FOR HEALTHCARE

With many of the patients in the UK now coming from sub-Saharan Africa, the issue of eligibility for medical treatment and social support is encountered more frequently. As the legislation in this area is subject to constant review, readers are advised to check with the appropriate authority and advocacy group. Eligibility for medical care is generally based upon residence rather than nationality, but the rules are complex. It can be an area where health professionals find that regulations are in conflict with personal ethical beliefs.

Management of common physical symptoms

Many of the symptoms in advanced HIV infection are similar to those seen in malignant disease (Table 14.1). The principles of symptom control are identical and an understanding of the likely pathophysiology allows selection of the most appropriate management. Ideally, treatment should be holistic, tailored to the individual with frequent review of benefits, side effects and the wishes of the patient. However, there is increased risk of drug toxicities (from long term combination antiretroviral medication) and of drug interactions.

Table 14.1 Common physical symptoms in AIDS [7].

Symptom	Patients (%)
Pain	60
—Neuropathic	22
—Pressure sore	12
—Visceral	10
—Headaches	8
—Epigastric/retrosternal	7
—Joint	7
—Myopathic	5
—Anorectal	4
General debility	61
Anorexia	41
Nausea	21
Confusion	29
Diarrhoea	18
Dyspnoea	11

Perhaps inevitably, some patients comment that their symptom control needs are not addressed in HIV clinics, where the emphasis is on their immunological response to treatment rather than their quality of life [10]. With the increasing complexity of antiretroviral medication, some patients perceive less time is available to them in busy and over-pressured clinics. Nevertheless, it is easy for patients to end up taking medication prescribed by several different clinicians—and in some cases without full awareness or adequate communication between the physicians involved. Time spent reviewing the patient's medication can reduce toxicity, interactions, adverse-effects and overall costs.

PAIN

Pain in HIV disease is common—and frequently both underestimated and under medicated [11, 12], particularly in women, less educated patients and injecting drug users. Pain is more common as the disease progresses. Common pain syndromes associated with HIV infection often involve the GI tract, nervous system (e.g. peripheral neuropathy) or the musculoskeletal system. The principles of pain control are similar to those in cancer care, based upon the World Health Organisation's three-step analgesic ladder (see Chapter 8).

PAINFUL NEUROPATHY

Peripheral nerve disorders are among the most common problems encountered, with a predominantly sensory polyneuropathy—generally distal and symmetrical—being most problematic. HIV itself may be responsible, but many of the nucleoside analogues (particularly stavudine and zalcitabine) can be responsible, due to inhibition of mitochondrial DNA-polymerase. Other causes (nutritional deficiencies such as vitamin B_{12}, pyridoxine or thiamine, diabetes, hypothyroidism, syphilis and other drugs—including vincristine, isoniazid and dapsone) should be excluded by appropriate investigation, and diagnosis can be confirmed by nerve conduction studies—which show abnormal sensory nerve amplitude and conduction velocity. However, in many centres this investigation is only available after a significantly long wait; analgesia should not be delayed waiting for this to take place.

Peripheral neuropathy may present as continuous or episodic pain, sometimes associated with an exaggerated pain response to other stimulus such as touch (clothes, bed covers, etc). Patients generally report the nature of the pain using terms such as 'burning', 'stabbing', 'aching' or 'cramping'.

Management of peripheral neuropathy (if simple analgesia has failed) often starts with tricyclic agents such as amitryptiline or lofepramine (which has fewer anti-cholinergic side effects). The dose may need to be increased gradually every 4–7 days—and the patient will need to be specifically reassured that the use of a drug that is also an antidepressant does not indicate that the physician feels that the patient is imagining the pain. If the patient fails to tolerate tricyclic antidepressants, or pain relief is inadequate, one normally considers anticonvulsants. However, both carbamazepine and phenytoin are contraindicated due to drug interactions, leaving gabapentin as the agent in most use, as it is generally well tolerated and has no interactions with antiretrovirals. Doses are generally the same as those used for epilepsy, but again careful dose titration is the general approach, since some patients will have tolerability problems. If using gabapentin, a starting dose of 300 mg once daily can be increased up to 2400 mg in gradual increments of 300 mg. Some palliative care physicians may take the daily dose up to 3600 mg.

Individual responses are variable in terms of agents, doses and serum levels. You should be open with your patient about the 'trial and error' nature of the approach and be prepared to monitor them regularly for benefits and side effects. The most common reasons for failure to achieve adequate pain control include early termination of treatment because of side effects from increasing the dose too quickly, starting at too high a dose or failure to reach a sufficient dose for that individual (yet with minimal adverse effects).

Some patients may benefit from a combination of tricyclic agents and anticonvulsants. In resistant peripheral neuropathy, specialist advice should be sought. Sometimes anti-arrythmics such as mexilitine may be considered. Finally, opiates are now used more often in the management of peripheral neuropathy than in the past, despite concerns about their use in patients who may live with the condition for many years. Methadone in particular, due to its wide range of receptor affinity, appears to be more effective than other opioids, and at relatively low doses (5 mg twice daily is often sufficient).

Topical agents including capsaicin and lidocaine can be of benefit in a few cases, and many physicians also advocate acupuncture.

If adequate relief from the symptoms can be obtained with relative ease, and the precipitating factor seems to have been a nucleoside agent, antiretroviral therapy may be continued without change. However, if the neuropathy is severe, disabling, not amenable to palliation or any combination of these, a change in antiretroviral therapy is desirable.

GASTROINTESTINAL TRACT PAIN

Odynophagia (pain on swallowing) may be caused by infection (e.g. candida or cytomegalovirus) or by malignancy (e.g. lymphoma). Abdominal pain may be caused by infection (such as CMV or MAI) or malignancy. Antiretroviral drugs can cause pancreatitis and constipation is generally drug-induced. Anorectal pain may be due to infection (herpes simplex or abscess), anal fissure or anal carcinoma. In all of these cases, investigation is essential to establish a cause.

NAUSEA AND VOMITING

It is important to establish an underlying cause and treat appropriately. A rational approach to anti-emetics should always be used, according to the emetic stimulus. A single agent is usually effective if this policy is followed, but if a second anti-emetic is necessary, it should be chosen for its different mode of action. Parenteral administration may rarely be necessary for the patient who cannot tolerate oral

Case study

'Tom' is a 32-year-old single man living alone in a flat in west London. Nigerian-born, his family has never fully accepted his homosexuality and relations with his parents are strained. He started on a social work degree but mental health problems (including admissions under the mental health act) have interrupted his studies. He has been HIV positive for 8 years and although he has tried combination antiretroviral drugs on several occasions, the side-effects have been unpleasant and he is unable to tolerate them now. He has made a decision not to try any others and has made this clear in an advance directive (living will). As a result, he is extremely immunocompromised and his weight has gone down from 90 kg to 63 kg.

He is reliant upon his primary care team to support him at home; his analgesia (methadone) and the specific treatment for his disabling neuropathy (gabapentin) are all provided by his GP in close liaison with the local HIV clinic. His GP is also prescribing Co-trimoxazole and Azithromycin which Tom takes as primary prophylaxis to prevent opportunistic infections such as pneumocystis pneumonia (PCP) and mycobacterium avium infection (MAC or MAI). He is supported by his local community nurse specialist who visits him weekly, and he has spent periods in the local hospice for respite care. His HIV clinic has encouraged a close relationship with his primary care team in anticipation of his request to die at home if possible.

medication. Drug-induced nausea is common, and many physicians will routinely prescribe anti-emetics to patients on the initiation of antiretroviral therapy. Other commonly prescribed drugs that may cause nausea include co-trimoxazole and dapsone, both in use as prophylaxis against *pneumocystis pneumonia*.

If the nausea and/or vomiting are associated with gastric stasis, a pro-kinetic drug (such as metoclopramide or domperidone) is most likely to be effective. Cyclizine is more likely to be effective if there is raised intracranial pressure, or vestibular problems, due to its action on the vomiting centre (emetic pattern generator). Haloperidol is the drug of choice for most chemical causes of vomiting (drug-induced, renal failure) as it acts principally on the chemoreceptor zone (area postrema); haloperidol is also useful for its long half-life, and is generally given at bedtime. Finally, levomepromazine reportedly has a broad spectrum of action and may be useful if there are several possible causes—or if other agents have failed.

From time to time, agents such as nabilone or ondansetron are used, but generally under specialist supervision.

DIARRHOEA

Diarrhoea is common. Whereas the cause for the majority of patients with diarrhoea in the early days of the epidemic was chronic infections such as cryptosporidium or microsporidium, for most patients nowadays, the antiretrovirals—especially the protease inhibitors—are the responsible cause. Nevertheless, investigations should always be undertaken to exclude infection, inflammatory bowel disease and/or malignancy in any case of altered bowel habit. Symptomatic treatment is crucial in improving quality of life, controlling hydration and weight loss, and improving adherence to antiretrovirals. Loperamide is effective for most patients; the dose should be flexible and titrated by the patient and physician in partnership. Doses of up to a maximum of 32 mg daily can be used (although this represents 16 tablets/capsules). It is more effective, and has fewer side effects than codeine or co-phenotrope.

Codeine phosphate is useful in those cases where loperamide is not successful, and where pain is an additional factor (at doses of 30–60 mg 4–6 hourly). Very few patients require oral morphine, but this may be used if the first two choices do not succeed. Finally, subcutaneous octreotide can be useful, but under expert guidance.

Other specific HIV related problems

ORAL PROBLEMS

Mouth ulcers and oral candidiasis may cause significant difficulty in eating for some patients. Topical steroids (triamcinolone in orabase or hydrocortisone pellets) may help relieve the painful ulcers, but beware of the possibility that an underlying herpetic infection or malignancy may be present. For some patients with candidiasis, treatment with antiseptic mouthwash and topical nystatin/amphotericin (2–3 hourly) may be sufficient. Others may need a course of oral fluconazole. Gingivitis is also a problem for the immunocompromised, and regular dental supervision is recommended. Hairy oral leukoplakia is a condition caused by Epstein-Barr virus, which results in adherent white lesions—usually on the lateral border of the tongue. A course of aciclovir can be helpful.

RESPIRATORY PROBLEMS

Pneumocystis carinii pneumonia (PCP) remains one of the commonest presentations of previously undiagnosed HIV related immunosuppression. Due to the often insidious onset, early diagnosis can be difficult.

A dry, non-productive cough with significant dyspnoea on exertion is the classic presentation. Unfortunately late presentation is still associated with death. Pneumothorax is a known complication. Cotrimoxazole (or alternative) is effective prophylaxis and should be continued in all patients with a cd4 lymphocyte count less than 200.

Mycobacterium tuberculosis (TB) is very common in this group of patients, and the emergence of multi-drug resistant tuberculosis (MDR-TB) has highlighted the importance of good infection control and the need for optimal adherence to a medication regime. Continued bacterial surveillance and resistance monitoring is also essential. TB should always be considered in any respiratory illness with cough, and the patient needs to be isolated until diagnosis is excluded (generally by smear examination of sputum). Any procedures that induce cough should only be undertaken in properly ventilated sealed areas to prevent spread of infection to others. Directly observed therapy helps compliance–particularly in those with chaotic lifestyles, visual impairment or cognitive difficulties.

Kaposi's sarcoma can cause extensive pulmonary lesions and carries a very poor prognosis. External skin lesions would also be present.

OPHTHALMIC PROBLEMS

Sight-threatening retinitis caused by cytomegalovirus is seen only in the severely immunocompromised, and is relatively uncommon nowadays in the developed world. Significant disability can follow since the damage to the retina is irreversible—and the patient may be at risk of sudden retinal detachment affecting the remaining sight.

Ophthalmic herpes zoster (with dendriform keratitis) and herpes simplex keratitis can also cause serious problems, and advice from an experienced ophthalmologist should be sought at a relatively low threshold.

DERMATOLOGICAL PROBLEMS

Dry skin is very common in HIV infection, and topical emollients (used liberally) are the recommended management. Yeast and fungal infections are also commonly seen and generally managed with topical combination steroid/antifungal preparations. Psoriasis can be more extensive and more aggressive.

Herpes simplex is likely to be more severe, and recurrences more frequent. Oral acyclovir may be given regularly (400 mg twice daily) as prophylaxis. Herpes zoster is also likely to be seen more often than in the immunocompetent and may affect more than one dermatome. Molluscusm contagiosum is caused by a poxvirus and presents as small umbilicated vesicles.

Scabies can be a problem as immunocompromised individuals may often be heavily infected before showing significant signs. Norwegian scabies in particular may be a problem in the institutional setting.

TUMOURS

Kaposi's sarcoma is seen mostly in patients who have acquired HIV sexually. It is caused by infection with the herpes virus KS–HV or HHV–8 and appears as nodular, purplish lesions commonly affecting the face, trunk or limbs. Antiretroviral treatment is generally extremely effective; as the immune system is restored, the lesions regress. Sometimes chemotherapy and/or local radiotherapy may also be necessary.

Non-Hodgkin's Lymphoma is seen significantly more common in those with HIV infection, and is treated with systemic chemotherapy. Prognosis is variable, but better than it was earlier. However, primary cerebral lymphoma is usually associated with an extremely poor prognosis.

NERVOUS SYSTEM

HIV related brain impairment (once known as 'AIDS dementia') is much less commonly seen, thanks to antiretroviral therapy. Progressive multifocal leucoencephalopathy ('PML') is a rapidly progressive condition with extensive cerebral demyelination associated with the reactivation of infection with the JC virus, which carries a very poor prognosis.

Issues relating to medication and HIV/AIDS in palliative care

ANTIRETROVITRAL THERAPY

In 1987 zidovudine (also known as AZT) was the first antiretroviral agent shown to improve survival in patients with AIDS. Now there are seventeen antiretroviral agents (see Table 14.2) licensed for prescription in the UK: seven nucleoside/nucleotide reverse transcriptase inhibitors (nRTIs), six protease inhibitors (PIs), two non-nucleoside reverse transcriptase inhibitors (nnRTIs) and most recently a fusion inhibitor. Clear benefit of combination antiretroviral therapy is now

Table 14.2 Antiretroviral drugs.

Nucleoside reverse transcriptase inhibitors	Protease inhibitors	Non-nucleoside reverse transcriptase inhibitors
Abacavir *Emtricitabine (FTC)* *Didanosine (ddI)* *Lamivudine (3TC)* *Stavudine (d4T)* *Zidovudine (AZT)* *Zalcitabine (ddC)*	*Amprenavir* *Indinavir* *Lopinavir* *Nelfinavir* *Ritonavir* *Saquinavir*	*Efavirenz* *Nevirapine*
Nucleotide reverse transcriptase inhibitor		**Fusion inhibitor**
Tenofovir		*T–20*

well established and even in late-stage disease they can achieve both immunological and clinical benefit with dramatic decline in HIV viral load. Benefit in terms of morbidity and mortality is demonstrated as well as in the immune markers.

Nevertheless, there will always be a small number of people who are diagnosed very late in the course of their HIV infection, or who cannot tolerate the drugs, or who have significant drug resistance, or who do not wish to take them (or any combination of these factors).

TOXICITY OF ANTIRETROVITRAL AGENTS

Long-term use of antiretroviral medication is associated with a number of abnormalities related to lipid metabolism, fat distribution and mitochondrial function. For peripheral neuropathy see earlier. Other problems include:

- Hypercholesterolaemia
- Hypertriglyceridaemia
- Insulin resistance and Type II diabetes
- Body fat loss (face, buttocks, legs)
- Body fat accumulation (abdominal, breast, buffalo hump)

Metabolic sequelae are treated with nutritional advice/support, exercise programmes, lipid regulating agents and diabetic agents, as appropriate. For subcutaneous fat loss, management is often supportive—but the body changes can lead to significant psychological consequences if severe. Injections of polylactic acid are available at some centres to provide bulk to the facial area where fat loss is most prominent and visible. Additionally, osteopenia has been reported in a few patients (and avascular necrosis of the hip).

CORTICOSTEROIDS

Practitioners are often reluctant to prescribe steroids to patients with HIV because of fears that this will accelerate the disease and predispose to opportunistic infections. However, the benefits of steroids in certain situations are clearly established and they may also be helpful in palliating non-specific symptoms by:

- lifting mood;
- reducing fatigue;
- improving anorexia resistant to anabolic steroids;
- acting as an adjuvant anti-emetic for nausea or vomiting;
- promoting weight gain with improved body image;
- modulating fever associated with HIV *per se*, lymphoma, or *Mycobacterium avium* complex (MAC) infection;
- reducing the oedema and pain from visceral Kaposi's sarcoma (KS);
- acting as an adjuvant to analgesia for patients with painful neuropathy or myopathy.

Short courses at a higher dose probably give more benefit than prolonged low-dose treatment. Patients need to be aware of the potential side-effects and offered an initial trial of treatment.

OPIOID MEDICATION

There is often concern about prescribing opioids for pain when treating patients with a current or previous history of drug abuse, and pain may be under-treated for this reason. In all stages of HIV, control of pain must be a priority. Additionally, patients who have been on maintenance methadone for many years are sometimes fearful of changing to an alternative opioid. For such a patient in pain the choices are:

1 To continue same dose of methadone and *add* morphine or some other opioid as an analgesic.

2 To increase dose of methadone: using it for both 'maintenance' and analgesia.

There is little evidence about the comparative efficacy of these methods but probably the first is the most satisfactory. Although the

GP may be prescribing both methadone maintenance and opioid analgesia, it is important that the patient is clear about the difference between the two.

Methadone equivalence with other opioids can be difficult to calculate owing to the comparatively longer half-life and broad-spectrum receptor affinity. Therefore a single 5-milligram dose may be equivalent to 7.5-milligrammes of morphine, but when given repeatedly, it may be 5–10 times more potent, gram for gram, than morphine [13].

The use of the additional opioid for *analgesia* should be fully discussed and clear guidelines, boundaries and a plan for review unambiguously drawn up with the patients and their carers and other professionals involved in the patient's care in order to prevent abuse. Many of these patients exhibit remarkable opioid tolerance and sometimes pain control may be achieved and maintained only with what may appear to be an alarmingly high opioid dose. Appropriate antiemetic and laxative agents should always be prescribed and, if needed, sedative agents.

Lastly, some drug users come from families where substance abuse is common, and times of stress, such as a relative dying, may precipitate excesses of drugs and/or alcohol with unpredictable behaviour during visits. Setting clear guidelines on visiting—both in the home and in the hospital/ hospice—and giving frequent and clear explanations about the patient's treatment plans and condition are crucial to avoid unpleasant confrontations around the dying patient.

Drug interactions

The antiretroviral drugs affect hepatic metabolism of many other drugs (either through inhibition or induction of the CYP3A/ cytochrome P450 pathway). For full up-to-date information, the reader is referred to the web site of Liverpool University (http:// www.hiv-druginteractions.org/) or the British National Formulary. Some important interactions concern nevirapine and methadone (reduction in methadone levels can lead to withdrawal syndrome in some patients), and drugs such as fluconazole, itraconazole, ergotamine derivatives, cisapride, phenytoin, phenobarbital and carbamazepine—all of which are contraindicated with various antiretrovirals. Finally, there are potential interactions with herbal remedies (including St John's Wort and Echinacea) that can affect the potency of antiretroviral drugs.

Complementary therapy

Acupuncture, aromatherapy, reflexology and massage can all be very beneficial for specific symptoms, as well as the general well being of a person living with symptomatic HIV infection. Many involve hands-on therapy with human contact that is much valued by the client—and the consultation time is often longer than that of the traditional services.

The end of life

In many cities, certain undertakers have established a good reputation for sensitivity in handling HIV related deaths. Patient support/advocacy groups or local HIV units should be able to give advice on this. There are no agreed guidelines on the use of body bags and practice varies considerably according to local practice. There is no reason why a body bag should be necessary for deaths in the community—apart from other considerations, the undertaker is very often not aware of the cause of death or the underlying illness.

Death certification

In the United Kingdom death certification continues to be a contentious issue largely for the reasons that a death certificate is a public document [13]. At the same time the law requires doctors to provide factual information—where available—about the cause of death. Add to this the fact that a doctor's duty of confidentiality to the patient continues beyond his or her death and it can be seen that several dilemmas can occur at this particularly sensitive time. Anticipation is the key.

Death certificates are problematic if, for example, surviving sexual partners or family members do not want to reveal that their relative has died from an HIV-related cause. In practice, many doctors at many treatment centres and hospices do not write HIV or AIDS on death certificates, but tick the box on the back of the certificate indicating that they can provide further information in confidence.

Unfortunately, this may not be 'best practice'. Where a doctor knows that HIV infection or AIDS has contributed to the death of the patient then this information must be stated on the certificate, whatever the views of the patient and/or family [14].

It must also be remembered that such documentation is also critical for HIV/AIDS statistics and ultimately public health—so it is everyone's duty to provide this whenever possible.

Where people die?

Since the early 1990s, the improved prognosis (in a relatively young group of patients) has naturally led to a more aggressive approach to treatment of those who become ill. Although the proportion of those who die in hospice has not changed significantly, fewer deaths occur at home, with more deaths occurring in an acute hospital setting.

Suicide

Suicide is reportedly more common in populations with AIDS than other terminal illnesses and much greater in those with inadequately treated pain [15]. However, it appears that much of this morbidity was present prior to an HIV or AIDS diagnosis.

Advance directives

Advance directives ('living wills') were once common in this group of patients [7]. However, nowadays, with the greatly improved prognosis, clinicians rarely address the issue in the early stages of infection. Many patients will, however, welcome the chance to discuss their desired level of medical intervention. Further advice and sample templates are still available from the Terence Higgins Trust.

Bereavement

Carers, family, friends and professionals may be at risk of difficult and abnormal grief in relation to deaths from HIV and AIDS. Chapter 7 discusses in detail the identification of risk factors and the prevention of problems. Table 14.3 gives a synopsis of risk factors associated with abnormal or a protracted bereavement process (taking into account that this is often such a personal issue that defining is normally difficult).

Conclusion

Defining the role of palliative care for people living with HIV and AIDS will always be a challenge as the advances in antiretroviral therapy bring an increase in life expectancy, yet associated drug toxicities and other problems connected with chronic illness. The divisions between aggressive/curative medical care and supportive/palliative care

Table 14.3 Risk factors for difficult bereavement in AIDS related deaths.

Multiple loss experiences
History of alcohol and drug abuse
Bereaved may also be ill
Denial of status as a lover/partner
Social isolation
Stigma of the disease
Stigma of their lifestyle
Undisclosed diagnosis
Family rejection
Anger
Powerlessness

are frequently unclear, and in most cases overlap. In the future, the extended survival and the importance of quality of life as well as length of life, places a different importance on the need to optimise symptom control for those living with HIV.

References

1 Gibb DM, Duong T, Tookey PA. Decline in mortality, AIDS, and hospital admissions in perinatally HIV-1 infected children in the United Kingdom and Ireland. *Brit Med J* 2003; 327: 1019–1024.
2 http://www.unaids.org: the website for the United Nations' fight against HIV infection and AIDS.
3 Kikule E A good death in Uganda: survey of needs for palliative care for terminally ill people in urban areas. *Brit Med J* 2003; 327: 192–194.
4 Sepulvida C, Habiyambere V, Amandua J et al. Quality care at the end of life in Africa. *Brit Med J* 2003; 327: 209–213.
5 Health Protection Agency, SCIEH, ISD, National Public Health Services for Wales, CDSC Northern Ireland and the UASSG. Renewing the focus. HIV and other sexually transmitted infections in the United Kingdom in 2002. London: Health Protection Agency, November 2003.
6 Singh S, Dunford A, Carter Y. Routine care of people with HIV infection and AIDS: should interested general practitioners take the lead? *BJGP* 2001: 51; 399–403.
7 Selwyn PA, Rivard M, Kappell D, et al. Palliative care for AIDS. *J Palliat Med*, 2003; 6(3), 475–487(13).
8 Sims R, Moss VA. *Palliative Care for People with AIDS*, 2nd edition. London: Arnold, 1995.
9 General Medical Council (Sept 2000): *Confidentiality: Protecting and Providing Information*. London, UK.
10 Cox S, Pickhaver K. The changing face of palliative care for AIDS. *Eur J Palliat Care*, 2002; 9(6).

11 Larue F, Fontaine A, Colleau SM. Underestimation and undertreatment of pain in HIV disease: multicentre study. *BMJ* 1997; 314: 23–28.
12 Breithcart W, Rosenfeld BD, Passik SD, et al. The undertreatment of pain in ambulatory AIDS patients. *Pain* 1996; 65: 243–249.
13 Twycross R, Wilcock A, eds. *Symptom Management in Advanced Cancer*, 3rd edition. Oxford: Radcliffe Medical Press, 2001.
14 *Guidelines and Best Practice for Referring Deaths to the Coroner*. February 2000. London UK: Coroner for Inner South District Greater London.
15 Sherr L. ed. *Grief and AIDS*. Chichester: Wiley, 1995.

Further reading

Brettle RP, Bisset K, Burns S et al. Human immunodeficiency virus and drug abuse: the Edinburgh experience. *Brit Med J* 1987; 294: 421–424.
Gazzard B ed. *AIDS Care Handbook* 2nd edition. London, UK: Mediscript, 2002.
Harding R, Stewart K., Marconi K et al. Current HIV/AIDS end-of-life care in sub-Saharan Africa: a survey of models, services, challenges and priorities. *BMC Public Health* 2003; 3: 33.
Healing TD, Hoffman PN, Young SEJ. The infection hazards of human cadavers. *Commun Dis Rep* 1995; 5.
Miller R., Murray D. *Social Work and HIV/AIDS–Practitioner's Guide*. Birmingham UK: Venture Press, 1998.
Pratt R. *HIV & AIDS — A Strategy for Nursing Care*, 4th edition. London, UK: Edward Arnold, 1995.
Quinn TC. Global burden of the HIV pandemic. *Lancet* 1996; 348: 99–106.
Sherr L ed. (1995) *Grief and AIDS*. Chichester: Wiley.
Singh S., Madge S. *Caring for People with HIV: A Community Perspective*. UK: Ashgate Publications, 1999.
UK Department of Health. *Guidance for Clinical and Health Care Workers: Protection Against Infection with HIV and Hepatitis Viruses*. London: HMSO, 1990.
Wood CGA, Whittet S, Bradbeer C. ABC of palliative care: HIV infection and AIDS. *BMJ* 1997; 315: 1433–1436 (29 November).

Appendix

What are universal infection control precautions?

Universal Infection Control Precautions means taking precautions with everybody. If the same precautions are taken by everyone, health care workers do not have to make assumptions about people's lifestyles and risk of infection. Health care workers have the right to be able to protect themselves against infection, whether it is HIV or Hepatitis.

The following universal infection control precautions are advised in the UK to help protect health care workers from blood-borne infections including HIV.

The following should be carried out for protection against any infection:

- Always wear gloves when handling blood and other body fluids.
- If you have cuts or other abrasions then cover them with a waterproof plaster.
- Mop up blood spills using gloves and paper towels and wash with either detergent or a chlorine solution made from NaDCC (sodium dichloroisocyanurate) tablets. For large spillages NaDCC granules should be available. An alternative is to use a 1% solution of sodium hypochlorite.
- 'Spill Kits' containing the above items may also be available in some districts for use in the community. In instances where NaDCC tablets are not available, diluted household bleach should be used.
- In hospital settings all linen with blood on it should be sealed in a water-soluble bag. This should then be placed in a red marked bag and labelled according to hospital procedures. Linen contaminated in the community should be washed on a hot wash cycle (approx. 70 degrees). If a machine is not available, contact should be made with the Infection Control Department.
- In domestic settings pads, sanitary wear and disposable nappies should be (double) wrapped in polythene bags and put in a lidded bin away from children, or put in an incinerator where available. Hands should be washed before and after changing nappies, or disposable gloves should be used.
- Terry nappies and protective plastic pants should be washed as normal (soaked in a bucket with nappy cleanser, rinsed and washed with hot water and detergent).

For further information

- HIV and AIDS: information and guidance in the occupational setting, http://www.hpa.org.uk/infections/topics_az/hiv_and_sti/hiv/occupational.htm
- HIV Post-Exposure Prophylaxis: Guidance from the UK Chief Medical Officers' Expert Advisory Group on AIDS, Department of Health, July 2000 (also accessible via the above web-site www.hpa.org.uk).

15: Palliative Care for Children

KEITH SIBSON, FINELLA CRAIG
AND ANN GOLDMAN

Introduction

The death of a child is recognized as one of the greatest tragedies that can happen to a family. The family's grief and distress are intense and long lasting and, now that death in childhood is so uncommon, parents can experience considerable isolation. In the developed world, parents' expectations and plans barely even acknowledge the possibility of a child dying and society as a whole has become unfamiliar and uncomfortable with death in childhood and the ways to offer support. This includes medical and nursing staff too, who are affected not only emotionally but often also by their lack of experience and confidence.

This chapter can only offer an overview of paediatric palliative care. It will identify the children for whom palliative care is appropriate, discuss some of their needs, particularly where these differ from the needs of adults, and consider how services can be provided for them. The aim of this chapter is to provide an insight into the problems of the sick child and their family, and to encourage those caring for the child to work together and with the family to provide as good a quality of life as possible.

Children needing palliative care

The nature of children needing palliative care differs significantly from that of adults and the number of anticipated deaths is very much smaller. Recent data indicate figures higher than those previously estimated. The annual mortality rate for children aged 0–19 with life-limiting conditions is 1.5–1.9 per 10 000 and the prevalence of such children requiring palliative care is 12–17 per 10 000 [1]. In a health district of 250 000 people, with a child population of 50 000, in any one year there will be 60–85 children known to have a life-limiting condition, of whom eight are likely to die: three from cancer, two from heart disease and three from other conditions [1].

Table 15.1 Main life-limiting conditions in childhood.

Malignant diseases
Severe cerebral palsy
Degenerative disorders
Inborn errors of metabolism
Neurodegenerative diseases
Cystic fibrosis
Duchennes muscular dystrophy
Organ failures
Heart
Liver
Kidney
HIV/AIDS

The range of life-limiting conditions that affect children is wide (Table 15.1). Palliative care needs to be considered for all these children, not just those with cancer. Most of the illnesses are specific to paediatrics and many are very rare; some are familial and many have a protracted course. Four broad groups can be identified [1]:

- Life-threatening conditions where curative treatment may be possible but may fail. Palliative care is needed in times of prognostic uncertainty or when cure becomes impossible. Cancer is an example.
- Conditions where there are long periods of intensive treatment aimed at prolonging life, but premature death is still inevitable. Cystic fibrosis and AIDS fit this pattern.
- Progressive conditions where treatment is entirely palliative and may extend over many years. Neurodegenerative diseases and many inborn errors of metabolism are examples.
- Irreversible but non-progressive conditions causing severe disability, such as severe cerebral palsy. These can lead to a susceptibility to health complications and the likelihood of premature death.

Providing services for the family

Paediatric palliative care is very much an evolving speciality, still defining and researching both the clinical care the children need and the best way to provide services. Significant developments have been made over the past few years in terms of service provision, with an increase not only in the number of specialist medical and nursing posts but also in children's hospices and community teams providing paediatric palliative care. At present, however, the care and support for children with life-limiting illnesses continues to be provided by a variety of professionals who have acquired their skills and knowledge in several different ways. It remains vitally important that the needs of each child and family are considered individually, both in the context of the illness and of what is available locally.

Accessing the services

When a child is diagnosed with a life-threatening illness, the family rapidly learns a great deal about the disease and its management. For some children, especially if the disorder is uncommon and/or intensive treatments are needed, care may seem to focus around in-patient or out-patient hospital management. Families may build up very close relationships with various members of the hospital staff and can become heavily reliant on them.

As a consequence of this, the primary health care team can easily feel superfluous and marginalised. This is exacerbated by the fact that most family doctors will see relatively few children with life-limiting illnesses, each of whom is likely to have a different, rare and complex illness. It is therefore difficult for the family doctor to gain experience and confidence in paediatric palliative care, and to define his or her role in the care of such a child. This can be misinterpreted by the family as lack of interest and concern, thereby perpetuating the lack of contact with the primary care team.

For other disorders, frequent hospital contact is unnecessary. This can lead to the contrasting situation of a child with long-term illness being cared for at home by the family, with very little or no hospital input. Here the primary health care team may at times feel overwhelmed, abandoned and unsupported by the hospital services.

Since most children and families prefer to spend as much time as possible at home, the active involvement of the primary health care team is vital. It is essential that the primary care team receives support from professionals with experience in paediatric palliative care as well as professionals with knowledge and experience of the child's underlying disorder.

Organisation of services

As stated, there are usually a number of professionals from different disciplines involved in a child's care, especially if the illness is prolonged over a number of years. It is therefore important to identify one member from this group of professionals to act as the key worker for the child and family, facilitating good communication and co-ordination of professional care. This ensures that all the family's needs are being met, without overlap or gaps developing, which minimises the chance of any part of the team becoming marginalised. In most situations the professional who fulfils this role most effectively is a nurse.

One established model of paediatric palliative care is for children with cancer. Here the child's care is likely to be shared between a children's cancer centre some distance from where they live, their local paediatric department and care at home. Paediatric oncology outreach nurse specialists are usually hospital based, but travel out into the community when required. They offer expertise and experience in symptom management, as well as psychosocial support. When the child is at home they liaise closely with the local paediatric community nurses and primary health care teams, who in turn provide most of the ongoing medical and nursing care of the child.

Children with other life-limiting diseases, especially those with a prolonged course where care is mainly home-based, have traditionally had less well-structured provisions for care. However, increasing numbers of districts have now developed multidisciplinary teams built up from local staff (e.g. community paediatricians, nurses, social workers, therapists and psychologists) who devote part of their time to providing appropriate palliative care for such children. Additionally, some specific paediatric palliative care nursing posts, as well as full teams, have been funded over recent years. However, there is still no uniformity of service provision throughout the United Kingdom; hence the service available to a child and family remains, to some extent, dependent on geographical location. There is still a risk that families may be either neglected or the focus of inappropriate or uncoordinated help.

Children's hospices

A number of children's hospices contribute to the facilities available. In the United Kingdom there were 27 children's hospices in 2003, with a further 10 in the planning stages [1, 2]. These are all charitable organisations and have developed in response to a perceived need by families, offering a markedly different service from adult hospices [3]. They provide small comfortable 'home-from-home' facilities with accommodation and support for siblings and parents as well as the sick child. They are staffed by those experienced and qualified in the care of children, and have excellent facilities for play, education and nursing support. The majority of children visiting the hospices have prolonged illnesses with considerable nursing needs, for whom respite care is important. Children with cancer are referred less commonly but those with a prolonged illness, such as brain tumours, or families with difficult social circumstances, may find the additional support valuable. Relatively few children die at the hospices as most families choose to be at home. Some families, however, arrange for their child to be moved to the hospice for a period of time after the death, so the child can remain in a cooled bedroom and the family can stay with the child or visit freely. Hospices also offer support through bereavement, even if there has been little contact prior to the death.

Palliative care needs

The principles of palliative care for children are similar to those for adults. The overall needs for children and their families have been summarized in the ACT Charter (Association for Children with life threatening or Terminal conditions and their families) (Figure 15.1) [4].

Location of care

It is important that families are given choices as to where their child is cared for, although most parents prefer to care for their child at home [5]. Other alternatives, such as hospital or hospice care, should be discussed, as for some this will be the preferred choice. Families should be given a realistic idea of what to expect with regard to the needs of their child as they deteriorate and the support that is available. Those who are at home need access to advice and support 24 hours a day and this should be planned so that professionals caring for the child have back-up from others with experience in paediatric palliative care. Families should also be given some flexibility, so they can move between home, hospital and hospice as they choose, without their care being compromised.

Parents bear a heavy responsibility for nursing and personal care of their child, and most take on the burden willingly. However, whilst viewing parents in their role as part of the caring team, it is important to acknowledge their need for support themselves. Siblings are especially vulnerable and their needs must also be considered.

ACT Charter for Children with Life-threatening Conditions and their Families

1 Every child shall be treated with dignity and respect and shall be afforded privacy whatever the child's physical or intellectual ability.

2 Parents shall be acknowledged as the primary carers and shall be centrally involved as partners in all care and decisions involving their child.

3 Every child shall be given the opportunity to participate in decisions affecting his or her care, according to age and understanding.

4 Every family shall be given the opportunity of a consultation with a paediatric specialist who has a particular knowledge of the child's condition.

5 Information shall be provided for the parents, and for the child and the siblings according to age and understanding. The needs of other relatives shall also be addressed.

6 An honest and open approach shall be the basis of all communication which shall be sensitive and appropriate to age and understanding.

7 The family home shall remain the centre of caring whenever possible. All other care shall be provided by paediatrically trained staff in a child-centred environment.

8 Every child shall have access to education. Efforts shall be made to enable the child to engage in other childhood activities.

9 Every family shall be entitled to a named key worker who will enable the family to build up and maintain an appropriate support system.

10 Every family shall have access to flexible respite care in their own home and in a home-from-home setting for the whole family, with appropriate paediatric nursing and technical support.

11 Every family shall have access to paediatric nursing support in the home when required.

12 Every family shall have access to expert sensitive advice in procuring practical aids and financial support.

13 Every family shall have access to domestic help at times of stress at home.

14 Bereavement support shall be offered to the whole family and be available for as long as required.

Association for Children with life threatening or Terminal conditions and their families
65 St Michael's Hill, Bristol, BS2 8DZ Tel: 0117 922 1556 Registered Charity No. 1029659

Fig. 15.1 The Charter of the Association for Children with Life-threatening or Terminal conditions and their families (ACT).

The role of children and families in symptom management

Parents fear the pain and other symptoms that their child may suffer and that they will not have the skills and confidence to relieve them. It is therefore important to provide them with detailed and honest information about the management of their child's current symptoms and any others that may be anticipated. Both they and the sick child need to take an active part in planning a practical and acceptable regimen of care, where possible retaining their confidence and control.

As death approaches parents will need and value further information, including what signs might suggest that death is imminent and the possible modes of death. Professionals can sometimes be reluctant to undertake such frank discussion, but knowing what to expect and having a clear plan of what to do as the situation changes can enable families to cope better. Indeed, it is essential if the child is being cared for at home.

Almost all families can be reassured that death will be peaceful, but if there are concerns about the possibility of sudden distressing symptoms (such as convulsions, acute agitation or bleeding) these should be discussed. The team should ensure that emergency drugs (i.e. anticonvulsants, strong analgesics and powerful sedatives) are available in the house, or are easily accessible if the child is in hospital. Suitable doses via appropriate routes must be calculated ahead of time, so that medication can be given as soon as it is needed. If the child is at home, the medication doses and the route of administration should be such that the parents will be able to give the drugs themselves, although there should always be a professional available who they can contact for additional support.

Symptom management

Many symptoms in palliative care are obviously common to a variety of illnesses. However when a child has an uncommon illness it may be difficult for the local doctor or family to anticipate which particular problems will develop as the disease progresses. Specialist paediatricians and nursing staff with more experience of the particular illness should be able to advise. There are also many disease-specific parent help groups for rare illnesses that offer information and practical advice.

Patterns of symptoms

Children dying from cancer are likely to have a final illness lasting only a few weeks or months, although brain tumours tend to have a more protracted course. These children often experience pain, depending on the site and spread of the tumour. Other problems include gastrointestinal symptoms such as nausea, vomiting and constipation. Bone marrow involvement is common in childhood cancer, so anaemia and bleeding are often concerns. Dyspnoea, anxiety, agitation and seizures may also occur.

In contrast, children with slower degenerative diseases suffer a different spectrum of problems, over a much longer period. Feeding difficulties, impaired intellect and communication, convulsions and poor mobility are common. These increase as the illness progresses and respiratory difficulties and excess secretions may develop. Pain is usually less prominent, although muscle spasms may be troublesome.

Assessment of symptoms

As in adults, thorough assessment of any symptom is essential before developing a plan of management. This can be particularly challenging in children. Since the experience of pain and other symptoms is subjective, ideally children should provide the information about their problems themselves. However, the ability of children to do this will vary in relation to their level of understanding, experience and communication skills. In preverbal children and those with severe developmental delay it can be particularly difficult [6].

The use of a variety of approaches can help towards building up a more complete picture. Firstly, much can be gained from observing a child's behaviour and comparing it to a time when symptoms were absent or different. Parents are particularly adept at this and their opinions should be sought and respected. When it comes to listening to the child, a range of assessment tools for different ages and developmental levels are available, but these are developed specifically for pain. They include body charts, pictures of faces and visual analogue scales [7]. Play specialists can also help to uncover a child's symptoms with the use of toys, puppets, art and music. The team should remember that psychological and social factors affecting the child and family are often significant and are an important part of the assessment (Table 15.2).

Making a plan

When planning treatment the preferences of the child and family need to be taken into account. Many find that taking a lot of medication is difficult, so complex regimens may not be possible. It is important to find the most acceptable route for the child and to be flexible to changing situations. The key issues in deciding on routes of administration are as follows:

- the oral route is often preferable;
- long-acting preparations are more convenient and less intrusive;
- the child should be allowed to choose between liquids and whole or crushed tablets;

Table 15.2 Assessing a child's pain.

Watch the child	
• Non-specific, but often enlightening;	
• Behavioural changes	– Crying, screaming, irritable, aggressive, head banging – Clinging, quiet, withdrawn, frightened look, reluctant to move
• Physiological changes	– Increased heart rate/respiratory rate/BP – Decreased saturations, change in colour, sweating
Ask the child	
• Difficult, dependent on age/developmental level/contributory factors	
• Use play, puppets, drawings, music (play specialists)	
• Specific assessment tools:	
• 3 years up	– Faces scales (e.g. Bieri, Wong & Baker, Oucher)
• School age	– Visual analogue scale (straight line, +/– numbers) – Colour body chart (different colours for different pains)
• Older child	– Any of the above – Numerical rating scales – Direct questioning
Ask the parents	
• They know their child the best	
• But they may lack confidence in their own assessment	
Consider contributory factors	
• Coping skills of the child and family	
• Past experience of the child and family	
• Anxiety and emotional distress levels in the child and family	
• Meaning of the pain and underlying disease to the child and family	

- as a child's condition deteriorates the treatment plan often has to be simplified, routes of administration altered, and priority given to those drugs that contribute most to the child's comfort;
- although rectal drugs are not popular in paediatrics, they can play a role; some children prefer them to using any needles, and they may be helpful in the final hours when the child's level of consciousness has deteriorated;
- if parenteral drugs are needed they are usually given by continuous subcutaneous infusion, not as bolus doses; alternatively an intravenous line can be used if it is already in place;
- intramuscular drugs are painful and not necessary.

Doses of drugs for children are usually calculated according to their weight. Generally neonates tend to need reduced doses relative to their size, whilst infants and young children may need comparatively higher doses and at shorter intervals than adults. Many of the drugs used in palliative care have not been recommended formally for use in children but a body of clinical experience has developed in the absence of many trials or extensive pharmacokinetic data [8]. In addition there are now several paediatric drug formularies available, the most widely used having been produced by the Royal College of Paediatrics and Child Health [9].

It should be remembered that medication is only one aspect of symptom management. Other simple measures include:

- care over positioning;
- maintaining a calm environment;
- distraction, imagery and relaxation techniques;
- play, art and music therapy.

Explaining the reason for the symptom and discussing a logical step-wise approach to management can also be extremely helpful, reassuring the child and family that the situation is not out of control. Adopting a holistic approach that addresses the psychological, social and spiritual concerns of the child and family is likely to achieve better symptom management than medication alone.

Pain

After thorough assessment of pain, a treatment regimen can be planned. This should consider the likely cause of the pain and whether this can be relieved by specific measures (e.g. radiotherapy for an isolated bony metastasis or antibiotics for a urinary tract infection). Symptomatic relief can be addressed by combining pharmacological, psychological and practical approaches, as discussed previously. Whilst analgesics often form the backbone to a plan, this combined approach is likely to be more successful.

The WHO ladder of analgesia is widely adopted for children, although recent evidence has shed some doubt on the routine use of codeine. Up to 10% of the population in the UK may be poor metabolisers of the drug (compared to morphine) rendering it of little or no benefit to them, whilst there may be very low efficacy in infants due to their immature enzyme systems [10].

Strong opioids

These are used extensively in managing pain in paediatric palliative care. When prescribing strong opioids for children, the following points should be borne in mind:

- long-acting morphine preparations are effective and particularly convenient;
- families should also have a short-acting preparation for breakthrough pain;
- where oral administration is difficult or impossible, the use of transdermal patches (e.g. fentanyl) has proved invaluable [11];
- if oral or transdermal routes are not appropriate, diamorphine is the drug of choice for subcutaneous/intravenous infusion due to its superior solubility;
- some children may have sudden onset of severe pain and may need breakthrough analgesia with a faster onset of action than oral morphine; for older children, fentanyl lozenges can fulfil this role, although they should be encouraged to try not to swallow the drug [12];
- studies of the pharmacokinetics of oral opioids and their metabolites suggest that in young children metabolism is more rapid than in adults and they may require relatively higher doses for analgesia;
- neonates and infants under 6 months of age, however, require a lower starting dose of opioids because of their reduced metabolism and increased sensitivity [8].

Side effects of opioids

Many doctors lack experience of using strong opioids in children, which often leads to unnecessary caution, under-dosing and inadequate pain control. Respiratory depression with strong opioids however, is not usually a problem in children with severe pain. In addition, side effects from opioids tend to be less marked than in adults. Nausea and vomiting are rare and routine antiemetics are not needed.

Constipation is probably the most common side effect and regular laxatives should always be prescribed. For some children relatively mild laxatives such as lactulose may be sufficient, but the majority will require a stimulant in addition to a softener.

Some children are initially quite sleepy after starting on opioids and parents should be warned about this or they may fear that the child's disease has suddenly progressed and that death is imminent. The drowsiness usually resolves within a few days. Itching may occur with morphine in the first few days but it is less common and if it occurs, it may respond to antihistamines. If either the somnolence or the pruritus remain troublesome, switching to fentanyl or hydromorphone (or a combination of the two) is usually effective [13].

Parental concerns over opioids

Parents may be reluctant for their child to have strong opioids. It is important to establish exactly what their concerns are, particularly as children can often be aware of their parents' reluctance and may, as a consequence, under-report their pain. Parents may be anxious about the side effects in which case it will be helpful to reassure them that these too can be treated. They may also be worried that if opioids are started 'too early' there will be nothing left for later. In such a situation it would be necessary to explain that there is no upper dose limit to strong opioids, and that other medications are available to treat different types of pain.

However, another common difficulty for parents is the feeling that by agreeing to start opioids they are acknowledging that their child is really going to die. They may even be concerned that this step represents them as giving up hope—something they would find unacceptable. This clearly requires sensitive discussion and support. It may be helpful to explain that death is unlikely to be imminent, and to gently encourage them to focus again on the immediate needs of the child. With this, in the vast majority of cases, their perception will change such that their child can again receive the analgesia that he or she requires.

Musculoskeletal pain

Non-steroidal anti-inflammatory drugs (NSAIDs) are often helpful for musculoskeletal pains, especially in children with non-malignant disease. Some caution is needed in children with cancer who have bone marrow infiltration because of the increased risk of bleeding. Selective Cox 2 inhibitors may be useful in such situations but there is no published data yet to support this practice in paediatrics. Meanwhile bisphosphonates are beginning to be used for the treatment of bony pain due to malignancy. Oral chemotherapy can also be of benefit in this situation.

Headaches

Headaches from central nervous system leukaemia respond well to intrathecal methotrexate. Headaches from raised intracranial pressure, associated with progressive brain tumours, are best managed with gradually increasing analgesics. Although steroids may seem helpful initially, the symptoms will inevitably recur as the tumour increases in size and a spiral of increasing steroid doses will then develop. The side effects of steroids in children almost always outweigh the benefits [14]. There is an increase in appetite (at a time when feeding may be difficult), dramatically changed appearance and often marked mood swings. Both parents and the children themselves find these symptoms distressing.

Other forms of pain

Neuropathic pain can often be helped by antiepileptic and antidepressant drugs. For severe pain unresponsive to these drugs, epidurals and nerve blocks may be considered. Painful dystonia or muscle spasms may improve with baclofen +/or diazepam. Treatment of possible gastro-oesophageal reflux should also be considered in such patients having episodes of pain associated with abnormal posturing, as reflux can mimic dystonia and is very common in patients with neurodevelopmental abnormalities. Physiotherapists and occupational therapists may also be able to help reduce this pain using exercises, positioning and physical aids.

FEEDING

For mothers and fathers, an inability to feed and to nourish their child is very upsetting and often makes them feel they are failing as parents. Also, sucking and eating are an essential part of a child development, providing comfort, pleasure and stimulation. Children with neurodegenerative diseases and brain tumours often have problems with eating because of neurological damage. Others, such as those with cancers, will lose their appetite. Nutritional goals aimed at restoring health often become secondary to comfort and enjoyment. Assisted feeding, via a nasogastric tube or gastrostomy, may be the entirely correct choice for those with slowly progressive disease, but inappropriate for a child with a rapidly progressing tumour.

NAUSEA AND VOMITING

These are quite frequent problems in a variety of diseases. As in adults, antiemetics can be selected according to their site of action and the presumed cause. Ondansetron, which is very helpful in the cancer patient undergoing chemotherapy, becomes far less useful in the palliative phase. Vomiting from raised intracranial pressure often responds well to cyclizine, while hyoscine patches are very useful in the child who cannot tolerate drugs enterally.

SEIZURES

Watching a child have a seizure is extremely frightening for parents and they should always be warned and advised about its management if there is any possibility that this may happen. Children with neurodegenerative diseases often develop seizures as part of their ongoing disease and will already be taking long-term anticonvulsants. These can be adjusted when the pattern of seizures changes. Sudden acute onset of seizures can be treated with rectal diazepam or, if the child or parents prefer, buccal midazolam. This has now been extensively studied in children and found to be at least as effective as rectal diazepam, well tolerated and highly acceptable to families [15]. Unfortunately at present syrup formation is not widely available so the parents need to be shown in advance how to draw up the i.v. preparation. Repeated severe or continuous seizures in a terminally ill child can be treated at home with a continuous subcutaneous infusion of midazolam, adding phenobarbital if necessary.

AGITATION AND ANXIETY

Agitation and anxiety may reflect a child's need to talk about his or her fears and distress (see below). In addition, drugs such as benzodiazapines, haloperidol, and levomepromazine may provide relief, especially in the final stages of life. These can be given via a variety of routes, as outlined previously.

RESPIRATORY SYMPTOMS

Dyspnoea, cough and excess secretions can all cause distress to children and anxiety for their parents. If the underlying cause of the symptom can be relieved, even temporarily, this may be appropriate. Palliative radiotherapy, for example, can bring good symptomatic relief to some children with malignant disease in the chest.

Where treatment of the underlying cause is unlikely to be beneficial, symptom relief can be addressed by combining drugs with practical and supportive approaches. Fear is often an important element in dyspnoea, and reassurance and management of anxiety may help to relieve symptoms. Simple practical measures such as finding the optimum position, using a fan and relaxation exercises may all help. The sensation of breathlessness can be relieved with opioid drugs, and small doses of sedatives such as diazepam or midazolam are often helpful in relieving the associated anxiety.

Children with chronic chest diseases causing gradually increasing hypoxaemia may suffer from headaches, nausea, daytime drowsiness and poor-quality sleep. Intermittent oxygen may help relieve these symptoms and can be given relatively easily at home. Children with dyspnoea in the later stages of malignant disease do not usually find oxygen helpful.

Excess secretions are often a problem for children with chronic neurodegenerative diseases as their illness progresses and they become less able to cough and swallow. This may also occur in other terminally ill children as they approach death. Oral glycopyrronium bromide, or hyoscine hydrobromide (given transdermally or subcutaneously) can help to reduce the secretions. Altering the child's position often provides temporary relief, but suction equipment is not usually so helpful.

ANAEMIA AND BLEEDING

The treatment of anaemia in the late stages of a child's life should be directed towards relief of symptoms rather than the level of haemoglobin. Transfusions are only helpful if they make the child feel better and it should be explained to the child and family that there is likely to come a point in the illness where they will stop finding transfusions beneficial. Blood counts are not routinely indicated but are sometimes helpful to support a clinical decision to transfuse.

Florid bleeding (e.g. severe haemoptysis or haematemesis) is extremely frightening for a child, distressing for the carers, and may leave the family with unforgettable painful memories. If this is a serious risk, such as in liver disease, emergency drugs should be readily available and include an appropriate analgesic and sedative, such as diamorphine and midazolam. Correct dosage should be calculated ahead of time and the drugs and syringes immediately accessible either at home or in hospital. In an emergency parents can give these drugs by the buccal route, but must be shown in advance how to administer them.

Many children with malignant diseases have widespread bone marrow infiltration and low platelets, but although petechiae and minor gum bleeding are common, serious bleeding is unusual. Minor gum/nose bleeding can be managed with tranexamic acid, either orally or by direct application to the bleeding point. In general, platelet transfusions are confined to bleeding that is severe or interferes with the quality of life. They are rarely justified solely on the basis of a low platelet count. A child with an established history of bleeding throughout the illness, however, may appropriately be treated with regular platelet transfusions.

Support for the child and family

Support for the child and family begins at the time of diagnosis and continues as the illness progresses, through the child's death and into bereavement. All the family—the sick child, the parents, siblings and the wider family—will be affected by the illness and may need help, both as a family unit and as individuals. A flexible approach, with time to listen and build up relationships, is important. A balance must also be sought in which the child's and the family's problems are recognized but not overemphasized to the point that the family are disabled and their own resources diminished.

Although all families will suffer emotional distress, the majority possess considerable strength and resilience and do find ways to continue to function effectively from day to day. A number of factors have been identified which can help predict a family's capacity to cope, and this knowledge can be helpful in identifying families who may be at extra risk and need particular support (Table 15.3). It is important to be aware of families and family members who have language difficulties or a different cultural approach to illness and death.

Table 15.3 Predicting how well a family will cope.

Positive	Negative
Cohesive family	Over-involved family
Supportive family	Unconnected family
Flexible approach	Rigid approach
Open communication in family	Closed communication in family
Open communication with staff	Closed communication with staff
Good record with past stress	Poor record with past stress
	Previous parental psychopathology
	Concurrent stresses (e.g. single parent, parental strife, financial problems)

AT DIAGNOSIS

The time of diagnosis of a life-threatening illness is one of great turmoil for the family. Their grief begins at this time. The way in which the diagnosis is given has a powerful impact and forms the foundation for communication in the future. The family's expectations and pattern of life are disrupted and, especially if frequent hospital admissions are involved, many practical difficulties arise in day-to-day living. It can be easy for the parents and other children to feel overwhelmed, helpless and out of control. Parents have a great need for information at this time and may value leaflets, contact with other parents in similar situations and links with self-help groups (see Resources and Useful Addresses). The sick children face the trauma of being in hospital and the experience of unpleasant and frightening investigations and treatment. They may be particularly confused as explanations and understanding of what is happening may be delayed whilst parents themselves are just learning about the illness. Some parents may be reluctant to discuss the diagnosis with their children and may need encouragement and help to do so.

AS THE DISEASE PROGRESSES

As the illness progresses the family has to live with the underlying conflict of maintaining some hope and semblance of day-to-day life in spite of persistent uncertainty. The parents may develop depression, anxiety and sleep disturbance although they are often reluctant to speak of these problems unless asked specifically. Marital discord and loss of libido are also common. Parents often find difficulty in handling the children, particularly in maintaining discipline and boundaries for the sick child, and in balancing their time and emotions between the sick child and well siblings [16]. If frequent hospital admissions are involved there are practical problems of travel, separation and finance. If the child has heavy nursing needs, with physical disability and/or developmental delay, the burdens of care can be considerable. Parents may have very little time to themselves or to devote to well brothers and sisters, and the opportunity for some respite care for the sick child, either at home or away from home, becomes essential [1, 17].

The sick child may continue to experience regular hospital visits and treatment, whilst developing increasing symptoms and disability. Trying to encourage as normal a life as possible—maintaining friendships, education and outside activities—within the confines of the illness—is a continual but important struggle. Children themselves are usually surprisingly keen to attend school as much as they can. However, as the illness progresses, extra support, special facilities and home education may need to be introduced.

Most families employ some avoidance and denial as part of their coping strategy, including avoiding discussion and reminders of the illness. This is normal behaviour that helps protect them from extremes of emotion. It allows them to live with the illness and function day to day, whilst coming to understand and recognize the situation gradually. This needs to be recognised and respected; frequent discussions about the disease at this time may prove burdensome rather than supportive. In addition to this, parents often want health professionals to maintain some hope (with them) as long as their child is alive. This has to be expressed in the context of honest information about the progression of the disease, but this is also what parents would expect [18]. However, it can prove very challenging to get the balance right for each individual family.

THE FINAL STAGES

Eventually it becomes clearer that not only is death inevitable but that the time of death is becoming quite close. This may be apparent from gradual deterioration in a long progressive illness or more abruptly, such as after a relapse in cancer. The emotional impact at this time may be dramatic for parents, particularly for those who have held a very positive and 'fighting' approach throughout the treatment. For others it is just a confirmation of what they have dreaded and known was inevitable all along. Sometimes there is a sense of relief that the uncertainty and suffering will soon be over, alongside the distress and sadness.

As well as information and discussion about the child's care, parents need an opportunity to explore their own feelings and express their emotions. They may be able to talk to each other openly and offer each other support, but more often they will cope in different ways and find that the whole experience is so physically and emotionally exhausting that they have little strength left to offer support either to each other or to their other children. Both the parents and well siblings often value the opportunity to talk to someone outside of the immediate family during this time [18, 19].

Many parents have never seen anyone die and will value the opportunity of talking about what may happen at the moment of death.

They also appreciate information about the practical details of what to do after a person has died. Most will have been anticipating the funeral in their mind and are relieved to be able to acknowledge this and make some plans before the child has died.

An important issue at this time for parents is what to discuss with the child who is sick and with their other children. Parents, understandably, are usually reluctant to discuss with their children that they are not getting better from their disease. Their aim in this is to protect their children from fear of death. However, it is clear that children understand and learn about their illness and its implications whether the parents and the professionals encourage it or not [20]. This can go unnoticed as it is common for the *children* to 'protect' their *parents* by keeping their worries to themselves. It is therefore important to provide opportunities for the sick child to discuss what is actually on his or her mind. Parents (and health professionals) can be surprised by the nature of the child's fears: rather than being scared of death per se it is more common that they are scared of situations that they can be genuinely reassured about. That is not to deny that open discussion with children, particularly when death is a real possibility, can be a daunting prospect and very difficult to establish in practice.

Communicating with children must take into consideration their level of understanding about illness and the concept of death [20, 21]. It also will be influenced by the child's previous experiences, the family's style of communication, and their own personal defences. Some approaches to helping families towards a more open and honest pattern of communication include:

- shifting the emphasis from 'telling' to 'listening';
- helping them identify the child's indirect cues as well as obvious questions;
- discovering the child's fears and fantasies;
- maintaining the child's trust through honesty;
- building up the whole picture gradually;
- explaining that communication need not rely on talking-drawings, stories, and play is often more effective and easier for children [22, 23].

In the same way it can be equally difficult for the parents to discuss the seriousness of the situation with their other children. Siblings may feel isolated and left out by their parents and, noticing the differential treatment they are receiving, can come to resent their sick brother or sister. They may also feel less worthy and develop low self esteem as a result. This is less likely if they have opportunities to talk about their feelings and are given honest answers to their questions about what is happening. They also benefit from being involved in the day to day care of their brother or sister, by having a role in planning and attending the funeral and by being allowed to keep some of their sibling's possessions [24, 25].

THE BEREAVED FAMILY

The grief suffered after the loss of a child has been described as the most painful, enduring and difficult to survive, and is associated with a high risk of pathological grief. Parents lose not only the child they have loved, but their hopes for the future and their confidence in themselves as parents. It puts an additional stress on their own relationship and alters the whole family structure. The brothers and sisters who are grieving may continue to feel isolated and neglected as their parents can spare little time or emotion for them.

Ideally the professionals who know the family well and have been involved throughout the sick child's life should continue to be available through their bereavement. Grief is likely to continue over many years, and its depth and persistence is often underestimated. Parents value continuing contact with professionals who have known their child and the opportunity to talk about the child and their grief when others in the community expect them to 'have come to terms with it' [18]. This support, initially more frequent and gradually decreasing, helps facilitate the normal tasks of mourning. Help can be offered for brothers and sisters and information provided about appropriate literature, telephone helplines and support organizations (see Useful Addresses). Most families will not need formal counselling but it is important to be able to recognize when there are signs of abnormal grief that may require referral for specialist help.

CONCLUSIONS

Helping to care for a child with a life-threatening illness, and for the family of such a child, is rarely easy. It presents many challenges both in terms of the professional tasks that may be required and to our own emotional resources. Though the task may seem daunting, families greatly value professionals who stay alongside them throughout their difficult journey, offering practical help and support in an almost intolerable situation. Parents will have a lasting memory of their child's death and as professionals we have the privileged opportunity to make this as good as it can be.

References

1 ACT/RCPCH. *A Guide to the Development of Children's Palliative Care Services*. Update of a Report by the Association for Children with Life- Threatening or Terminal Conditions and Their Families (ACT) and the Royal College of Paediatrics and Child Health (RCPCH). ACT/RCPCH, 2003.
2 ACT. *ACTPACK—Children's Hospices*. Bristol: Association for Children with Life Threatening or Terminal Conditions and Their Families, 1998
3 Dominica F. The role of the hospice for the dying child. *Br J Hosp Med* 1996; 38(4): 334–343.
4 ACT. *ACT Charter*. Bristol: Association for Children with Life Threatening or Terminal Conditions and Their Families, 1998.
5 Goldman A, ed. *Care of the Dying Child*. Oxford: Oxford University Press, 1994.
6 Hunt A, Mastroyannopoulou, Goldman A, Seers K. Not knowing—the problem of pain in children with severe neurological impairment. *I J Nurs Stud* 2003; 40: 171–183.
7 Mathews JR, McGrath PJ, Pigeon H. Assessment and measurement of pain in children. *Pain in Infants, Children and Adolescents*. Baltimore: Williams & Wilkins, 1993: 97–112.
8 McGrath P, Brown S, Collins J. Paediatric palliative medicine . *Oxford Textbook of Palliative Medicine*, 3rd edition. Oxford: Oxford University Press, 2004: 775–797.
9 Royal College of Paediatrics and Child Health. *Medicines for Children*, 2nd edition, 2003.
10 William DG, Hatch DJ, Howard RF. Codeine phosphate in paediatric medicine. *Br J Anaesth* 2001; 86(3): 413–421.
11 Hunt A, Goldman A, Devine T, Phillips M; FEN-GBR-14 Study Group. Transdermal fentanyl for pain relief in a paediatric palliative care population. *Palliat Med* 2001;15(5): 405–412.
12 Wheeler M, Birmingham PK, Dsida RM, Wang Z, Cote CJ, Avram MJ. Uptake pharmacokinetics of the fentanyl oralet in children scheduled for central venous access removal. *Paediatr Anaesth* 2002; 12(7): 594–599.
13 Goodarzi M. Comparison of epidural morphine, hydromorphone and fentanyl for postoperative pain control in children undergoing orthopaedic surgery. *Paediatr Anaesth* 1999; 9(5): 419–422.
14 Watterson G, Goldman A, Michalski A. Corticosteroids in the palliative phase of paediatric brain tumours. *Arch Dis Child* 2002; 86(Suppl 1): A76.
15 Scott RC, Besag FM, Neville BG. Buccal midazolam and rectal midazolam for treatment of prolonged seizures in childhood and adolescence: a randomised trial. *Lancet* 1999; 353 (9153): 623–626.
16 Bluebond-Langner M. *In the Shadow of Illness: Parents and Siblings of the Chronically Ill Child*. Princeton: Princeton University Press, 1996.
17 Miller S. Respite care for children who have complex health care needs. *Paediatr Nurs* 2002; 14(5): 33–37.
18 Laakso H, Paunonen-Ilmonen M. Mothers' experience of social support following the death of a child. *J Clin Nurs* 2002; 11(2): 176–185.
19 Martin TL, Doka KJ. *Men Don't Cry... Women Do: Transcending Gender Stereotypes of Grief*. Philadelphia: Brunner/Mazel, 2000.

20 Bluebond-Langner M. *The Private Worlds of Dying Children.* Princeton NJ: Princeton University Press, 1978.
21 Stevens M. Psychological adaptation of the dying child. *Oxford Textbook of Palliative Medicine*, 3rd edition. Oxford: Oxford University Press, 2004: 799–806.
22 Wellings T. Drawings by dying and bereaved children. *Paediatr Nurs* 2001; 13(4): 30–36.
23 List of age appropriate books: www.winstonswish.org.uk
24 Foster C et al. Treatment demands and differential treatment of patients with cystic fibrosis and their siblings. *Child Care Health Dev* 2001; 27(4): 349–364.
25 Pettle Michael SA, Lansdown RG. Adjustment to death of a sibling. *Arch Dis Child* 1986; (61): 278–283.

16: Palliative Care for Adolescents and Young Adults

DANIEL KELLY AND JACQUELINE EDWARDS

Introduction

> Laura was 15 when she was diagnosed and 19 when she died and during that time she struggled hard with her emotions and matured at an alarming rate leaving her friends behind, as they too struggled to come to terms with her illness—how she desperately fought the treatment and would not allow them to see her ill—she was such a clever actress never allowing many people to see the real Laura—in pain, vomiting, weak, high temperature, mouth full of ulcers—I could go on and on ... [1]

This aim of this chapter is to highlight the particular needs of adolescents and young adults who are faced with a life-threatening illness. It is important to emphasise at the outset that there has been a lack of research and policy developments addressing the needs of this patient group. Attention has only slowly shifted towards the care of those who can no longer be considered children, but who are neither fully independent adults. A recent working party set up to explore this issue concluded:

> "The needs of this age group are specific and different from both children and adults." [2]

The chapter will examine the nature of some of these specific needs to help professionals, families or friends to understand the needs of young people whose lives are shortened by serious illness. It is not our intention to review the medical management of common symptoms that are covered elsewhere. Instead, the emphasis is placed on the *appropriate application* of such interventions—ensuring that the necessary medication is employed in line with the expectations of young people themselves.

Young people facing a serious illness may, for instance, want to maintain some degree of control over their lives—as they become more ill their focus is likely to shrink to involve events and people in their immediate environment. At the same time they will also need help to cope with a number of debilitating symptoms such as pain, breathlessness, nausea and fatigue. A fine balance will need to be struck between becoming dependent on professionals for some things and retaining a degree of independence. A common example of this concerns the provision of analgesia, which may need to be matched with a young person's wish to remain awake for certain visitors or events with special significance. Achieving this balance can challenge even the most experienced parent or health professional, as frustration and exhaustion take their toll. In addition, related concerns such as being able to access appropriate expertise when at home (especially if symptoms suddenly worsen) or having skilled psychological support available when it is needed, are practical concerns that need to be addressed. They assume even greater importance as time is recognised as a valuable resource that cannot be wasted. The challenges of providing effective palliative care for young adults are magnified as their condition deteriorates and they are faced with a range of inter-related physical, emotional and existential needs.

The challenge of providing palliative care for young people

Providing appropriate palliative care for young people presents professionals with a series of complex challenges. Firstly, the dawning realisation that a young person is unlikely to reach adulthood is likely to provoke a crisis. Strong emotions, including anger and disbelief may be expressed by the young persons themselves, as well as by family and friends [3]. The roots of such responses can be traced to social and cultural expectations about death and illness over the lifecourse. Socially, we are poorly prepared to comprehend the death of those who are on the threshold of adulthood, and for whom the future usually holds promise. The focus of the resulting anger and confusion may often be the professionals involved in the young person's care—especially when delays or similarly frustrating events that characterise hospital life combine to provoke the expression of pent-up feelings.

When caring for young people who are very ill, professionals may also experience strong emotional reactions—especially if they have had limited exposure to death in this age group during their career. For some, there may be a risk of over-identifying with the young patient's or the parent's situation as they relate closely to them and their suffering [4]. In such a situation it is easy for personal/professional boundaries to become blurred and some form of debriefing, supervision or staff support should be available [5, 6]. One of the benefits of developing specialist centres for young people (such as teenage cancer units) is that expertise will be developed to deal with the complex issues of death and dying. On the other hand, such centres may be so few in number that the young person has to travel so far that they become further isolated from their friends and family and transference of skills into the community is more limited [7].

Wherever palliative care is provided it is crucial that decisions are taken by involving the patient, family and friends in ways that are meaningful to them. Towards the end of life it is especially important that effective communication is promoted between all members of the health care team to minimise misunderstandings and the frustrations within what is likely to be an already highly emotional situation. This relies on hospital staff passing on the history and care goals to primary care colleagues who will become more closely involved in provision of palliative care. At this stage it is crucial that general practitioners, district nurses, Macmillan nurses and social workers work together to make the final phase of life as acceptable as possible. Importantly, this will require professionals to confront the poignancy of an adolescent or young adult facing the end of their life. An understanding of the underlying psychology of this patient group is, therefore, essential.

In health, the transition from adolescence to young adulthood is characterised by growth, development and the challenging of social norms [8]. The rate of such development varies widely between individuals, however, and is often unpredictable [9]. Particular cognitive functions, such as abstract thinking develop at different rates—as do the physical changes associated with puberty itself. Chronological age, therefore, may not always be the most appropriate indicator of whether a 'young adolescent' with cancer would best be admitted to an adult or paediatric ward for a highly specialised surgical procedure. Similarly, age does not always correspond to physical or cognitive maturity. As the opening quotation suggests, young people facing a life threatening illness often develop wisdom beyond their years, and they can usually detect when professionals are trying to avoid certain topics, or trying to protect them from bad news. Regardless of where such care is provided, the main concern is the provision of appropriate psychosocial care. For the purpose of this chapter, a range of 13 to 24 years has been adopted as this has also been applied elsewhere [2]. However, flexibility is often needed in practice and open dialogue may offer the best approach when decisions are made with young people about their individual care needs.

The psychology of adolescence and young adulthood

The range of developmental changes that occur between adolescence and young adulthood means that this patient population will present with diverse support needs. A life-limiting condition brings about a change in the perceived natural order of events and the challenge for palliative care services is to respond appropriately whilst remaining aware of the young person's stage of development. By the time palliative care is required, those involved will already have faced the disappointment of failed treatments and, possibly, a gradual realisation that they are likely to succumb to their disease. This process takes time and will have occurred alongside the normal developmental tasks of adolescence and young adulthood (see Tables 16.1 and 16.2). It is little wonder that those who find themselves in such a situation will express a wide range of emotions. At the same time as their body and mind are developing, they are become increasingly dependent on others and face the possibility of death itself.

From health to illness—a series of transitions

The experience of cancer for a young person has been described as a process of transition [1, 10]. Edwards [10] suggests that there are two dimensions of this transition. These are:

1 The transition from a state of perceived health to living with a life-threatening illness.

2 The transition from active treatment to palliative care—essentially moving from a *life-threatening* illness to a *life-limiting* one.

Table 16.1 Developmental tasks of adolescence.

- Forming a clear identity
- Accepting a new body image
- Gaining freedom from parents
- Developing a personal value system
- Achieving financial and social independence
- Developing relationships with members of both sexes
- Developing cognitive skills and the ability to think abstractly
- Developing the ability to control one's behaviour according to social norms
- Taking responsibility for one's own behaviour

Based on Havinghurst work, Russell-Johnson (1996), in Joint Working Party on Palliative Care for Adolescents and Young Adults, 2001, Joint Working.

Table 16.2 Stages of adolescent and young adult development and the impact of a life-threatening/life-limiting illness.

Age	Early adolescence 12–14 years (female) 13–15 years (male)	Middle adolescence 14–16 years	Young adult 17–24 years
Key issues and characteristics	Focus on development of body Most Pubertal changes occur Rapid physical growth Acceptance by peers Idealism mood swings, contrariness, temper tantrums Day-dreaming	Sexual awakening Emancipation from parents and figures of authority Discovery of limitations by testing limitation/boundaries Role of peer group increases	Defining and understanding functional roles in life in terms of; • Career • Relationships • Lifestyle
Social relationships, behaviours	Improved skills in abstract thought foreseeing consequences, planning for future Physical mobility prominent Energy levels high Appetite increases Social interaction in groups Membership of peer group important	Relationships very narcissistic Risk-taking behaviour increases Intense peer interaction Most vulnerable to psychological problems	Increasing financial independence Planning for the future Establishment of permanent relationships Increasing time away from family
Impact of life-threatening illness	Concerns about physical appearance and mobility Privacy all-important Possible interference with normal cognitive development and learning (school absence, medication, pain, depression, fatigue). Comparison with peers hindered, making self-assessment of normality difficult Possible lack of acceptance by peers Reliance on parents and other authorities in decision-making Hospitals perceived as very disturbing	Illness particularly threatening and least well tolerated at this stage Compromised sense of autonomy Emancipation from parents and authority figures impeded Interference with attraction of partner fear of rejection by peers Limited interaction with peers may lead to social withdrawal dependence on family for companionship and social support Hospitalisation, school absences interfere with social relationships and acquisition of social skills non-compliance with treatment	Absences from work, study Interference with plans for vocation and relationships difficulties in securing employment and promotion at work Unemployment hinders achieving separation from family and financial independence Discrimination in employment, health cover and life insurance Loss of financial independence and self-esteem Concerns about fertility and health of offspring

Adapted from work of Joint Working Party on Palliative Care for Adolescents and Young Adults, 2001.

Major life events such as these will impact on all aspects of a young person's experience. For example, symptoms arising as a result of disease or treatment will mean time being lost from education or work. This, in turn, will mean less contact with peers whilst being more dependent on professionals or family. Once again it is clear that serious illness impacts as much socially as it does physically for a young person [11]. Advancing symptoms will also result in changes such as skin breakdown, the insertion of central venous catheters and weight loss or gain, which further threatens self-esteem and sense of personal control [12].

An example from practice helps to illustrate these points:

> Mary was 19 years old when she was diagnosed with Acute Myeloid Leukaemia (AML). Prior to this she had taken a year out from her studies and had travelled the world. She enjoyed partying with friends and was due to return to university when she suddenly became unwell. The leukaemia chemotherapy treatment schedule was intense, which meant that very little time was spent out of the hospital environment. Side effects from the treatment left her feeling exhausted; she experienced weight loss and had to have a central venous catheter inserted. Gradually she refused to see her friends because she felt more and more like a 'freak'. At the same time she became so dependent on her mother that she asked her to stay with her in hospital every night.

The development of appropriate helping strategies in such a situation requires an awareness of the environmental, cultural and historical factors as well as the biological, psychological and social phenomena that are now impacting on the young person's life. One of the most fundamental concerns is the place of medical technologies on an already changing body. Having to expose the body for physical examinations or during activities such as washing and defaecating can also be painfully undignified and embarrassing to a young person. Some may find having to be examined by a member of staff of a different gender particularly distressful—having a parent present may also be upsetting for some, whilst helpful for others.

Sexuality and fertility are also notoriously difficult issues for any young person to discuss with their parents [8]. Whilst sexuality may be considered a taboo subject by some, early adolescence and young adulthood are times of intense sexual activity and development [13]. A life threatening disease does not necessarily halt this process. Instead, sexual function can become a focus of concern for young people as a result of the disease, its treatment or side effects. For instance, failing to menstruate may be seen as a highly significant loss for some young women. Such concerns may be coupled with a lack of sexual experience prior to diagnosis and may result in resentment towards healthy peers who are developing in this way. Discussing such topics can be very difficult for parents, especially as friends and peers are the usual first choice [1].

Despite the presence of serious illness some aspects of physical and emotional development will continue and strong feelings and attractions may be experienced for the first time. Such feelings may be directed towards those closest to the young person, including those providing medical or nursing care. This can be problematic when the boundaries between personal and professional relationships become blurred and attention is invested in one 'special' caregiver. Once again, clinical supervision or some method for debriefing is essential to help health professionals recognise and manage such situations appropriately.

Different concerns may arise for young adults, particularly as they may be involved in established relationships and, as a result of their illness or treatment, will never have the opportunity to produce, or raise, their own children. As the illness progresses, some may wish to leave something tangible behind for their children, such as a book of memories or a tape recording (see Winston's Wish: Useful Addresses).

Another important consideration is the promotion of intimacy and supportive personal relationships during the later stages of serious illness. The provision of privacy and space may be difficult in hospital settings, or may be easily overlooked [14]. Young adults may also seek 'normality' in other ways, such as seeking to return to a working role in which they felt productive and useful. A mother, in Grinyer [1], recounts the following account of her son Steve's experience:

> "Work was always so important to you Steve, especially when your life was threatened. Work was a place where customers asked you for help and didn't ask you about the cancer ... Now I am reliving the last three months, exactly twelve weeks to the day when we knew it had really got you and was in your bones, back to normality while you could. How sensible, how mature ... Your pain is unbearable, you can only work for short bursts, but as you say at least on the shop floor people treat me normally, they ask me for help. You go on, what strength you have." (p. 51)

The desire to retain their individuality is not uncommon in young people facing imminent death. Eventually, however, there will also be a need to provide practical help as their symptoms increase.

Towards end of life care

The slow trajectory towards death is a highly subjective one and a variety of reactions and needs should be anticipated. No two people will react in the same way, regardless of their age, background or situation. The realisation that cure is no longer possible is a crucial point when it is important to be aware of feelings of abandonment and failure—patients may feel they have somehow 'failed' those working to cure them and professionals may find it difficult to acknowledge that their interventions have been unsuccessful. Not all individuals, however, will have the emotional capacity to comprehend the enormity of the situation [11]. Importantly, this can impact on the way that frightening symptoms such as pain, anxiety and restlessness are experienced. An individual's willingness to engage in decisions about symptom control is likely to mirror their own, and their family's, coping strategies. Some may ask for every detail to be explained, whilst others prefer deferring to professional opinions.

The following case study illustrates some of the end-of-life issues that arose with Mark, a young man with advanced cancer:

Mark was 16 years old and the only child of Janet (a housewife) and Charlie (a businessman). He was diagnosed with a pelvic sarcoma three years previously and since then his disease had metastasised to his lungs despite conventional and experimental therapy. The medical team had informed him that his life was now severely limited. He seemed to feel reassured in the hospital environment where he was well known to the staff and had not attended school on a regular basis since his diagnosis.

Mark began to experience a pain in his leg that caused him to walk with a limp. This also led to him being unable to sleep at night. A transdermal Fentanyl patch was applied with directions that Oramorph could be taken for breakthrough pain as required. Mark also found Entonox therapy helped, as and when required.

Whilst at home Mark removed the Fentanyl patch saying that the pain was improved and that the cancer was obviously better. The following day he was found to be excessively sleepy. During the night he had experienced excruciating pain and had applied three Fentanyl patches to try and obtain

Continued

Continued

some relief. It was explained that this dose was too high and was reduced. Over the following 24 hours Mark became anxious and requested re-admission to hospital. Mark's parents were keen for him to die at home, and had discussed this option with him; however, he was reluctant to stay and asked to go to back to hospital to get on top of his pain better and then return home. Mark's parents felt that he was denying the seriousness of his condition. Each time they, or the staff, tried to talk about his illness he would become angry or buried his head under a pillow.

On re-admission Mark immediately asked for Entonox, stating this was the only thing that eased his pain. His parents, however, felt that the Entonox was used when he felt out of control.

Over the next two days Mark's condition deteriorated. He became increasingly agitated and confused. He received intravenous Diamorphine for pain and Midazolam for agitation. His parents and the nursing staff found his restlessness difficult to witness as he was experiencing vivid hallucinations—including speaking to deceased members of his family. He muttered and rolled around the bed. His parents were advised to speak to him reassuringly and to promote a calming environment by playing his favourite music. Mark died ten hours later with his parents present.

Although similar difficult situations are likely to arise in both adult and paediatric palliative care practice, there are key issues that merit specific consideration. They include the following:

- The importance of negotiation between patient, family and health care professionals.
- Respect for patient autonomy, while at the same time fostering a family-centred approach to care.
- Partnership and collaboration between the patient, family and professionals.
- Flexibility within service provision.

The role of negotiation between the patient, family and health care professional at the end of life

Increased levels of negotiation may be required about the use of experimental drugs as well as the management of symptoms at the end of life. Patient involvement in clinical decision-making at this time has been found to be an essential element in the delivery of effective patient-and-family-centred care. Research findings suggest that there are two key issues that benefit those assisting young people and their families in making end-of-life decisions. The first is clarity and honesty when information is being imparted. The second involves trust in, and having the support of, the health care team [6]. From interviews with bereaved parents, adolescents and staff, key concerns included knowing that all that could be done had been done to achieve a cure; no acceptable treatment options remained untried and, as a result, long-term survival was unlikely. Decisions made by parents and families were judged according to the balance struck between quality of life, treatment toxicity and other adverse outcomes, as well as estimations of suffering and the patient's individual preferences. Such findings may be helpful in practice—especially when the boundaries between cure and care, or between experimental therapy and palliation, become blurred.

Respect for patient autonomy whilst fostering family-centred care

Young people's preferences for specific treatment interventions will be influenced by social and emotional maturity, as well as past experiences and cultural and spiritual beliefs. While some wish to be involved in decision-making throughout their illness, others may prefer to rely upon carers to decide on their behalf. Some may also wish to be involved in some areas of care but not others. This situation can result in family discord as protective instincts may challenge the young person's need to remain independent. Professionals need to be sensitive to the dynamics and tensions in such situations, and adopt practical strategies such as encouraging both parties to spend time away from each other. End of life care for adolescents and young adults (whether provided in the home or hospital/hospice setting) requires openness, honesty, flexibility and responsiveness in order to meet the many individual needs that will arise in each situation.

Professionals involved in supporting families need to ensure that they are open to questioning their own practice, especially if they have had limited experience of this patient group. District nurses working closely with Macmillan colleagues, for instance, can make sure that relevant information is shared and that visits are planned in a way to minimise overlap. Ensuring that a summary care plan, essential equipment, emergency supplies of medication and the telephone numbers of relevant contacts in a patient's home can also help prevent problems or delays in the final days of care. This may be especially helpful when such professionals are asked to visit who do not know the patient well.

Partnership and collaboration between patients, families and professionals

Negotiation and partnership between young people, families and professionals are also necessary to achieve an acceptable transition towards end-of-life care. Many young people will prefer to seek advice and accept care from professionals with whom they have developed trusting relationships. This relates in part to the fact that new and unfamiliar situations may be especially stressful to people at the end of life, [15] and emphasises the importance of effective collaboration between the different agencies involved. Rather than transferring end-of-life care from one team to another, members of the multi-disciplinary teams from the speciality, working in partnership with palliative care services and community staff can deliver a coordinated package of supportive care [10].

An important aspect of adolescence and young adulthood that is often stressed is the forming of independent relationships apart from the family unit. For those young people with a life-limiting illness this may often be difficult to achieve due to deteriorating health. Such disruption can result in frustration and conflict. Support from family members, however, is also crucial at other times. Researchers have found that informal support from family members was directly linked to the illness experience of young adults aged between the ages of 19 and 30 years [16]. They describe a situation that required balancing the challenge of living with cancer and its treatment with relationships, careers and other life events. Those supported by family members felt more able to cope with such demands. It is likely that family members will also be experiencing significant life events and transitions. One theoretical approach for assessing family functioning in such situations is presented below [17, 18]:

Vulnerable families tend to show the following characteristics:

- Serious illness occurring alongside other major life transition can result in a loss of individual and family coherence/adaptability.
- The greater the match between the social character of the family and the developmental needs of its members, the better likelihood there is of adapting to serious illness.
- Middle-aged families with adolescents living with a chronic illness may show less family unity or achievement of developmental tasks.
- The older the family, the less the likelihood of disruption when a member becomes ill.

Despite the fact that variation should be anticipated, guidelines such as these may help to focus attention on the nature of family relationships in end-of-life care situations. Individual or family counselling may also be helpful for the young person and their family when necessary [19].

Flexibility within service provision

Symptom management at the end of life can be particularly challenging with adolescents or young adults, as the meanings attached to symptoms will vary. This will, in turn, determine what is meant by effective symptom management.

Adolescence and young adulthood can be a time of contradict ions—seeking ways to be understood may be opposed by a reluctance to express feelings [20]. The desire to maintain control and independence whilst experiencing physical deterioration can be demoralising, frustrating and confusing. A deteriorating physical condition can also result in being treated in a child-like way.

Carers who witness a young person's suffering yet feel unable to provide adequate relief may also experience frustration [21]. Understanding the importance placed on symptoms can help direct care planning. For instance, pain control may be less important to some than remaining lucid as long as possible. Similarly, symptoms that seem distressing to those witnessing them, such as restlessness or agitation, may be explained in order to share lucid moments before sedatives are employed. The significance of symptoms should not be under-estimated as this has been found to be linked with how life-limiting illness is perceived by young people and their families [22–25].

A situation in which pain signifies disease progression, as it did for Mark, needs to be appreciated and appropriate strategies adopted. Negotiation and flexibility are, once again, essential features of effective end of life care for this patient group.

A recent study suggests that there is also a need to consider the place of death as a measure of the quality of supportive and palliative care [26]. There were 3197 cancer-related deaths for children and young people up to the age of 24 between 1995 and 1999. It was found that home deaths were less likely to be achieved for those lower in the social scale, or for those with leukaemia or lymphoma rather than solid cancers. This raises important questions about the quality of palliative services for these patient groups, and suggests the need to devote further attention to their needs. Similarly, areas in inner London (with higher rates of child poverty) were less likely to achieve home deaths than more 'affluent' areas of England. Young people with brain tumours were also more likely to die in a hospice setting.

Conclusions

This chapter has suggested that adolescents and young adults present particular challenges for professionals providing effective palliative care. Awareness of developmental needs, as well as the disruption that serious illness causes at this stage of life, may help to ensure that we respond appropriately to this unique patient group. An issue of crucial importance is the need for channels of communication between the family, hospital and primary care professionals to ensure that all parties are working together to achieve the same goals [27]. Practical expertise needs to be combined with appropriate education and research to ensure that adolescents and young adults who are facing death are provided with the support that their situation merits.

References

1 Grinyer A. *Cancer in Young Adults: Through Parents' Eyes* Buckingham: Open University Press, 2002.
2 Joint Working Party on Palliative Care for Adolescents and Young Adults. *Palliative Care for Young People Aged 13–24*. Bristol: Association for Children with Life-Threatening Conditions and Their Families, 2001. ISBN 1 898447 06 3.
3 Grinyer A, Thomas C. Young adults with cancer: The effects on parents and families. *Int J Palliat Nurs* 2001; 7: 162–170.
4 Evans M. Interacting with teenagers with cancer. In: Selby P, Bailey C, eds. *Cancer and the Adolescent*. London: BMJ Publishing Group, 1996: 251–263.
5 Papadatou D, Anagnostopouros F, Mouros D. Factors contributing to the development of burnout in oncology nursing. *Br J Med Psychol* 1994; 67: 187–199.
6 Hinds P, Quargnenti A, Hickey S. A comparison of stress response sequence in new and experienced paediatric oncology nurses. *Cancer Nurs* 1994; 17: 61–71.
7 Kelly D, Mullhall A, Pearce S. Adolescent cancer: The need to evaluate current service provision in the UK. *Eur J Oncol Nurs* 2002; 7: 53–58.
8 Brannen J., Dodd K., Oakley K., Storey, P. *Young People, Health and Family Life*. Buckingham: Open University Press, 1994.
9 Silverman R P. *Never Too Young to Know. Death in Children's Lives* Oxford: Oxford University Press, 2000.
10 Edwards J. A model of palliative care for the adolescent with cancer", *Int J Palliat Nurs* 2001; 7: 485–488.
11 Eiser C. The impact of treatment: adolescents' views." In: Selby P, Bailey C, eds. *Cancer and the Adolescents*, London: BMJ Publishing Group, 1996: 264–275.
12 Ritchie M A. Psychosocial functioning of adolescents with cancer: A developmental perspective. *Oncol Nurs Forum* 1992; 19: 1497–1501.

13 Muuss R E. *Theories of Adolescence*, 6th edition. London: The McGraw-Hill Companies, Inc.
14 Searle E. Sexuality and people who are dying. In: Heath H,White I, eds.*The Challenge of Sexuality in Health Care*, London: Blackwell Science, 2002.
15 Peterson A C, Leffert N. Developmental issues influencing guidelines for adolescent health research: a review. *J Adolesc Health* 1995; 17: 298–305.
16 Lyman J M. Supporting one another: the nature of family work when a young adult has cancer. *J Adv Nurs* 1995; 22: 116–125.
17 Rankin S H, Weekes D P. Life-span development: a review of theory and practice for families with chronically ill members. *Sch Inq Nurs Prac* 2000; 14: 355–273.
18 Weekes D P, Rankin S H. Life-span developmental methods: application to nursing research. *Nurs Res* 1988; 37: 380–383.
19 Rose K, Webb C, Waters K. Coping strategies employed by informal carers of terminally ill cancer patients. *J Clin Nurs* 1997; 1: 126–133.
20 DeMinco S. Young adult reactions to death in literature and life. *Adolescence* 1995; 30: 179–185.
21 Hinds P S, Oakes L, Furman W, Quargnenti A., Olson M S, Foppiano P, Srivastava D K. End-of-life decision making by adolescents, parents, and health care providers in pediatric oncology, *Cancer Nurs* 2001; 24: 122–135.
22 Woodgate R M S. Symptom distress in children with cancer: the need to adopt a meaning-centred approach" *J Pediatr Oncol Nurs* 1998;15: 3–12.
23 Woodgate R L, Degner F. Nothing is carved in stone!: uncertainty in children with cancer and their families. *Eur J Oncol Nurs* 2002; 6: 191–202.
24 Woodgate R L, Degner F. A substansive theory of keeping the spirit alive: The spirit within children with cancer and their families. *J Pediatr Oncol Nurs* 2003; 13: 61–71.
25 Weekes D P. Application of the life-span developmental perspective to nursing research with adolescents. *J Pediatr Nurs* 1991; 6: 38–48.
26 Higginson I, Thompson M. Children and young people who die from cancer: epidemiology and place of death in England (1995–99). *Br Med J* 2003; 327: 478–479.
27 George R, Hutton S. Palliative care in adolescents. *Eur J Cancer* 2003; 39: 2662–2668.

17: Palliative Care in Advanced Heart Disease

GILLIAN HORNE AND STEPHANIE TAYLOR

Introduction

Most patients with advanced heart disease who require palliative care suffer from heart failure and there is now an increasing recognition of their needs [1–3]. The National Service Framework for Coronary Heart Disease [4] has endorsed this. However, the organisation and provision of palliative care for heart failure lags far behind the need and many patients with advanced heart failure experience a poor quality of life with worsening symptoms, frequent emergency hospital admissions and poorly coordinated care [5, 6].

What is heart failure?

Chronic heart failure (CHF) is not a single disease but "a clinical syndrome in which heart disease reduces cardiac output, increases venous pressures, and is accompanied by molecular abnormalities that cause progressive deterioration of the failing heart and premature myocardial cell death" [7]. In affluent countries coronary artery disease (CAD) is the commonest underlying cause of heart failure. When the cardiac pump fails, it triggers a complex neurohumoral response, which has both short-term adaptive effects and long-term maladaptive effects. This neurohumoral response involves physiological and inflammatory changes and modifies myocardial cell growth and death. A common description of the severity of symptoms in heart failure is given in The New York Heart Association (NYHA) Classification (see Box 17.1).

Epidemiology

CHF is a common condition with a crude prevalence of 3 to 20 per 1000 in the general population [9]. Both the incidence and prevalence of heart failure rise sharply with age and the condition affects 10% of those aged 80 to 89 years [10]. Most patients with heart failure

Box 17.1 The stages of heart failure—The New York Heart Association (NYHA) Classification [8]

- **Class I** (Mild): No limitation of physical activity. Ordinary physical activity does not cause undue fatigue, palpitation or dyspnoea (shortness of breath).
- **Class II** (Mild): Slight limitation of physical activity. Comfortable at rest, but ordinary physical activity results in fatigue, palpitation, or dyspnoea.
- **Class III** (Moderate): Marked limitation of physical activity. Comfortable at rest, but less than ordinary activity causes fatigue, palpitation or dyspnoea.
- **Class IV** (Severe): Unable to carry out any physical activity without discomfort. Symptoms of cardiac insufficiency at rest. If any physical activity is undertaken, discomfort is increased.

are elderly, the mean age at first hospital admission is 74 years [11]. The condition carries a dismal prognosis. In a recent study of Scottish data the median survival time after a first admission with CHF was 16 months and the 5-year survival rate was just 25% [12]. In the same study, of all the common malignancies in both sexes only lung and ovarian cancer had worse 5-year survival rates. The condition also has a profound impact on patients' quality of life [13].

Patients with heart failure may experience frequent hospital admission. In one study 44% of patients admitted with CHF were readmitted within 6 months [14]. CHF patients commonly have other serious medical problems. A national study of CHF in patients aged 65 years or older in the United States found that 55% also had CAD, 38% had diabetes, one third had chronic obstructive pulmonary disease and 18% had previous history of a stroke [15]. In another study 30% of patients were clinically depressed on screening 4–6 weeks after discharge from a hospital admission for heart failure [16].

CHF patients are generally managed with complex medication regimens and lifestyle advice, although a very small number of patients with advanced heart failure will also be on a waiting list for heart transplantation.

Coordination and organisation of care

In a recent qualitative study of general practitioners and secondary care doctors in England, barriers to practising the palliative care approach were identified as:

- organisational barriers including a lack of continuity of care and poor support in the community;
- the unpredictable course of the disease;
- doctors' understanding of the roles and responsibilities of others [5].

Against this rather pessimistic backdrop, new models of care for CHF are emerging [17]. For example, there is evidence that coordinated multidisciplinary care of heart failure patients in hospital and extra support during the first week after discharge may reduce readmissions and improve survival without hospital readmission [18]. Other studies suggest that specialist nurse interventions could also improve survival without hospital admission [19] and reduce unplanned hospital readmissions [19] or reduce readmissions for heart failure [20]. Specialist heart failure clinics do not seem to be effective [21, 22] and they are unlikely to be a feasible option for heart failure patients [22]. The education of patients and carers about CHF and the involvement of a heart failure specialist nurse are typical components of most of the new disease management interventions. In the UK, the British Heart Foundation has promoted heart failure specialist nurses utilising a similar model of nursing to that in cancer care.

One way to promote a palliative care approach to CHF is to have a 'key worker' to oversee and co-ordinate care [5]. The key worker could be a general practitioner, a community geriatrician or a district or practice nurse with an interest in heart failure management. Where a specialist heart failure nurse is in post they would seem to be an ideal candidate for this role.

Palliative care teams have a wealth of knowledge to share with such key workers. CHF patients are often denied access to conventional palliative care because prognosis is less predictable than in cancer. However, if health care professionals adopt a coordinated approach in which palliative care runs alongside active treatment from diagnosis [23] then palliative care may have a place much earlier on in the disease trajectory. Joint consultation between cardiologists and palliative care team members is recommended [24]. Early referral and access to specialist palliative care teams for advice on relief of symptoms and supportive care may improve patients' quality of life and allow coordination of effective end-of-life care.

Common physical symptoms in patients with advanced heart failure

Patients with advanced heart failure may present with a variety of symptoms [25], which are similar to patients with advanced cancer. Patients often experience six or seven symptoms at any one time [26].

A detailed history, physical examination, investigations and establishment of patient priorities will help in the management of their symptoms and improvement of quality of life. An accurate drug history is important due to the nature of complex drug regimens. The difficulties of coping with unwanted drug side effects may cause patients to be afraid to report their non-concordance [27], which may precipitate hospital admission. Common physical symptoms are listed in Box 17.2.

Box 17.2

- Fatigue
- Breathlessness
- Pain
- Oedema
- Dizziness
- Cachexia
- Anorexia
- Nausea
- Insomnia
- Difficulty in walking
- Constipation

Management of symptoms

Optimised cardiac drug therapy for this patient group is needed before considering prescribing from palliative care formularies. Patients may be on sub-optimal doses of ACE inhibitors, beta-blockers and diuretics [27]. Titration of medications under the care of cardiologists or heart failure nurse specialists may relieve many of the patient's symptoms and improve quality of life. Collaboration between cardiology and palliative care teams in the management of symptoms is highly recommended. When the patient's cardiac drugs are optimised and their symptoms still remain, the use of palliative care drugs may be beneficial. The management of many physical symptoms has already been discussed in Chapters 8, 10 and 19. The following symptoms are discussed with specific reference to heart failure.

Breathlessness

This is the most distressing symptom that patients complain about and often causes patients to be admitted to hospital [24]. Breathlessness can also cause patients to wake up at night and many patients resort to sleeping in a chair.

> *"I used to go to bed and, oh, I couldn't breathe. I were up and downstairs" male, age 70.*

Breathlessness is commonly caused by pulmonary oedema due to failing left ventricular function or sometimes due to anaemia. Other causes such as chest infection should not be overlooked. Anxiety, depression and inactivity can also contribute to breathlessness. Increasing diuretics is the first line treatment for breathlessness due to increasing congestion. Cardiologists or heart failure nurse advice is needed when patients do not respond to increased diuretics as patients may benefit from reduction in their beta-blockers, or the addition of spironolactone, metolazone or digoxin [28]. Morphine 2.5–5 mg given every 4 hours around-the-clock may be helpful for breathlessness not relieved by increased diuretics [29]. Home oxygen may be useful for patients with daytime low blood-oxygen saturations. The use of breathing and relaxation exercises can help reduce the anxiety, which often accompanies breathlessness. Further research is needed in the use of complementary therapies for the treatment of this and other symptoms in advanced heart failure.

Fatigue

Fatigue is the one of the most common symptoms experienced by patients with heart failure and many feel constantly tired and lacking energy. The main factors contributing to fatigue are: abnormalities in skeletal muscle due to reduced perfusion and neurohumoral changes; the side effects of medications; reduced activity; anaemia; lack of appetite and muscle wasting (cardiac cachexia).

Fatigue causes reduced quality of life because it severely restricts the patient's activities and creates difficulties in walking and getting out of the house [30, 24].

> *"I'm more tired all the time. I get out of bed in a morning and I feel as though I want to go back to bed" male, age 60.*

In the last stages of heart failure even managing personal hygiene and dressing can be difficult. Fatigue induced inactivity may lead patients to feel they are a burden to their carers and society. Fatigue can also compound other physical symptoms such as constipation, oedema and pain. Access to exercise programmes may be of benefit to reduce fatigue and can give patients a greater sense of well being [31]. Explanation to the patients and their carers about the physiological causes of fatigue can help them understand what they are experiencing and referral to occupational therapy or physiotherapy for advice on energy conservation and exercise can be useful. Education about healthy eating and correcting anaemia can also be beneficial. However, there is a dearth of research evidence on the management of fatigue in patients with advanced CHF.

Pain

Patients with advanced heart failure frequently experience pain [32]. This may be chest pain related to angina, pericarditis, mechanical implants, food or musculoskeletal pains. Oedematous limbs can also cause pain and discomfort. Patients may also experience chronic pain not specifically related to their underlying disease but from co-morbidities such as osteoarthritis, or as a result of previous heart surgery [24].

In addition to its use in dyspnoea, morphine can be used to treat pain not relieved by simple analgesics (Chapter 8). Non-steroidal anti-inflammatory drugs are not advised in this patient group due to the retention of sodium, which potentiates fluid overload. Doses of morphine should be titrated to the patient's individual pain. Ideally immediate release morphine should be given every 4 hours around the clock and then converted to a slow release preparation. In our experience, complementary therapies may also be helpful in managing pain such as aromatherapy, massage, TENS, relaxation and visualisation although there is little published research evidence to support this.

Case study 1

Paul is 48-year-old married man and father of three who has a history of five myocardial infarctions and two coronary artery bypass grafts. He has advanced CHF (NYHA Class IV) and is awaiting a heart transplant. Paul is admitted to hospital because of unrelieved chest pain, which occurs 4–6 times a day. He is on sustained released morphine and requires frequent

Continued

> ***Continued***
> intermittent doses of intravenous diamorphine. Paul is tense and feels low in mood.
>
> How would you assess Paul's pain and how would you plan to help Paul manage his pain?
> (see discussion below)

Case study 1: Discussion

Paul was given an opportunity to discuss his feelings about his illness and any other concerns. He was assisted to describe his pain using a visual analogue scale. After detailed assessment Paul's regular dose of morphine sulphate tablets (MST) was increased and his breakthrough medication dose was prescribed as one sixth of his daily dose. Within 24 hours Paul had significant improvement in his pain and did not require further intravenous diamorphine. Paul was offered relaxation exercises using visualisation to help relieve his tension. He responded well so relaxation scripts and a tape were left for him to use at home. After discussion with the primary care team involved in Paul's care, he could be discharged later that day.

Oedema

Oedema occurs predominately in the lower limbs or manifests as ascites, hepatomegaly or pulmonary oedema. Patients are advised to monitor their weight to watch for early signs of fluid retention and inform their health care professionals. Some of the factors leading to oedema are fluid overload, renal failure, non-concordance with diuretic therapy and inactivity. Accurate clinical assessment is needed to exclude other causes of oedema such as venous thrombosis.

Increased doses of diuretics are used to reduce oedema and hospitalisation may be necessary to give intravenous diuretics and monitor electrolyte balance. Patients need to be taught good skin care when oedema is present to prevent abrasions and subsequent infection. Heavy limbs can often become painful therefore adequate analgesia is also an important aspect of management.

Common psychological symptoms

Diagnosis of heart failure may trigger emotional stress. Depression, anxiety, social isolation and loneliness are common symptoms experienced by patients with advanced heart failure [6, 24]. The lack of emotional and social support is an important predictor of morbidity [33] and when patients become isolated and lack the ability to cope with their disease, this can also be a significant predictor of their mortality [34].

A patient's experience of depression is often compounded by their physical symptoms [26]. Psychological symptoms are debilitating and can reduce quality of life. Patients complain of being informed that '*nothing more can be done*' for them, which can hinder hope for the future. When opportunities are given to patients they often talk about dying. Fears of how they may die, of pain and of leaving others behind are common [24, 26].

Case study 2

Mr Brown is a 69-year-old man with advanced heart failure and a history of repeated hospital admissions for increased breathlessness. He lives alone and has one sister living nearby. During his latest admission he was told by the hospital team that no further surgery or medical interventions could be offered. After his discharge from hospital Mr Brown requests a home visit from you. He appears to be very anxious and tells you he was informed he could die at anytime. He complains of insomnia and depression.

How would you begin to manage Mr Brown's insomnia and depression? Could Mr Brown's psychological symptoms have been prevented? What support systems may be needed?
(see discussion below)

Case study 2: Discussion

An important aspect of Mr Brown's management is exploring his understanding and feelings about his illness. He does not sleep at night because he is frightened he may not wake up and believes nothing further can be done for him. Providing support through effective communication skills may prevent fear and loss of hope in patients with advanced disease (see Chapter 8). Feelings of being a burden on the family are common. Exploring concerns about the future can provide opportunities to discuss death and preferences for end-of-life care. Good palliative symptom management, psychological, spiritual and social support will provide hope and reassurance. Teaching relaxation techniques and other complementary therapies are also helpful (see Chapter 23). He may benefit from a referral to social services and district nursing. Liaison between his primary care team and the local palliative care team is strongly recommended and Mr Brown could be given contact numbers for the palliative care services. Hospice day-care for further social support and respite may be beneficial.

Management

Emotional support is important for patients with advanced heart failure. Effective communication with patients and their carers is needed from diagnosis and throughout the course of the illness. The process of breaking bad news similar to that used with cancer patients [35] is advocated. To maintain hope, patients can be offered good palliation of their symptoms and exploration of their preferences for care. Information needs to be available about the disease process, common feelings experienced and local social support services. Referral to psychology services or counsellors may be required and some patients may benefit from an antidepressant. Tricyclic antidepressants are not usually advised due to their pro-arthymic side effects. Selective serotonin reuptake inhibitor antidepressants (e.g. fluoxetine 20 mg once daily) are more commonly prescribed.

Social and practical needs of patients and carers

Patients with advanced heart failure and their carers need help to access the following:

- Information about the disease process, treatment and general advice on what to do and what not to do. This information needs to be accessible early in the disease trajectory because in the advanced stages patients cannot get out of their home to access information. Carers also require written and verbal practical guidelines for providing care at home; this is often lacking [6].
- Social services to provide equipment such as stair lifts, ramps, commodes and information about packages of care.
- District nurses for assessment of symptoms and support. District nurses are often not aware of patients living with advanced heart failure until they become hospitalised.
- Community physiotherapy and occupational therapy for assessment and advice on exercise, energy conservation and home adaptations to aid in activities of daily living.
- Benefits advice—patients may be eligible for Disability or Attendance Allowance.
- Access to the palliative care team and to respite for carers.

Resources

- British Heart Foundation
  This charitable organisation provides funding for research into heart diseases, education for patients and the public, patient information leaflets, a national help-line and funding for some heart failure nurses posts.
- Carers National Association
  This charity provides information, advice and support to informal carers.

Terminal care

Many patients with advanced heart failure will die suddenly, often from arrhythmias or coronary thromboses. However, there will be some patients who have a more predictable death. Those patients who slowly decline have repeated admissions to hospital without regaining previous return of function. There are certain factors which can help predict death such as: low serum sodium, high creatinine levels [36]; raised plasma cytokines [37] repeated hospital admissions with decompensated heart failure and patients' self-awareness of their approaching death.

Quality of life and eliciting patient preferences is important in planning terminal care. Discussion with the patient about not attempting resuscitation should be done preferably before the patient enters the terminal phase. For patients who have Internal Defibrillators (ICDs) and their carers a discussion about the benefits versus potential problems of ICDs in the last days is needed to prepare patients that ICDs can sometimes cause pain or discomfort and may need to be deactivated. Specialist advice is recommended if ICDs are reducing patient's quality of life.

Intravenous inotropes are sometimes used as an attempt to treat the patient's worsening symptoms; however, evidence is limited on their usefulness in the terminal phase. Quality of life is not improved by infusions of inotropes [38] and their use may even increase mortality [39].

In contrast to patients with advanced cancer, patients with severe heart failure may warrant continuation of their cardiac medications to treat symptoms and help maintain some quality of life. However drugs aimed at longer term prevention such as statins should be stopped. In the terminal phase joint consultation is advised between cardiology, general practitioners and palliative care teams in medicine management.

Patients' symptom management and support needs in the terminal phase are similar to patients with other life threatening diseases (see Chapter 21). Care pathways such as the Liverpool Care of the Dying Pathway are often helpful [40].

Conclusion

- Heart failure is a common condition associated with poor survival and a poor quality of life. Patients are usually elderly and often have other serious medical conditions. Few CHF patients currently access palliative care specialist services.
- Lack of continuity of care, poor support in the community and the unpredictable course of the disease itself are potential barriers to a palliative care approach.
- Better coordination of care and the adoption of a 'key worker' approach could improve patients' access to appropriate palliative care.
- Good communication between all those caring for the patient in both primary and secondary care is essential.
- Consideration of palliative care should begin early on in the disease and should run alongside treatment.
- Emerging disease management models for CHF could be a useful vehicle to promote a palliative care approach for CHF patients.
- Specialist palliative care teams have a role to play in heart failure, both in providing expert advice and support to those managing the patient and in providing patient care when symptoms are difficult for other health care professionals to manage.
- Patients with heart failure often experience a multitude of symptoms; in particular they may experience breathlessness, fatigue, pain and oedema. Their management is discussed in this chapter.
- Depression, anxiety and social isolation are also common problems for patients.
- Many patients with heart failure experience sudden death, but for others the final decline will be more gradual and their needs will be similar to those of patients dying from other terminal diseases.

References

1 Gibbs LME, Addington-Hall J, Gibbs JSR. Dying from heart failure: lessons from palliative care. *BMJ* 1998; 317: 961–962.

2 Stewart S, McMurray JV. Palliative care for heart failure. *BMJ* 2002; 325: 915–916.

3 Ward C. The need for palliative care in the management of heart failure. *Heart* 2002; 87: 294–298.
4 Department of Health. National Service Framework Coronary Heart Disease, 2000.
5 Hanratty B, Hibbert D, Mair F, May C, Ward C, Capewell S, Litva A, Corcoran G. Doctors' perceptions of palliative care for heart failure: focus group study. *BMJ* 2002; 325: 581–585.
6 Murray SA, Boyd K, Kendall M, Worth A, Benton TF, Clausen H. Dying from lung cancer or cardiac failure: prospective qualitative interview study of patients and their carers in the community. *BMJ* 2002, 325: 929–933.
7 Katz AM. *Heart failure pathophysiology, molecular biology and clinical management*. Philadelphia: Lippincott Williams & Wilkins, 2000.
8 Heart Failure Society of America www.abouthf.org/questions_stages.htm accessed 19.12.2003.
9 Cowie MR. Annotated references in epidemiology. *Eur J Heart Fail* 1999; 1: 101–107.
10 Kannel WB, Belanger AJ. Epidemiology of heart failure. *Am Heart J* 1991; 121: 951–957.
11 Cleland JGF, Gemmell I, Khand A, Boddy A. Is the prognosis of heart failure improving? *Eur J Heart Fail* 1999; 1: 229–241.
12 Stewart S, MacIntyre K, Hole DJ, Capewell S, McMurray JJV. More 'malignant' than cancer? Five-year survival following a first admission for heart failure. *Eur J Heart Fail* 2001; 3: 315–322.
13 Stewart AL, Greenfield S, Hays RD, Wells K, Rogers WH, Berry SD, McGlynn EA, Ware JE Jr. Functional status and well-being of patients with chronic conditions. Results from the medical outcomes study. *JAMA* 1989; 262: 907–913.
14 Krumholz HM, Parent EM, Tu N, Vaccarino V, Wang Y, Radford MJ, Hennen J. Readmission after hospitalization for congestive heart failure among Medicare beneficiaries. *Arch Intern Med* 1997; 157: 99–104.
15 Havranek EP, Masoudi FA, Westfall KA, Wolfe P, Ordin DL, Krumholz HM. Spectrum of heart failure in older patients: results from the National Heart Failure project. *Am Heart J*. 2002; 143: 412–417.
16 Friedman MM, Griffin JA. Relationship of physical symptoms and physical functioning to depression in patients with heart failure.*Heart & Lung: The Journal of Acute and Critical Care* 2001; 30: 98–104.
17 Riegel B, LePetri R. Heart failure disease management models. In: Moser DK, Riegel B, eds. *Improving Outcomes in Heart Failure an Interdisciplinary Approach*. Maryland: Aspen, 2001: 267–281.
18 Rich MW, Beckham V, Wittenberg C, Leven CL, Freedland, KE, Carney RM. A multidisciplinary intervention to prevent the re-admission of elderly patients with congestive heart failure. *N Engl J Med* 1995; 333: 1190–1195.
19 Stewart S, Marley JE, Horowitz JD. Effects of a multidisciplinary, home-based intervention on unplanned readmissions and survival among patients with chronic congestive heart failure: a randomised controlled study. *Lancet* 1999;354: 1077–1083.
20 Blue L, Lang E, McMurray JJV, Davie AP, McDonagh TA, Murdoch DR, Petrie MC, Connolly E, Norrie J, Round CE, Ford I, Morrison CE. Randomised

controlled trial of specialist nurse intervention in heart failure. *BMJ* 2001; 323: 715–718.
21 Cline CM, Israelsson BYA, Willenheimer RB, Broms K, Erhardt LR. Cost effective management programme for heart failure reduces hospitalisation. *Heart* 1998; 80: 442–446.
22 Ekman I, Andersson B, Ehnfors M, Matejka G, Persson B, Fagerberg B. Feasibility of a nurse-monitored, outpatient-care programme for elderly patients with moderate-to-severe, chronic heart failure. *Eur Heart J* 1998; 19: 1254–1260.
23 Gibbs J, McCoy A, Gibbs L, Rogers A, Addington-Hall Living with and dying from heart failure: the role of palliative care. *Heart* 2002;88: ii36–ii39.
24 Horne G, Payne S, Removing the boundaries: palliative care for patients with heart failure. *Palliat Med,* 2004; 18(4): 291–296.
25 Nordgren L, Sorensen S. Symptoms experienced in the last six months of life in patients with end-stage heart failure. *Eur J Cardiovasc Nurs* 2002; 2: 213–217.
26 Friedman MM, Griffin JA. Relationship of physical symptoms and physical functioning to depression in patients with heart failure. *Heart & Lung: The Journal of Acute and Critical Care* 2001; 30: 98–104.
27 Quaglietti S, Atwood J, Ackerman L, Froelicher V. Management of the patient with congestive heart failure using outpatient, home and palliative care. *Prog Cardiovasc Dis* 2000; 43: 259–274.
28 NHS National Institute for Clinical Excellence. *Compilation Summary of Guidance issued to the NHS in England and Wales* 2003. Issue 7. London: NICE.
29 Johnson MJ, McDonagh TA, Harkness A, McKay SE, Dargie, HJ. Morphine for the relief of breathlessness in patients with chronic heart failure—a pilot study. *Eur J Heart Fail* 2002; 4: 735–756.
30 Martensson J, Karlsson J, Fridlund B. Male patients with congestive heart failure and their conception of the life situation. *J Adv Nurs* 1997; 25: 579–586.
31 Lloyd-Williams F, Mair F, Leitner M. Exercise training and heart failure: a systematic review of current evidence. *Br J Gen Prac* 2002; 52: 47–55.
32 McCarthy M, Lay M, Addington-Hall J. Dying from heart disease. *J R Coll Physicians Lond* 1996; 30: 325–328.
33 Krumholz H, Butler J, Miller J, Vaccarino V, Williams C, de Leon C, Seeman T, Kasl S, Berkman L. Prognostic importance of emotional support for elderly patients hospitalized with heart failure. *Circulation* 1998; 97: 958–964.
34 Murberg T, Bru E. Coping and mortality among patients with congestive heart failure. *Int J Behav Med* 2001; 8: 66–79.
35 Kaye P. *Breaking Bad News: A 10 step Approach.* Northampton: EPL Publications, 1996.
36 Kearney MT, Fox KAA, Lee AJ, Prescott RJ, Shah AM, Batin PD, Baig W, Lindsay S, Callahan TS, Shell WE, et al. Predicting death due to progressive heart failure in patients with mild-to-moderate chronic heart failure. *J Am Coll Cardiol* 2002; 40: 1801–1808.
37 Rauchhaus M, Doehner W, Francis DP, Davos C, Kemp M, Liebenthal C, Niebauer J, Hooper J, Volk HD, Coats AJ, Anker SD. Plasma cytokine parameters and mortality in patients with chronic heart failure. *Circulation* 2000; 102: 3060–3067.

38 Scott, L. Care giving and care receiving among a technologically dependent heart failure population. *Adv Nurs Sci* 2000; 23: 82–97
39 Felker G, O'Connor C. Inotropic therapy for heart failure: An evidence-based approach. *Am Heart J* 2001; 142: 393–401.
40 Ellershaw J, Ward C. Care of the dying patient: the last hours or days of life *BMJ* 2003; 326: 30.

18: Palliative Care in Renal Disease

ALISTAIR CHESSER

Introduction

Chronic renal failure is a progressive and incurable disease. Palliative care should ideally commence at the time of diagnosis, and assume increasing importance as the disease becomes more advanced. However the availability of dialysis means that technically nobody in the developed world needs to die of renal failure. Renal replacement therapy (dialysis and/or transplantation) makes end-stage renal disease (ESRD) treatable, but not (yet) curable.

For all patients with advanced chronic renal failure, a decision has to be made as to whether to commence dialysis. When the prognosis of the patient is poor, irrespective of the renal problems, the best decision may be to continue with symptomatic management. Patients already on dialysis may also face circumstances that prompt them to decide to withdraw from dialysis treatment. While many of these decisions are made in conjunction with the renal unit, the primary care team often is also closely involved in the management of these patients.

For the primary care team, palliative care in patients with ESRD is a challenge. Often many different teams in primary and secondary care are involved in the management of the patient. Professionals more experienced in the management of malignant disease may feel uncomfortable when dealing with the less familiar problems of the patient dying with renal failure. However, the role of the GP and primary care team is crucial, both in ensuring that the patient is offered and receives care which is appropriate, and in coordinating the different aspects of that care.

Chronic renal failure

Deciding whether to commence dialysis treatment

Case scenario A (Part 1): Mr A is a 62-year-old man who has a history of ischaemic heart disease, having had an MI five years ago. Two years ago

Continued on p. 346

Continued

he had a stroke, which has left him with a mild hemiparesis. He needs help with walking and usually has a wheelchair when he goes out of the house. His wife has mild but progressive dementia, though she still cooks and shops for him. They have two daughters, one of whom lives close by and pops in most days to help and check that they are well. Mr A has slowly declining renal function secondary to renovascular disease. His kidneys are likely to reach end stage within the next few months and a decision has to be made as to whether to commence dialysis at this time.

The use of dialysis to treat chronic renal failure is relatively novel. Dialysis was not available until the 1960s and at first was used only to treat patients thought to have reversible acute renal failure. As technology advanced it became possible to offer dialysis to a few patients with ESRD. These patients had to be selected (they were usually young patients who were otherwise well), and all other ESRD patients had no choice but to die. This is no longer the case, as in recent years a number of factors have combined to widen access of dialysis treatment for patients with ESRD. These include technical advances in dialysis delivery, improvements in techniques for vascular and peritoneal dialysis access, increasing expertise in looking after older and sicker patients on dialysis treatment, increasing public and political expectations and increased financial input. It is generally recognised that dialysis should be offered to all patients who need and want it, and the decision not to commence dialysis should be made by the patient (or carer) in conjunction with the nephrologist.

The decision to commence dialysis is often straightforward, such as when the patient has no significant co-morbidity, a good quality of life and wishes to remain alive. But dialysis is physically and psychologically demanding, especially for those patients who reach ESRD with co-morbidity. Data from a dialysis unit in the UK shows that 17.5% of all patients commencing dialysis treatment for ESRD die within the first 12 months [1]. The alternative to commencing dialysis in these patients is to offer conservative management of the kidney failure. There is evidence that in selected patients this planned non-dialytic management offers a better quality of end-of-life care without significantly reducing the length of survival [2]. Thus thought and discussion should take place when counselling the patient with multiple medical problems on whether to commence dialysis treatment. The key question to be addressed is whether dialysis is going to prolong the length and quality of life of the patient, or whether it will merely prolong the dying process. If the latter is the case then the patient who has full understanding of the likely prognosis may wisely elect not to embark on renal replacement therapy.

> Case scenario A (Part 2): Mr A does not want to die. Previous abdominal surgery makes peritoneal dialysis impossible and he would therefore have to undergo haemodialysis. This would mean travelling to the local haemodialysis centre three times a week, and being out of the house for up to 8 hours on each occasion. His daughter arranges to see his GP with Mr A, and expresses her anxiety about how her father will cope with this regime and particularly how her mother will cope alone in the house for so long. The GP contacts the renal unit and passes on these concerns. A meeting is arranged between Mr A, his daughter and the nephrologist to discuss the way ahead.

The United States Renal Physicians Association and the American Society of Nephrology have drawn up a guideline to assist doctors in the decision-making process about withholding and withdrawing dialysis [3, 4]. It contains nine recommendations (summarised in Box 18.1), 15 prognostic tables and 302 references. They can be applied to the patient who is deciding whether or not to commence dialysis, or equally to the patient who is already receiving dialysis treatment and is contemplating withdrawal from treatment.

> **Box 18.1 Summary of guidelines for withholding or withdrawing dialysis therapy in patients with chronic renal failure** [3, 4]
>
> Shared decision making
> Informed consent or refusal
> Estimating prognosis
> Conflict in resolution
> Advance directives
> Withholding or withdrawing dialysis
> Special patient groups
> Time limited trials
> Palliative care

Shared decision-making and informed consent

These concepts underpin the process. Patients should never have the decision to commence dialysis (or not to commence dialysis) foisted upon them, and ultimately the will of the patient is of paramount importance. But equally, the patient should not feel alone when faced with such a decision and the physician should be in a position to guide and support the patient and carers. With good communication between patient and doctors, it is usual for a decision to be made with which all are comfortable. Usually the patient will want the family and/or carers to be involved in these discussions, and it may be helpful for other members of the professional team to contribute (with the consent of the patient). If the patient does not have the mental capacity to make such a decision, then the legal agent of the patient should be involved. All parties need to know what is available and how having dialysis would impact on the quality of daily life. Time should be spent explaining the different types of dialysis which may be most suitable (e.g. haemodialysis versus peritoneal dialysis), how much travelling to and from the dialysis centre would be required, what surgery or other preparation for dialysis would be needed, and what possible complications might occur with and without dialysis.

Different religious and ethnic groups have differing approaches to the withholding and withdrawal of dialysis treatment. The patient may find it helpful to receive expert advice from a religious or spiritual guide.

Before accepting a decision by the patient not to commence dialysis, the professional carers should be satisfied that the patient is competent to make such a decision. The decision should be made over a sustained period of time and the patient should remain consistent in that decision, understand the consequences of not starting dialysis and have the ability to rationalise the decision in a logical way. As part of the process it is important that depression or other psychological or psychiatric problems are ruled out, if necessary with the help of a psychiatrist or counsellor.

Estimating prognosis

If the burden of co-morbidity is heavy, the prognosis on dialysis for the patient with ESRD may be no better than with conservative management. Predicting survival on dialysis depends more on the level of co-morbidity and functional isolation than on the age of the patient [5]. Doctors should try to estimate the prognosis of the patient, acknowledging that such an estimate may be very imprecise, in order to allow the patient to make an informed decision. The patient may end up balancing quality of life against quantity of life. These value judgments are intensely personal, but can only be made when armed with the correct information. The RPA document [4] provides useful tables that can be used to provide a guide to the patient on the likely length of life once dialysis is commenced. These tables combine information about the age of the patient with important indicators of co-morbidity to provide prognostic data. They do not allow one to combine different co-morbidities which may be unique to that patient, and variability between patients still makes it difficult to predict accurately the early death of any individual patient commencing dialysis [6]. Nevertheless, prognostic tables are helpful for informative discussions.

There are patients who do not wish to discuss their prognosis. It is incumbent on the team to explore why this is the case, and to use sensitivity in the discussion. The doctor may only need to provide enough information, delivered in a compassionate and understanding way, to show the patient that survival on dialysis is not likely to be long. If the patient does not wish to be involved in the decision-making process, then the doctor should ask the patient whom the patient wants to be involved.

Conflict in resolution

Occasions do arise when concordance is not reached. Disagreement on the best way forward may occur between the patient, the multidisciplinary team and/or the patient's carers or representatives (see Figure 18.1).

While the views of the patient should ultimately determine the course of action, it is important that all parties in this process try and

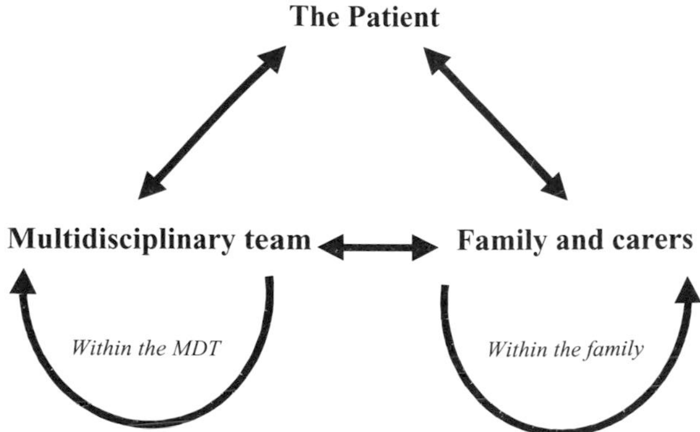

Fig. 18.1 Possible sources of conflict in decision-making about dialysis therapy.

understand and respect the position of those who disagree. With good communication and discussion of the prognosis and of the choices available, resolution should be possible. Differences of opinion may also occur within the multi-disciplinary team, or between the team and the patient and/or the family. Where conflict persists, it may be appropriate to commence and continue with dialysis until these issues have been completely ironed out.

Advance directives

The severely uraemic patient is in no position to make any decision about anything. Thus the above discussions and decisions need to be made relatively early in the course of chronic renal failure. If the issue of possible future dialysis is likely to become important for any patient, early referral to a nephrologist is advised. These decisions need time in order to be made properly and reconciled, and the patient needs to be well enough to make them. One study has shown that after referral specifically for dialysis to a nephrologist, 25% of referred patients eventually elected not to commence dialysis [7]. Late referral may make it necessary to dialyse the patient by default until he or she is well enough to understand the implications of withdrawal from treatment, thus generating unnecessary morbidity and suffering.

Written advance directives may facilitate decision-making on behalf of the patient when a crisis point is reached, either when deciding whether to start dialysis or whether to withdraw it. Advance directives are also recommended for patients already on dialysis. Despite this, a minority of severely ill dialysis patients make advance directives. In one study in the United States of dialysis patients with severe co-morbidity, only 32% had a living will [8]. GPs and dialysis staff need to be comfortable while discussing these issues and to encourage patients to include advance directives for when withdrawal from dialysis might occur [9, 10].

Withholding or withdrawing dialysis and special patient groups

The informed patient who has decision-making capacity and who decides not to commence dialysis, or to withdraw from dialysis, should have that decision respected. Equally the patient who no longer has decision-making capacity but who has previously indicated that he or she would not like to commence dialysis, or whose legal representative refuses dialysis, should not be dialysed. There is also consensus that the patient with profound neurological impairment who lacks signs of purposeful thought, sensation or behaviour should not be forced to undergo dialysis.

Patients who have a terminal non-renal illness, or those with co-morbid disease that makes dialysis technically demanding or impossible, are likely to have a poor prognosis if dialysis is commenced. In these patients it is hoped that with good communication a shared decision can be made not to commence dialysis.

Time-limited trials

It is possible to offer a patient to commence dialysis for a set time period, for example a month or two, and then to review the situation and decide whether it is appropriate to continue. While opting for this course may avoid conflict if there are differences of opinion on the best course of action, it should not be used as a substitute for making hard decisions that ultimately may be in the best interests of the patient. Stopping dialysis is usually a more difficult concept for a patient and the family than not starting it, and in such circumstances it may be better never to start at all. In reality, time-limited trials of dialysis usually are terminated by the onset of a complication or another illness that makes continuing dialysis unfeasible.

Case scenario A (Part 3): After discussion with his family, the GP and the renal team, Mr A eventually confirms that he would like to commence dialysis when necessary. His daughter remains concerned at how the disruption to family life may impact on her mother, but is prepared to go along with her father's wishes.

He commences dialysis and manages reasonably well at first. Several months later he develops an ulcer on his right foot, which becomes infected. He has an angiogram and angioplasty, but ultimately a right below knee amputation is required. Mr A does not feel that he would have any quality of life if he were to lose the right foot, and after long discussion with his family and carers decides that he would like to refuse this operation and withdraw from dialysis treatment.

For those patients who are already on dialysis, the development of terminal disease will occur at some point. The principles of palliative care for these patients are in many ways no different than for any other patient, but the decision about when and if to withdraw dialysis treatment adds another layer of complexity to the management. As with the decision on whether to commence dialysis, this is a decision that should ultimately be made by the patient whenever possible, guided and advised by the medical team. Dialysis withdrawal allows the care of the patient to concentrate on symptom control and maintenance of dignity, and for the place and manner of death to be peaceful and planned. It is a common event. In one study, death following withdrawal from dialysis therapy accounted for 23% of all deaths in a dialysis population [11].

Palliative care for the patient with end-stage renal disease

Case scenario B: Mrs B is an 82-year-old widow who lives alone. She has widespread osteoarthritis, which has left her virtually unable to get out of the house. She also has progressive chronic renal failure secondary to chronic glomerulonephritis and exacerbated by use of non-steroidal anti-inflammatory drugs. Her renal function is close to end-stage and a decision is required as to whether to commence dialysis. She has no immediate family, and seeks advice from her GP. Together with the renal team, a decision is taken not to commence dialysis but to continue with conservative management at home.

It is important that the patient should understand that opting not to receive dialysis is not synonymous with opting out of other aspects of care. In contrast, there are many supportive and palliative treatments that can greatly enhance the quality of life. For this patient the GP is likely to be at the hub of the care process. The nephrologist should also remain involved, even if one step removed (if travel to hospital clinics is not easy), and expert help should also be sought, if appropriate, from the palliative care team, the hospice and other sources of medical, psychological, social and spiritual support. In end-stage renal disease, attention to specific aspects of symptom management may be highly beneficial.

Treatment of anaemia

If anaemia is present, then deficiency of haematinics should be checked for and corrected if present. Once this has occurred, it may be appropriate to commence erythropoietin treatment. Patients with sepsis, malignancy or other inflammatory conditions may not respond well to erythropoietin, but a therapeutic trial may be helpful. If erythropoietin is not successful then intermittent blood transfusion may be the most appropriate treatment.

Management of fluid balance

A feature of ESRD is the loss of ability to regulate salt and water balance. Patients may be polyuric, and require encouragement to drink more fluids. More commonly fluid retention occurs. This can be uncomfortable and unpleasant. Increasing doses of diuretics may be required with a restriction on oral intake. Thiazides tend to be less effective in renal impairment, and loop diuretics are the treatment of choice. However if loop diuretics are used in combination with a small dose of a thiazide, the effect is synergistic and a diuresis may be established. Eventually fluid overload may become unresponsive to all pharmacological treatment. Pulmonary oedema may be the terminal event, and in these circumstances a small dose of opiate can be highly effective in controlling the distress of hypoxia. Isolated ultrafiltration can be used to treat pulmonary oedema (if vascular access for dialysis is in place), in which salt and water are removed but no dialysis is given.

Acidosis

Another possible cause of shortness of breath in ESRD is worsening metabolic acidosis. The result can be a subjective feeling of breathlessness as well as a general malaise and loss of energy. Sodium bicarbonate can be given to correct the acidosis, though the high sodium load may worsen problems of salt and water retention. Judicious balancing of bicarbonate and diuretic prescriptions may be required.

Diet

Protein restriction may delay the onset of uraemic symptoms, though this needs to be offset against the dangers of inadequate nutrition in the palliative care setting. Advice from a dietician on a low phosphate diet, and prescription of phosphate binders, may help in the management of pruritus, which is a common and distressing symptom in advanced uraemia. Potassium restriction may also be advised if hyperkalaemia is a problem. In the terminal stages of the disease, anorexia is usual and dietary restrictions become inappropriate.

Pain

Pain is often considered not to be a feature of the uraemic syndrome, but pain has been reported as occurring in the last 24 hours of life in 42% of patients who are dying with ESRD [12]. Pain control should be approached in the same way as with any other patient with some important provisos. Non-steroidal anti-inflammatory drugs are contra-indicated in these patients (unless death is imminent anyway), as there is a realistic prospect that even a small dose will have significant adverse effects on remaining renal function. Opiates are effective and safe in renal failure, but the team should be aware that the breakdown products of morphine accumulate when there is renal dysfunction and other opiates may have fewer side effects (e.g. fentanyl). The result of this accumulation may be to prolong the effect of opiates, including side-effects. Unrecognised severe toxic effects may develop, with increasing drowsiness, twitching and depressed respiration.

GI symptoms

Constipation is common when opiates are used, and stool softeners and laxatives may be required. Nausea and vomiting may also occur and should be treated symptomatically, though dose reduction of drugs may be required in renal failure.

Fits

It is estimated that only 10% of patients with terminal uraemia have convulsions [13]. Anti-convulsant prophylaxis is therefore not recommended for all such patients. If a patient has a convulsion, then further convulsions might be expected. In these circumstances it is appropriate to consider the use of an anti-convulsant. Phenytoin is often used, though therapeutic level monitoring is advised if usage is to continue for more than a few days, as dose reduction is necessary in renal failure.

Agitation, confusion and distress

Many patients with end-stage symptoms do not become distressed. Confusion progresses with drowsiness. If patients do become agitated, then benzodiazepines or haloperidol can be used judiciously, though dose reduction is required in renal failure. Benzodiazepines can also be used as palliative treatment for myoclonic jerks (which are common) and physical agitation (which is not).

End-of-life care

The patient may have a clear desire to die in a certain place, and these wishes should be respected whenever possible. For the patient withdrawing from dialysis, length of time until death is usually 8–12 days, and the prognosis for patients who develop uraemic symptoms who are not given dialysis is similar (though sudden death as a result of cardiac arrhythmias may occur). Withdrawal or withholding of dialysis facilitates the focus of care being on symptom control, spiritual and psychological care. The necessity of regular blood tests and maintaining dialysis treatment are removed and the timing of death can, to a certain extent, be predicted. Respect for religious and spiritual needs should be shown, and cultural or ethnic aspects should also be understood by the carers. One study [12] has reported that in patients withdrawing from dialysis treatment 15% had a 'bad death', 38% a 'good death' and 46% a 'very good death'. As expertise develops it is hoped that these percentages will improve.

Palliative care in the renal transplant recipient

Most renal transplant recipients either die with a functioning graft or lose their graft and go back on to dialysis. The management of those who require palliative care when the transplant continues to function depends on the level of function. If the transplant continues to work well, then the situation is virtually analogous to a non-renal patient (though nephrotoxic drugs should be avoided). One important difference is that the transplant patient will be taking immunosuppressive drugs, and at some point a decision may be made to taper down the immunosuppression, especially if sepsis or malignancy have developed. In these circumstances a judgement has to be made with the patient, weighing up the potential benefits on slowing the development of malignancy, or treating infection against the potential risks of losing transplant function. Some patients would rather die than lose their transplant and have to go back on dialysis treatment, while others would sacrifice the graft if there were some chance that this might prolong life in a meaningful way. Drug dosages in renal transplantation may require reduction depending on the level of renal function.

References

1 Walters G, Warwick G, Walls J. Analysis of patients dying within one year of starting renal replacement therapy. *Am J Nephrol* 2000; 20(5): 358–363.
2 Smith C, Da Silva-Gane M, Chandna S, Warwicker P, Greenwood R, Farrington K. Choosing not to dialyse: evaluation of planned non-dialytic management in a cohort of patients with end-stage renal failure. *Nephron Clin Pract* 2003; 95(2): c40–c46.
3 Galla JH. Clinical practice guideline on shared decision-making in the appropriate initiation of and withdrawal from dialysis. The Renal Physicians Association and the American Society of Nephrology. *J Am Soc Nephrol* 2000; 11(7): 1340–1342.
4 Renal Physicians Association and American Society of Nephrology. Shared decision-making in the appropriate initiation of and withdrawal from dialysis. *Clinical Guideline Number 2*, Rockville, MD: RPA 2000.
5 Chandna SM, Schulz J, Lawrence C, Greenwood RN, Farrington K. Is there a rationale for rationing chronic dialysis? A hospital based cohort study of factors affecting survival and morbidity. *BMJ* 1999; 318(7178): 217–223.
6 Barrett BJ, Parfrey PS, Morgan J, Barre P, Fine A, Goldstein MB, et al. Prediction of early death in end-stage renal disease patients starting dialysis. *Am J Kidney Dis* 1997; 29(2): 214–222.
7 Hirsch DJ, West ML, Cohen AD, Jindal KK. Experience with not offering dialysis to patients with a poor prognosis. *Am J Kidney Dis* 1994; 23(3): 463–466.
8 Weisbord SD, Carmody SS, Bruns FJ, Rotondi AJ, Cohen LM, Zeidel ML, et al. Symptom burden, quality of life, advance care planning and the potential value of palliative care in severely ill haemodialysis patients. *Nephrol Dial Transplant* 2003; 18(7): 1345–1352.
9 Perry E, Swartz R, Smith-Wheelock L, Westbrook J, Buck C. Why is it difficult for staff to discuss advance directives with chronic dialysis patients? *J Am Soc Nephrol* 1996; 7(10): 2160–2168.
10 Holley JL, Hines SC, Glover JJ, Babrow AS, Badzek LA, Moss AH. Failure of advance care planning to elicit patients' preferences for withdrawal from dialysis. *Am J Kidney Dis* 1999; 33(4): 688–693.
11 Neu S, Kjellstrand CM. Stopping long-term dialysis. An empirical study of withdrawal of life-supporting treatment. *N Engl J Med* 1986; 314(1): 14–20.
12 Cohen LM, Germain M, Poppel DM, Woods A, Kjellstrand CM. Dialysis discontinuation and palliative care. *Am J Kidney Dis* 2000; 36(1): 140–144.
13 Neely KJ, Roxe, D.M. Palliative care/hospice and the withdrawal of dialysis. *J Palliat Med* 2000; 3: 57–67.

19: Management of Lymphoedema

DENISE HARDY

Introduction

Lymphoedema is a progressive condition that results from insufficiency or failure of the lymphatic system, with or without co-existing venous insufficiency [1]. It results in the accumulation of protein-rich fluid in subcutaneous tissues. It can cause considerable distress, particularly if left untreated when it can become a crippling handicap to patients who are perhaps already weakened by advanced cancer. A heavy, oedematous limb has serious physical and psychological effects and may impair mobility, independence and quality of life.

As palliative care should be integrated into disease management from the time of diagnosis, early assessment and management of lymphoedema should be implemented in order to minimize debility [2]. For those in the UK who are uncertain about local services, the *Directory of Lymphoedema Services* is a useful reference point (www.lymphoedema.org/bls). It identifies specialist centres, referral details and outlines appropriate management techniques [3, 4].

Aetiology

Lymphoedema occurs when there is a disturbance of the equilibrium between the transport capacity of the lymphatic system and the load of lymph to be cleared [5]. This may be due to impaired lymphatic drainage, increased lymphatic load or gravitational effects.

Impaired lymphatic drainage

Lymph node irradiation or excision restricts lymphatic drainage routes and may result in the remaining vessels becoming overloaded. Patients at particular risk of developing lymphoedema are therefore those with breast, genital or pelvic tumours who may have undergone surgery and/or irradiation to a major group of lymph nodes. If local disease advances, established lymphoedema may progress due to local tumour/metastases obstructing the venous or lymphatic systems.

Lymphoedema may also result from congenital abnormalities of the lymphatics.

Increased lymphatic load

Increased lymphatic load can result from venous insufficiency or venous hypertension or acute tissue inflammation. Initially the lymphatic system will respond by increasing lymph flow, but if the increase in load continues, drainage fails as the vessels become overloaded.

Gravitational effect

Dependent or gravitational oedema arises because of a lack of propulsion to blood and lymph flow in a limb. Palliative patients who may have neurological damage or who are immobile for other reasons are therefore at high risk.

Other contributory factors

The following factors can also contribute to the formation of oedema in the palliative care setting [1, 2]:

- hypoprotemaemia;
- heart failure;
- fluid-retaining drugs (e.g. NSAIDs, steroids, some hormone therapies).

Characteristics of lymphoedema

In the early stages lymphoedema is soft, pitting and reduces with elevation. The onset of swelling may be gradual or sudden, depending on the aetiology. Exacerbation of the swelling may occur following an infection of the limb or be a result of disease progression.

Protein accumulation in the tissues results in fibrosis and thickening of subcutaneous tissues. Pitting of the skin becomes increasingly difficult and limb swelling does not reduce with elevation.

Typical changes of chronic lymphoedema are [6]:

- enhanced skin folds;
- hyperkeratosis (warty, scaly skin changes);

- lymphangiomata (blisters on the skin surface);
- papillomatosis (a 'cobblestone' change to the surface of the skin).

Assessment of a patient with lymphoedema

Assessment of a patient with lymphoedema includes consideration of all possible aetiologies (see above), the physical effects on the patient (including functional impairment), and the psychological and social effects on the patient and their carers. Comprehensive evaluation is essential with advanced disease as there may be many new or progressive factors. It is essential to identify any treatable aspects of the swelling such as anaemia [2, 7].

Evaluation

The examination of a swollen limb involves identifying the signs and extent of lymphoedema, which is an important factor in choosing appropriate treatment.

A thorough history should elicit the associated symptoms and will determine other possible aetiologies. The examination will look for clinical signs and evidence of complications such as infection or increased venous pressure (patients with advanced cancer may develop DVT even when wearing compression garments). See section on 'Blood circulation'.

The following investigations may also be useful in the palliative setting if the patient's general condition allows [7]:

- Full blood count;
- Plasma electrolytes, urea and creatinine concentrations;
- Plasma albumin concentration;
- Ultrasound, CT or MRI to determine disease status and lymphadenopathy;
- Colour Doppler ultrasound or venogram to evaluate venous function.

SKIN CONDITION

The changes of chronic lymphoedema should be noted and the skin checked for dryness, fungal infections, acute inflammatory episodes (AIE), and lymphorrhoea (leakage of lymph). The latter may be associated with rupture of lymph blisters, or fungation/ulceration and can cause much distress to patients.

Predisposition to AIE (commonly known as cellulitis) is increased in advanced disease and is particularly important to recognize and treat. It is not only a troublesome complication of lymphoedema, but can result in further swelling. Antibiotics should be commenced immediately. Phenoxymethylpenicillin (penicillin V) is the antibiotic of choice (erythromycin for those allergic to penicillin). A change of antibiotic may be necessary if a response does not occur within three days of commencing treatment.

Ulceration (usually uncommon in lymphoedema) may become a more prominent feature in advanced cancer due to fragility of the skin, fungating tumours, concurrent venous disease and the formation of lymph blisters (lymphangiomas).

BLOOD CIRCULATION

Signs of venous hypertension in limbs should be noted (i.e. distension of veins/cyanosis of limb), since venous obstruction or incompetence can influence the outcome of lymphoedema treatment. Should a deep vein thrombosis form in an already oedematous leg, compression treatment with hosiery or bandaging is usually postponed until 8 weeks after anticoagulant therapy has started [8]. This does not apply, however, to upper limbs where compression is often commenced in combination with anticoagulants. It is thought that veins in the arm have a small calibre and any emboli will not produce significant morbidity [1, 5].

Arterial insufficiency is an absolute contraindication for the use of elastic compression. Assessment by Doppler studies may be important before garments are applied.

FUNCTION AND MOBILITY

Functional assessment is essential since a swollen limb often reduces function and mobility, affects posture and balance and makes the limb uncomfortable to use. The resultant reduced function will perpetuate swelling, stiffness and discomfort. This may be exacerbated by weakness caused by advanced malignancy.

Many patients may complain of numbness or discomfort following surgery or radiotherapy. It is important to differentiate this from neurological deficit due to tumour infiltration, since this can cause progressive or complete loss of limb function and severe neuropathic pain. The skills of the multi-disciplinary team will often be required to relieve discomfort and maximise function within the limitations imposed by the condition [9].

PAIN

Lymphoedema does not cause acute pain. Most patients complain of tightness and aching due to the skin stretching over the swollen limb, and for some the weight of the limb can put a considerable strain on supporting joints and muscles causing aching and discomfort. When pain is more severe, it is important to consider the possibility of other complications and disease progression. In advanced disease, pain may certainly be exacerbated by inflammation, infection and DVT.

Patients' perceptions

Perceptions of body image are often affected by a swollen limb and can result in much psychological distress. It is crucial therefore to gain an insight into an individual patient's experiences so that the therapist and patient may join in partnership to make decisions about future management. Patients with advanced cancer may have numerous problems of which the lymphoedema may have less importance than the others. A thorough assessment will enable likely outcomes to be established and an appropriate, realistic and individualised treatment plan to be developed [1, 7, 9].

Management

Management should begin early if good results are to be achieved but should be considered even when advanced disease is apparent. Management aims include:

- Reduction
- Control
- Palliation.

It is important to involve the patient as much as possible in setting realistic goals for treatment and in optimising adherence to treatment; however, the burden of treatment must not exceed benefit. Education, advice and information about the swelling should also be discussed [2, 9].

Management employs a combination of skin care, external support or compression, manual/simple lymph drainage and exercise.

Intensive or reduction phase

Intensive treatment usually lasts 2–4 weeks and will require specialist help. The indications for intensive treatment are highlighted in Box 19.1. For cancer patients who do not have a locally recurrent disease and whose life expectancy is more than a few weeks, reduction and control of the swelling is appropriate.

Box 19.1 Indications for the intensive phase of treatment [8]

Long-standing or severe lymphoedema
Awkwardly shaped limb
Deep skin folds
Damaged or fragile skin
Lymphorrhoea
Swollen digits

SKIN CARE

Care of the skin is a fundamental part of any management programme for patients with lymphoedema (see Box 19.2). Impaired local immunity (by removal of lymph nodes) and the presence of static protein-rich lymph in the swollen limb makes the patient prone to infection, which in turn can lead to further fibrosis and scarring of lymphatics. Keeping the skin intact and supple will reduce the risk of infection. Equally, reduction in the limb size will lessen the risk of infection by reducing the amount of static lymph.

Box 19.2 Management of skin problems

Dry flaky skin	Daily wash with soap substitutes Daily application of bland moisturising products, e.g. aqueous cream
Hyperkeratosis	Moisturizing ointment to lift hard skin Diprosalic ointment for small areas Hydrocolloid dressings with steroid ointment for larger areas
Contact dermatitis	Avoid irritant substance Wash with bland emollients Topical steroid ointments

Continued

Box 19.2 ***Continued***

Fungal infections	Strict daily hygiene Topical antifungal cream/powder Use of Tea Tree Oil as a preventative measure Keep area cool and dry Long term treatment, if required with half strength Whitfields ointment
Acute inflammatory episodes (cellulitis)	Penicillin V 500 mg q.d.s. 2 weeks (or erythromycin if patient is allergic to penicillin) Analgesia to relieve pain and fever Rest and support of limb Avoid compression in acute phase
Lymphorrhoea	Non-adherent sterile dressing to leaking area Application of multi-layer short stretch bandages for 24–48 h, changing as necessary

EXTERNAL SUPPORT

External support in the reduction phase is achieved by the daily application of multi-layer, inelastic bandages. Applying a rigid support to the limb raises interstitial pressure, reduces lymph formation and provides a firm outer casing for the limb muscles to work against.

Low (short) stretch bandages (providing a low resting pressure and a high working pressure) are applied by a specially trained therapist whose experience ensures that the bandage provides even pressure around the limb. In awkwardly shaped limbs this can be achieved using soft foam or padding to smooth out the skin folds and promote a suitably smooth profile prior to bandage application. Bandages are replaced on a daily basis to ensure maintenance of appropriate pressure and to check skin condition. The resulting improvement of the limb shape then enables the fitment of containment hosiery (see section on 'Maintenance or control phase').

EXERCISE

Exercise is important to promote the drainage of lymph and discourage pooling in the limbs. The most significant effects of exercise are highlighted in Box 19.3. Referral to a physiotherapist should be made if there is evidence of functional deficit or poor range of movement of a joint. The use of slings should be discouraged unless required to relieve pain or support flail limbs.

Box 19.3 The value of exercise

Increases lymphatic drainage by stimulating the muscle pump
Maintains and/or improves joint mobility
Improves posture and facilitates functional activities
Points to remember:
Hosiery should always be worn during exercise
Movements should be slow, rhythmical and well controlled
Discourage over-exertion (this increases vasodilation/lymph production)

MANUAL LYMPATIC DRAINAGE

Manual lymphatic drainage (MLD) is a very gentle form of massage used to encourage the flow of lymph from congested oedematous areas of the body to areas where it can drain normally [10]. If performed correctly, skin surface massage encourages the drainage of lymph. It is particularly useful for facial and truncal lymphoedema where external support or compression is not appropriate. Unless congestion is removed from the root of the limb, reduction in the limb itself will not be achieved.

A simplified form of this massage, simple lymph drainage (SLD), must be taught to patients and carers to ensure continued improvement (see Box 19.4).

Box 19.4 Simple lymphatic drainage—practical guidelines

Simple lymphatic drainage (SLD) is based upon the principles of manual lymphatic drainage (MLD)

It is used within a lymphoedema treatment programme, particularly in the maintenance phase, and is designed to be taught to patients and their families

Simplified hand movements stimulate contraction of the skin lymphatics. This 'milking' action improves superficial lymphatic drainage

Movements are very slow, gentle and rhythmical, with just enough pressure to move the skin over the underlying tissue

SLD starts in the neck and unaffected lymphatics before working on the affected area. This ensures movement of fluid towards functioning lymphatics

SLD is concentrated in the neck and truncal area, although the limb itself may be treated if required

Daily treatments are required over a period of several months. Creams and oils are not used during the SLD

Maintenance or control phase

Once effective reduction of the swelling has been achieved, the maintenance or control phase of treatment is implemented. The aim is to prevent regression of the swelling using a combination of exercises, simple lymph drainage and strong compression (elastic) hosiery. Routine measures for continuing care are outlined in Box 19.5.

Box 19.5 Daily skin and general health care

Protect the limb against trauma. Avoid sunburn
Avoid injections/blood sampling in the affected limb
Keep the limb spotlessly clean using soapless cleanser
Moisturize the skin daily to avoid dryness
Report signs of infection immediately—have antibiotics at hand
Do not carry heavy bags/shopping with the swollen arm
Avoid standing for long periods if the leg is swollen
Use the swollen limb normally—avoid strenuous exercise
Wear loose clothing to prevent further restriction
Keep weight within normal limits—a normal, healthy balanced diet
Do not restrict fluids. Limit salt intake
Do not ignore a slight increase in swelling size—contact the therapist as soon as possible

Hosiery is an important element in this phase of lymphoedema management. Any improvement gained through intensive bandaging, exercise or manual lymph drainage is lost if containment hosiery is omitted.

There is a wide range of hosiery available, with varying compression classes. These range from class 1 (20–30 mmHg at the ankle) to class 3 (40–50 mmHg at the ankle). It is important to note that the European-manufactured hosiery has stronger compression than the equivalent class of British-manufactured hosiery. Lymphoedema usually requires the stronger variety. Guidelines for use of compression hosiery are given in Box 19.6.

Box 19.6 Containment hosiery–general information

It must be evenly distributed and graduated, providing the most pressure at the hand/foot
It must be firm fitting and comfortable
It must never be too tight or painful

Continued on p. 366

Box 19.6 *Continued*

Never fold over the top of the garment
Wear all day—remove at night
Avoid fitting following bathing or after moisturizing

Palliative phase

Reduction of swelling is, unfortunately, unrealistic for patients with locally recurrent advanced cancer, particularly when the trunk is congested. In these circumstances treatment of the limb will only result in an increase of oedema centrally. The palliative phase of lymphoedema management uses modified conventional treatments to address an individual's need and improve the quality of their life. Regular monitoring is required to adjust treatment to meet changing needs as the disease progresses.

Swelling often increases as tumour infiltrates into the skin and further compromises lymphatic drainage. Tissues can become very tense, hard and indurated, and the skin is often discoloured and inflamed in appearance. Skin breakdown, ulceration/fungation and lymphorrhoea are common. Swelling often extends beyond the root of the limb into the trunk and may involve the neck, head or genitals.

Application of external support (in the form of modified support bandaging and appropriate wound dressings for those with areas of skin breakdown, shaped Tubigrip or containment hosiery (particularly flat-knit custom made garments) will counteract feelings of pressure within the limb. Patient comfort will dictate the pressure used.

Although diuretics play no role in pure lymphoedema, a venous element to the swelling may well respond to diuretic therapy. When lymphatic/venous obstruction occurs due to recurrent tumour, a combination of high-dose steroid (dexamethasone 4–12 mg daily) and diuretics is worth considering to reduce peritumour oedema and pain.

Patients who are weak and debilitated and those with neurological dysfunction, such as spinal cord compression, are particularly at risk of dependent oedema. Gentle regular, active or passive exercise will enhance lymph flow as well as preventing joint and muscle stiffness. Manual lymph drainage will help to ease truncal swelling and relieve tension in the affected limb.

Dependent oedema responds well to pressure and if there is no limb distortion, appropriate compression hosiery may be fitted as part of a plan alongside exercise and skin care. Pneumatic compression pumps (Flowtron, Centromed) may also be used for this scenario, provided the oedema does not extend into the trunk. These are particularly useful for softening longstanding fibrosis and reducing oedema. Appropriate compression hosiery should always be fitted afterwards.

Injury to tissues, infection and discomfort are common features of this condition, and attention to them may make a difference between the patient preserving what little mobility remains, or becoming bedbound [1].

Conclusions

There is no doubt that the earlier lymphoedema treatment is introduced, the more successful it is. However, it is unlikely to resolve completely, particularly if there is evidence of progressive disease. As more patients spend longer time in the advanced stages of cancer, the prevalence of lymphoedema will increase [2] and it is therefore essential that early signs of oedema are actively sought and that intervention instigated as soon as possible. Ideally this should include an early referral to a local lymphoedema specialist.

References

1 Badger C. Lymphoedema. In: Penson J, Fisher R, eds. *Palliative Care for People with Cancer*, 2nd edition. London: Arnold, 1995: 88–90.
2 Cheville A. Lymphoedema in the palliative care. *Scope Phlebol Lymphol* 2000; 9 (2): 368-372.
3 British Lymphology Society. *Directory of Lymphoedema Treatment Services*, 3rd edition. Caterham, Surrey: BLS Publication, 2001. http://www.lymphoedema.org/bls/
4 British Lymphology Society. *Definitions of Need Document.* Caterham, Surrey: BLS Publication, 2001.
5 Badger C, Twycross R. *Management of Lymphoedema: Guidelines.* Oxford: Sir Michael Sobell House, 1988.
6 Veitch J. Skin problems in lymphoedema. *Wound Manage* 1993; 4(2): 42–45.
7 Keeley V. Oedema in advanced cancer. In: Twycross R, Jenns K, Todd J, eds. *Lymphoedema* Oxen: Radcliffe Medical Press, 2000: 338–358.
8 Badger C. Palliation or reduction? A guide to selecting treatment for oedema in advanced disease. *Palliat Matters* 1996; 6: 1, 4.
9 Woods M. Lymphoedema. In: Cooper J, eds. *Stepping into Palliative Care.* Oxen: Radcliffe Medical Press, 2000: 81–88.
10 Mortimer PS, Badger C. Lymphoedema. In: Doyle D, Hanks G, Cherny N, Claman K, eds. *Oxford Textbook of Palliative Medicine*, 3rd edition. Oxford: Oxford University Press, 2003: 640–647.

Further reading

Farncombe M, Daniels G, Cross L. Lymphoedema: the seemingly forgotten complication. *J Pain Symptom Manage* 1994; 9(4): 269–276.

Foldi E, Foldi M, Weissleder H. Conservative treatment of lymphoedema of the limbs. *Angiology* 1985; 36: 171–180.

Leverick JR. *An Introduction to Cardiovascular Physiology*. London: Butterworth, 1991.

Regnard C, Badger C, Mortimer P. *Lymphoedema: Advice on Treatment*, 2nd edition. Beaconsfield: Beaconsfield Publishers, 1991.

Thomas S. Bandages and bandaging. The science behind the art. *Care Sci Pract* 1990; 8(2): 56–60.

Woods, M. Patients' perceptions of breast cancer related lymphoedema. *Euro J Cancer Care* 1993; 2: 125–128.

Foldi M, Foldi E, Kubik S. *Textbook of Lymphology for Physicians and Lymphoedema Therapists*, 1st edition. München: Urban & Fischer, 2003.

20: Pressure Area Care and the Management of Fungating Wounds

MARY WALDING

Introduction

This book focuses on the holistic nature of palliative care, exploring the impact that a limited prognosis may have on an individual and their family. Physical symptoms cause great distress, which can increase the psychological impact. This is particularly true of pressure ulcers and fungating wounds. Not only can they cause pain and discomfort, but they are also a visible reminder of the impact of the disease upon the individual. It is difficult to ignore such an obvious reminder of one's illness, and developing a wound may precipitate grieving for what a patient is losing.

Denial is often associated with coping with this loss, and individuals may resist pressure-relieving strategies, or present with advanced fungating tumours that have previously been ignored. Treatment should respect the physical and psychological consequences and should always be what is acceptable to the individual. Box 20.1 identifies some of the factors to consider when assessing a patient's needs. The aim is to provide appropriate care that respects the patient's wishes and causes minimal disruption to their lifestyle.

Box 20.1 Possible impact of skin damage on patients who are dying

Physical	Psychological
Pain	Anxiety
Fatigue	Depression
Odour	Grief
Immobility	Feeling that the wound dominates their life
Lifestyle restrictions	Fear

Pressure ulcers

Pressure ulcers are also sometimes known as decubitus ulcers, pressure sores or bed sores. No term accurately describes the pathology involved and for clarity of purpose this text will use the term 'pressure ulcer', as used by the National Institute for Clinical Excellence (NICE) in their guidelines. A pressure ulcer is an area of localised damage to the skin and underlying tissue. It is difficult to assess the extent of the problem in the community, but the incidence of pressure ulcers in the general hospital population is 4–10% [1], but of greater concern is the rate in palliative care where studies have highlighted incidences of 15–43% [2]. This is due to the multiple factors involved in the maintenance and healing of normal skin that are compromised in the individual who is seriously ill.

A pressure ulcer arises as a result of pressure, friction and shearing. They rarely occur in those who are healthy because an individual will react to discomfort and alter position.

Propensity to develop pressure ulcers is related to:

- reduced mobility or immobility;
- sensory impairment;
- acute illness;
- level of consciousness;
- extremes of age;
- vascular disease;
- severe chronic or terminal illness;
- previous history of pressure damage;
- malnutrition and dehydration.

Development of pressure ulcers is exacerbated by some medications and moisture to the skin. Extrinsic forces on the skin, i.e. pressure, shearing or friction, are also a factor in their development [3]. Areas of the skin most likely to develop a pressure ulcer are those which tend to be in contact with support surfaces:

- heels;
- sacrum;
- ischial tuberosities;
- femoral trochanters;
- elbows;
- temporal region of the skull (including ears);
- shoulders;
- back of head;
- toes.

Signs of incipient pressure-ulcer development include persistent erythema; non-blanching hyperaemia; blisters; discolouration and localised heat, oedema or induration. NICE recommend that all health care professionals are aware of these signs and document and act upon them [3].

Using knowledge of aetiology of pressure ulcers, assessment tools have been developed to enable health care professionals to identify those most at risk. As with all checklists, their value is primarily as aides-mémoire and as guides for allocation of resources, rather than as comprehensive indicators. Most assessment tools will differentiate between low-, medium-, and high-risk categories.

Within palliative care, most patients will be indicated as at 'high risk' of developing a pressure ulcer. It is important that these scores are related to the clinical picture rather than merely reacting to the score. Preventative care plans are vital, ensuring that these are realistic and acceptable to the patient. It may not be possible to persuade a patient with a short prognosis to comply with all care, particularly when they only see a health care professional for a brief time at home. However, they have a right to be given the information required in order for them to make an informed decision.

Measures that can be employed to reduce the risk of pressure ulcers will depend on the needs and circumstances of the individual patient, but may include:

- nutritional support (consider involving the dietician);
- a mobility assessment by a physiotherapist;
- a review of manual handling procedures (how do the family manage?) Work with the physiotherapist to recommend moving and handling techniques;
- pain control (as this may improve mobility);
- skin hygiene;
- assessment and treatment of any incontinence problems (this may require a specialist referral);
- assessment of need for pressure-relieving support surfaces;
- regular observation of vulnerable pressure-points, as possible;
- review of medication.

Areas vulnerable to pressure-ulcer development are those which are in contact with a support surface. One of the ways of reducing the risk of developing pressure ulcers is to move the patient regularly. However, there is no evidence as to how often this should take place; traditionally nursing has taught that an immobile patient should be turned every two hours, but there is no evidence to support this. It has been suggested that an individual will automatically shift their position every 20 minutes if able, but it is unrealistic to disrupt a patient this regularly, and virtually impossible in the community setting.

A standard hospital mattress offers no pressure-relieving properties, neither is there evidence to suggest that soft mattress overlays are useful in preventing pressure sores. NICE guidelines state that all individuals assessed as being vulnerable to pressure ulcers should, as a minimum provision, be placed on a high-specification foam mattress with pressure-relieving properties [4]. It is important that patients at risk of pressure-ulcer development also have a seating assessment undertaken by a physiotherapist or occupational therapist [3].

Pressure relieving devices are either low-tech, using a conforming support surface to distribute body weight over a large area; or high-tech, using alternating inflatable cells [1]. These can be categorised as:

- High-specification foam mattresses: there is consistent evidence of effectiveness with these, but they are not the ideal support surfaces for immobile patients.
- Static air-filled: these can usually be adjusted so that the amount of air present in the mattress is appropriate for the individual in order to distribute the body weight evenly over a large area. However, this must be done by an appropriate health care professional, usually a physiotherapist or occupational therapist. It is possible to get low-air-loss mattresses that maintain cell inflation at a constant low pressure. Fluid-filled mattresses also work on the same principle, but have the disadvantage of weight and subsequent immobility.
- Alternating pressure: these consist of a system of cushions which are inflated and deflated in a preset alternating pattern, the cycle lasting several minutes. This relieves pressure and creates a pressure gradient that enhances blood flow. A wave-like motion may occasionally be felt, which can distress nauseated patients.
- Air-fluidised systems: these suspend the individual on a cushion of air, creating low interface pressure. They tend to be large, expensive and cumbersome, but are effective if an individual is bed-bound and immobile. The systems tend to be either cushion-based or bead-based. Whilst the individual will require assistance to move on bead-based beds, the advantage is great if a patient has a wound that produces a lot of exudate, or if incontinence is a problem, as fluids will sink to the bottom of the bed and be removed later without infection risks. Maintenance costs and storage problems mean that most units will hire these when needed. It is unlikely that these will be used in the community setting.

The price and sophistication of these mattresses varies widely and the most expensive is not necessarily the best. Each choice should be individual for the patient, taking into account their needs, abilities and expectations. It is helpful to use a risk assessment tool (mentioned earlier) in order to prioritise need, for example:

- low risk score: foam mattress (although few patients requiring palliative care will be in this category);
- medium risk score: high specification foam mattress;
- high risk score: alternating-pressure air mattress.

Treatment of pressure ulcers

The aim of wound care is to minimise patient distress and discomfort, and where possible promote healing. This can only be achieved through a holistic approach that considers the psychological and social issues discussed earlier alongside the physical problems.

Pain is often a problem associated with pressure ulcers and it should be addressed regardless of other proposed treatment options. Patients will often require extra analgesia about half an hour in advance of a dressing procedure. Some patients who experience extreme pain and anxiety may find the use of nitrous oxide gas during the procedure gives relief.

It should not be assumed that pressure ulcers in a palliative care population will not improve; they have been seen to heal even in individuals who were within weeks of death [2]. However, many of the systemic factors that support pressure ulcer development also inhibit wound healing [5] and care should be given to improve these factors and to maximise the environment suitable for healing to occur. The patient's care record should contain a detailed assessment of the status of all wounds, which is updated regularly. This should include:

- location;
- size (width, length, depth);
- presence of any sinuses;
- colour and type of wound tissue;
- exudate (amount and colour);
- odour;
- condition of wound margins;
- condition of surrounding skin;
- pain;
- dressing management;
- patient perceptions of wound and wound management.

Box 20.2 suggests dressings that are suitable for certain wound criteria. The recommendations may also be useful for wounds that are similar in nature, but not seen as pressure ulcers.

Wounds should not be routinely cleaned during dressing changes as this can cause physical damage, which disrupts the healing process. If debris or old dressing material needs to be removed this should be through irrigation with warmed isotonic (0.9%) sodium chloride [6].

Box 20.2 Suggested dressings for pressure ulcers

Appearance	Treatment
Intact skin; discoloured, erythema	Consider using a hydrocolloid dressing for protection. If it is possible to avoid pressure/friction and contact with urine or faeces, a transparent film may suffice.
Damaged epidermis; slight damage to dermis	Hydrocolloid dressing. Leave *in situ* for 5–7 days if possible. If bleeding occurs, use an alginate dressing and a film dressing. Change daily.
Full thickness, skin loss	Fill cavity with a hydrocolloid paste and cover with a hydrocolloid dressing.
Slough or necrotic tissue	Autolysis may be facilitated by maintaining a moist wound environment. Use a collagen or hydrogel.
Highly exuding wounds	Use hydrophilic foam sheets or cavity dressings. Use extra padding and film dressings to contain exudate. Wound drainage bags are also available.

NB: Hydrocolloid dressings are contraindicated in infected wounds.

Wounds are often colonised by a variety of bacteria, but this only constitutes an infection if there is evidence to suggest that the body's own defence systems cannot cope with the bacterial load—for example, there is increased erythema, increased exudate, malodorous exudate, pain or pyrexia [6]. The decision to swab a wound in order to identify appropriate antibiotic therapy should only be taken if the patient's prognosis indicates this or if the effects of the infection are difficult for the patient.

Fungating wounds

A fungating or malignant wound is a condition of proliferation and ulceration, which arises when malignant tumour cells infiltrate and erode through the skin [7]. They develop most commonly from the following cancers: breast, head and neck, skin and genital cancers. The incidence of these wounds in cancer patients is poorly recorded, but it has been estimated that 5–10% of patients with metastatic cancer will develop a fungating wound [8].

The spread tends to be through tissues that offer the least resistance—between tissue planes, along blood and lymph vessels and in perineural spaces [9]. Abnormalities in tissue growth in fungating tumours lead to areas of tissue hypoxia and consequent infection of the non-viable tissue. It is this that results in the characteristic malodour and exudate of fungating wounds.

It may be possible to control tumour growth in order to prevent further problems associated with an invasive tumour. The options include:

- radiotherapy;
- chemotherapy;
- hormone manipulation;
- low-powered laser therapy;
- surgery.

However, tumours do not always respond to palliative treatment and in these situations it is necessary to manage the wound to minimise its impact upon the patient. As indicated in the introduction, it is vital that the care of these wounds encompasses a full and holistic approach to the patient. A fungating wound will impact on social, emotional, mental, spiritual and sexual well-being and the psychological impact for the patient and family may be great. Health care professionals must work with the patient and family as a team, in order to comprehensively assess needs and provide a plan of care. There are likely to be many health professionals involved and it is often helpful to identify a key worker to link with the patient so that information is shared appropriately and efficiently.

Whilst not wanting to distract from the holistic treatment of the patient with a fungating tumour, it is important that the physical manifestations are controlled as well as possible. A summary of symptom control considerations for fungating wounds is provided in Box 20.3.

Box 20.3 Summary of symptom control approaches for fungating wounds

Aim	Action
Control tumour growth	Consider radiotherapy, surgery, chemotherapy, low-powered laser therapy, hormonal treatment.
Control malodour	Use occlusive dressings and charcoal pads. Consider the use of antibiotic therapy. Consider de-sloughing the wound. Use an air freshening unit and pleasant aromas. Consider the use of aromatherapy.

Continued on p. 376

Box 20.3 *Continued*

Control pain	Review analgesia, consider the need for co-analgesics. Consider use of TENS. Involve complementary therapists.
Control exudate	Use highly absorbent dressings and padding. Occlude wound if possible. Consider the use of wound drainage (or ileostomy) bags. Consider the use of radiotherapy.
Control bleeding	Consider radiotherapy. Consider using adrenaline 1:1000 soaks. Use padding and haemostatic dressings. Consider the use of silver sulfadiazine or sucralfate paste. Is there a risk of tumour infiltrating a vessel? If so, consider potential patient and family needs.

Fungating wounds are not going to heal, so conventional treatments to aid wound healing are less important than the priority of controlling odour and exudate. However, this is difficult to achieve, with many wounds requiring frequent dressing changes in order to control the symptoms. These wounds are also complicated by their rapidly changing nature; therefore dressing plans will need to be flexible.

As with all wounds, it is important to document an assessment of a fungating wound, so that all health professionals who are involved are aware of the state and requirements of the wound. This also allows changes in the wound status to be noted and the effectiveness of dressing regimes to be evaluated.

Dressings used for fungating wounds should be occlusive as this will help to control odour and exudate. This can be difficult to achieve as the wounds are not of a uniform size and shape, often being difficult to dress. It is important that the dressings which are used do not adhere to the wound. If a fungating wound produces little exudate, a hydrocolloid dressing may be useful. However, the problem is usually control of the exudate, in which case useful dressings include hydrophilic foam; alginates; hydrofibre dressings and semipermeable film dressing.

Large amounts of padding with absorbent materials is sometimes helpful, as is the use of wound drainage or colostomy bags if the wound can be contained and the bags will adhere. It can be helpful to use medical adhesive (and remove with a suitable solvent).

It is important that the skin surrounding the fungating wound is well protected. It is vulnerable to breakdown through infiltration, maceration due to the wound exudate and damage caused during removal of dressings. Cutting a thin hydrocolloid sheet to fit around the wound may provide protection, or consideration may be given to some of the barrier preparations used around stomas. Stoma therapists are skilled in protecting skin around stoma sites and are a useful resource if difficulties are encountered.

The malodour associated with fungating wounds can cause great distress as the individual feels permanently unclean and may isolate themselves for fear of offending others. It may also cause nausea and associated problems with appetite. Whilst the problem may be helped greatly through the use of occlusive dressings, other strategies may also need to be used, including the use of charcoal dressings, which will neutralise the odour.

The odour is caused by the anaerobic bacteria, which inhabits hypoxic and necrotic tissue. A successful treatment option is the use of metronidazole 200 mg orally t.d.s. However, the incidence of nausea associated with this drug often reduces compliance and there is a possibility that effective dosage may be compromised by inconsistent vascular perfusion of the wound. It may be more effective to apply the antibiotic topically in the form of a gel. The disadvantage of this is cost, and the fact that this mode of application may be of little use when there are large quantities of exudate.

De-sloughing the wound, i.e. removing the devitalised tissue, is also worth considering [10], although this should be done with extreme caution as de-sloughing may uncover further problems, such as bleeding, in a fungating wound.

It is often helpful to provide an air-conditioning unit for individuals with fungating wounds, or consider the use of air fresheners or aromatherapy oils.

Fungating wounds are usually vascular and are thus prone to bleeding. The padding that is often necessary to contain exudate also has a useful protective function. If there is localized capillary bleeding then one of the following may be used:

- alginate dressings (these have some haemostatic properties);
- topical adrenaline 1:1000, applied to a dressing pad;
- silver sulfadiazine (should be avoided during radiotherapy as it can disperse the rays);

- sucralfate paste (crush a 1g tablet and mix with hydrogel to an appropriate consistency);
- prophylactic use of tranexamic acid 1 g t.d.s.

Fungating wounds can rarely cause the rupture of a major blood vessel. The team caring for the individual should be aware of this and consideration given to the need to inform the patient and their family, particularly if cared for in the community. It is sensible to follow precautions similar to any situation where a haemorrhage may be considered likely: to have a dark or red blanket to hand; to have gloves and pads; and to ensure there is adequate sedation and analgesia prescribed as required.

Fungating wounds are often associated with pain that is difficult to control. The pain may be potentiated by the impact of the tumour and the experience for an individual. It is important to involve the wider multidisciplinary team, including the complementary therapists.

The patient may require large doses of opiates, plus the use of adjuvant drugs such as the non-steroidal anti-inflammatory drugs (see Chapter 8: The Principles of Pain Management). If pain is uncontrolled it is possible to apply opiates directly to the wound, using a 0.1% solution dissolved in a carrier hydrogel (1 mg morphine to 1 ml hydrogel) [11]. However, this has limitations in highly exuding wounds and is not always effective. The pain may also have a neuropathic component, due to the effect of the tumour distorting nerve tissue. Tricyclic antidepressants and transcutaneous electronic nerve stimulation (TENS) can be helpful. The latter is also of use in relieving the pruritis related to some fungating wounds.

Conclusion

The management of both pressure ulcers and fungating wounds is one of the major challenges of modern palliative care. Control of other symptoms is often so effective that wounds may be seen as the most obvious indicator of an individual's disease. However, as explored in this chapter, there are strategies available to reduce the impact on the patient and family. The use of creative, patient-centred, multidisciplinary management can maximize effectiveness of health care professionals in this area.

References

1 Cullum N, Nelson EA, Flemming K. et al. Systematic reviews of wound care management. *Health Technol Assess* 2001; 5(9).

2 Walding M, Andrews C. Preventing and managing pressure sores in palliative care. *Prof Nurse* 1995; 11(1): 33–38.

3 National Collaborating Centre for Nursing and Supportive Care *The Use of Pressure Relieving Devices (Beds, Mattresses and Overlays) for the Prevention of Pressure Ulcers in Primary and Secondary Care.* National Institute for Clinical Excellence, 2003.
4 National Institute for Clinical Excellence. *Pressure Ulcer Risk Assessment and Prevention (Guideline B)*, 2001.
5 Hess C.T, Kirsner R.S. Uncover the latest techniques in wound bed preparation *Nurs Manage* 2003; 34(12):54–56.
6 Thomas S. *Wound Management and Dressings.* London: The Pharmaceutical Press, 1990.
7 Mortimer P. Skin problems in palliative care: medical aspects. In: Doyle D, Hanks G, Macdonald N, eds. *Oxford Textbook of Palliative Medicine*, 2nd edition. Oxford: Oxford Medical Publications, 1997.
8 Haisfield-Wolfe M, Rund C. Malignant cutaneous wounds: a management protocol *Ostomy Wound Manage* 1997; 43(1):56–66.
9 Grocott P. The palliative management of fungating malignant wounds. *J Wound Care* 1995; 4 (5):240–242.
10 Enck R. The management of large fungating tumours. *Am J Hospice Palliat Care* 1990; 7 (3):111–112.
11 Naylor W Malignant wounds: aetiology and principles of management *Nurs Stand* 2002; 16(52):45–53.

Further reading

Grocott P. *Educational Leaflet 8(2) The Palliative Management of Fungating Wounds.* Huntingdon: The Wound Care Society, 2001.
Hollinworth H *Educational Leaflet 7(2) Pain and Wound Care.* Huntingdon: The Wound Care Society, 2000.
Ivetic O, Lyne P. Fungating and ulcerating malignant lesions: a review of the literature. *J Adv Nurs* 1990; 15 (1):83–88.
Mortimer P. Skin problems in palliative care: medical aspects. In: Doyle D, Hanks G, Macdonald N, eds. *Oxford Textbook of Palliative Medicine*, 2nd edition. Oxford: Oxford Medical Publications, 1997.
Ribbe MW Van Marum RJ. Decubitus: pathophysiology, clinical symptoms and susceptibility. *J Tissue Viability* 1993;3(2):42–47.
Surgical Materials Testing Laboratory. *A Prescriber's Guide to Dressings and Wound Management Materials.* Cardiff: VFM Unit, 1996.
Twycross R. *Symptom Management in Advanced Cancer.* Oxford: Radcliffe Medical Press, 1995.

21: Terminal Care and Dying

CHRISTINA FAULL AND BRIAN NYATANGA

Introduction

Patients who are entering the last phase of their illness and for whom life expectancy is especially short, require particular focus and expertise to meet their heath needs. Professionals need to draw on all their palliative care skills, in order for patients to achieve a transition towards death that fulfils the wishes of the patient and of those close to them. A combination of a rapidly changing clinical situation and considerable psychological demands, pose professional challenges that can only be met through competence, commitment and human compassion. It is important to remember that the nature of the terminal phase and subsequent death has particular consequences for the bereaved (see Chapter 7). Enabling patients to die with dignity, in comfort and in the place of their choice is a very valuable skill, which can in addition bring immense professional satisfaction.

> *We celebrated his life by singing "All You Need is Love" by the Beatles. Palliative care helped him to die entirely on his own terms. I felt honoured to be involved in his care* [1].

This chapter is concerned with how to care for patients whose health has deteriorated to the point when death is imminent. It includes how to recognize the terminal phase and how to manage the physical, psychological, and social needs of patients and their carers including reference to the use of an integrated care pathway. A summary of physical symptom management is given in Figure 21.1.

Helping people to die in the place of their choice

Patients can be looked after in various settings; each has inherent advantages and disadvantages (see Table 21.1). Although it appears most people would prefer to die at home [3], unfortunately this is, for a wide range of reasons not achieved in many cases. Key factors enabling people to stay at home are:

- family or other carers;
- adequate nursing care;

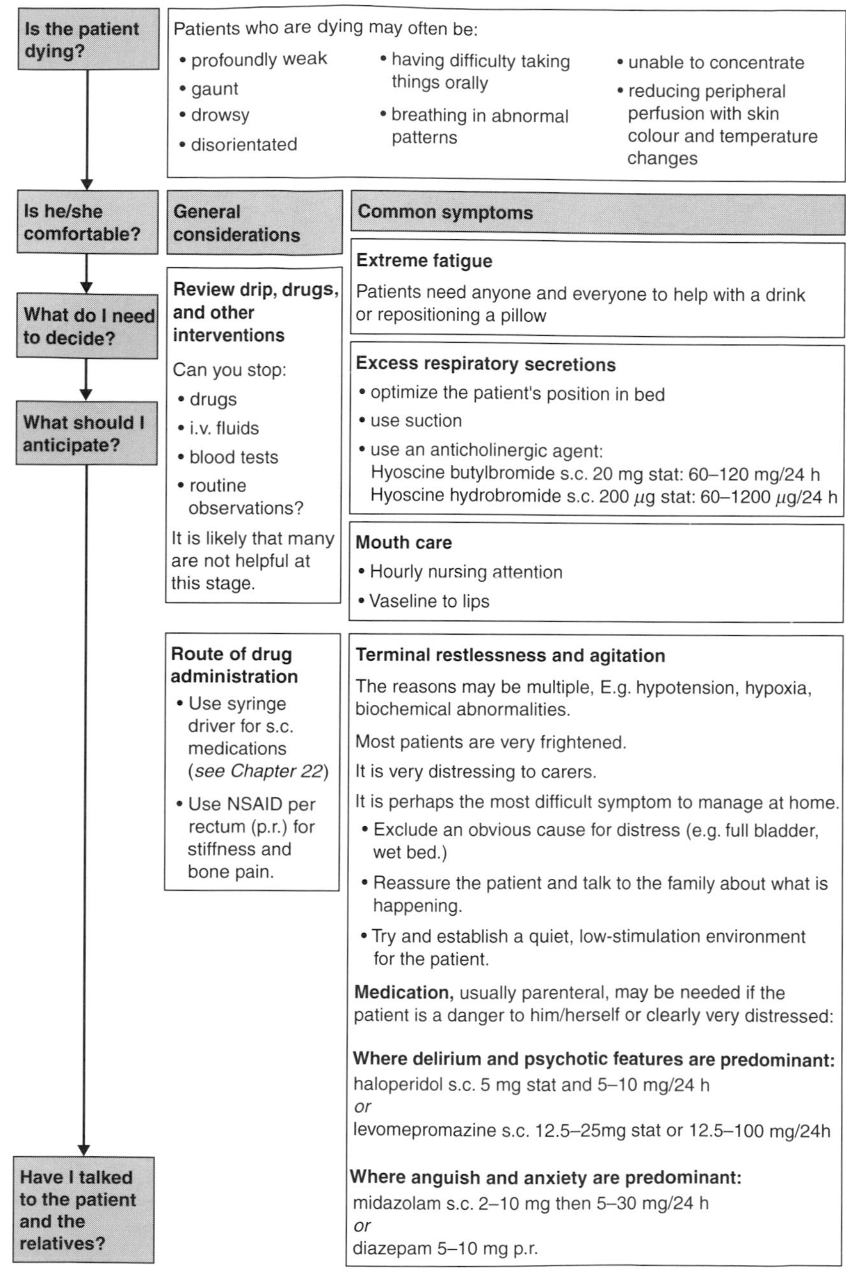

Fig. 21.1 A summary of the management of physical symptoms in the dying patient. (Adapted from Faull C, Woof R 2002: *Palliative Care: An Oxford Core Text* with permission from the publishers Oxford University Press)

Table 21.1 Advantages and disadvantages of different settings of patient care.

Setting	Number of deaths [2]	Advantages	Disadvantages
Home	• 29% of cancer deaths • 22% of non-cancer deaths	• Often preferred by patients [3] • Familiar surroundings and a non-medical environment • Family life maintained • Patient in control (e.g. decisions, visitors, cultural/ spiritual needs) • Home is generally a more peaceful environment • Familiar with medical staff (GP and District Nurse)	• Pain control may be inadequate [4] • Specialist palliative care services not always available for non-malignant disease • Professional help not as accessible • Patients may not be protected from unwelcome visitors • Burden of caregiving falls upon the relatives and friends who may be unable or unwilling to cope • Disruption of family life • Financial consequences to care at home • Critically ill patients may need intensive support (e.g. daily or twice daily visit by GP)
Nursing/ residential home	• 7% of cancer deaths • 16% of non-cancer deaths	• Immediate access to nursing care (except in residential care) • The family is relieved of the burden of care • Familiar GP will have ongoing responsibility for medical care	• Financial implications for patients and families • Standards of care may be variable, being limited by resources • Surroundings are unfamiliar • Families may experience guilt; 'don't put me in a home' • Staff knowledge on symptom control may be limited • Families may feel there is a lack of specialist medical and nursing attention [5]

Continued

Table 21.1 *Continued*

Setting	Number of deaths [2]	Advantages	Disadvantages
Hospital	• 50% of cancer deaths • 57% of non-cancer deaths	• Medical and nursing expertise is readily available • Burden of care is removed from the family • Patients and families may feel safe knowing that doctors and nurses are available	• Patients may feel isolated on a busy unit • Nursing care may be limited by resources • Symptoms may be poorly controlled • Care is more orientated to cure • Unfamiliarity with staff • Family may not be encouraged to participate in the care of the patient • Visiting hours may be restricted
Hospice	• 13% of cancer deaths • < 1% of non-cancer deaths	• Immediate access to specialised staff, within a multidisciplinary team • Palliative care philosophy is widely applied (see Chapter 1) • Most have a higher staff ratio of qualified nurses • Generally less noisy, more peaceful environment than hospitals • Bereavement support is generally more available	• Hospices may be perceived as 'a place to die' •Unfamiliar surroundings • Some hospices may be perceived as being too 'religious' • Many hospices may not meet the needs of patients from ethnic minority groups (although this could be true of other settings)

- night sitting service;
- good symptom control;
- confident committed GPs;
- access to specialist palliative care;
- effective coordination of care;
- financial support;
- education of health care professionals;
- effective out-of-hours medical services.

For example, patients referred to a hospice service in Japan were more likely to die at home than other patients if: they expressed the desire for receiving home care at referral; the family caregiver's desire was the same; they had more than one family caregiver; they had the support of their family physician; they were never re-hospitalised; they received more home visits by the home hospice nurse during the stable phase; and they were in the greatest functionally dependent status during the last week prior to death [6].

Is home 'best'?

It appears that people change their minds depending on the reality of the situation for both themselves and their carers. Dying can, despite great symptom management and lots of support, turn out to be much more difficult than people anticipate. Our understanding of this time and its struggles for patients and carers is becoming more sophisticated. For example:

The palliative care provided for patients with cancer or cardiopulmonary disease was studied in two Leicestershire practices [7]. Roughly 1:5 people died at home and 1:2 people in hospital. Fifteen per cent of cancer patients died in the hospice but none of the patients with cardiopulmonary disease. In this retrospective study 41% of relatives indicated that the patients had expressed a preference in where they wanted to die, 95% indicating home. Although less than half of those that expressed a preference were able to achieve this, 77% of carers felt that, on balance, the place that the patient had died had been the best place for them to die, irrespective of whether it was their preferred place of death or not.

Other significant factors in this 'home is best' debate are:

- Although many people may have clear views about their choice of place they may be unwilling to believe that they are dying here and now.
- The views of many patients cannot be established [8].

However, even allowing for change of heart and the difficulties of accurate prognostication there is a big gap between what patients seem to want and what is achieved.

When is a patient terminally ill?

Terminal care is an important part of palliative care, and usually refers to the management of patients during the last

> *few days, weeks or months of life, from a point when it becomes clear that the patient is in a progressive state of decline* [9].

Although useful, this definition highlights the difficulty of characterising the terminal phase, as it depends on a clinical assessment of subtle physical signs in order to predict a prognosis. Professionals require clinical acumen to discern between inevitable decline and potentially reversible deterioration. This dilemma is perhaps most pronounced in patients with non-malignant illness where episodic, life-threatening deterioration is the disease pattern (e.g. heart failure and chronic obstructive airways disease). These are difficult decisions, need experience and expertise and should be shared with the team.

> **Key point:**
>
> **Recognising that a patient is probably dying is perhaps THE most important factor in enabling achievement of all the factors we associate with a 'good death'.**

It is useful to observe for the following signs as indicators of irreversible decline. This process is often gradual, but progressive:

- Profound weakness;
- Gaunt appearance;
- Drowsiness;
- Disorientation;
- Diminished oral intake;
- Difficulty taking oral medication;
- Poor concentration;
- Skin colour changes;
- Temperature change at extremities.

Principles of management

The care of people who are dying often requires a change of gear [10]. To provide quality terminal care, the principles outlined in Chapter 1 need to be applied rigorously and intensely at this stage. Dying people require a truly holistic approach to their care. Physical comfort is essential but so too is consideration of place (where would they choose to be?) and environment of their care and their need for religious ritual or prayer.

Consider the patient plus their family and friends as the unit of care, and encourage participation from all of these people. It is vital

Box 21.1 Physical assessment checklist: what to look for:

- Pain
- Shortness of breath
- Nausea/vomiting
- Agitation/restlessness/confusion
- Myoclonus and epilepsy
- Noisy breathing
- Urinary incontinence or retention
- Constipation
- Pressure areas/skin care
- Dry/sore mouth
- Difficulty in swallowing
- Reversible complications/co-morbidity

to frequently offer information and support to patients and families. Every effort should be made to reduce the morbidity due to bereavement among family and friends.

A clinical pathway approach has been shown to be particularly effective in enabling high quality care. The Liverpool *Care Pathway for the Dying Patient* is a systematic approach to defining and monitoring the needs of patients, together with guidance for intervention that are commonly required [11, 12]. However the use of such a tool should not be mistaken or seen as reducing dying to a tick-box exercise.

Perform a systematic physical assessment (see Box 21.1) and relieve the patient's physical symptoms promptly. Consider the multifactorial nature of many symptoms, and remember the psychosocial component (e.g. fear) of certain symptoms. Avoid unnecessary medical intrusion—'First do no harm'. Stop all unnecessary drugs.

Follow-up, continuity and 24-hour emergency cover are key. Plan thoroughly as a team for future problems, in what is likely to be a rapidly changing clinical picture. Involve all necessary resources for extra support at an early stage and ensure good communication, especially with out of hours services.

How to assess the needs of a terminally ill patient

Ideally, needs should be defined by the patient and be managed in terms of quality of life. However, in terminal care it is not always feasible to make exhaustive assessments. In addition, communication with the patient may be difficult and accounts from carers can be inaccurate. Skills in non-verbal assessment of pain and distress are important [13] but a high degree of uncertainty may exist. Professionals therefore have to share greater responsibility when making difficult decisions in these situations. This can make practitioners feel outside of their 'comfort zone' and be a key factor leading to inappropriate and unwanted hospital admissions. The wise practitioner is able to use professional experience combined with knowledge of the patient (previous symptoms, concerns, wishes) to perform a sensitive, problem-focused assessment.

Psychosocial needs

Needs of patients

When assessing patient need, it is important to remember that some psychosocial problems may present as poorly controlled physical symptoms (e.g. total pain, terminal agitation, sick with fear). Some of the common problems experienced are outlined in Box 21.2.

Also, factors such as personality, relationships and coping mechanisms are important to consider. Giving patients time and encouraging them to express their feelings is particularly important. Some, however, will not appreciate unrequested 'counselling' and should be allowed the option of denial as a legitimate coping mechanism.

In responding to patient concerns and providing emotional support, it is helpful to use the following guidelines:

- Where does the patient want to die and is this likely to be possible?
- Involve the patient as long as possible in decision-making.
- Answer patients' questions honestly. Give them time. Explanations may need to be repeated on several occasions.
- Patient confidentiality should be assured.
- Allay any fears about dying (uncontrolled symptoms, prolonged process, being alone, lack of warning).

Box 21.2 Psychosocial needs: what to look for:

- Fear, e.g. the diagnosis, mode of death, drug side-effects
- Guilt, e.g. becoming a burden, past life experiences
- Anger, e.g. loss of dignity, missed opportunities, loss of independence
- Uncertainty, e.g. spiritual questions, prognosis, the future of the family
- Depression (often as a consequence to the above)

- Space and privacy should be provided if the patient wishes.
- Consider the patient's spiritual needs. Respect culture and religious views.

- Reassure patients that their family will be offered bereavement support.
- Do not let the medical process obstruct the expression of affection between loved ones.
- Make careful enquiries about the patient's will and 'affairs'.

Needs of family/friends

The team members may be so focused on the patient that family and friends have little opportunity to express concerns. Often, all that is required is a recognition of the family's position and an expression of understanding. However, in certain circumstances it is important to explore difficulties at a greater depth. This assessment should cover physical (e.g. fatigue), psychological (e.g. depression) and social (e.g. finances) needs.

The family and/or friends should have access to professionals, both for information and to meet their own health needs. Information should be given, whenever patient confidentiality allows, even if this feels somewhat repetitious to the professional. Explain to the family or friends what they should do in an emergency, and confirm the 24-hour availability of professional care. The strain on the family and carers should be acknowledged and support offered as appropriate. It may be helpful for team members to determine the family's previous experience of death.

If the patient is not at home, families and carers often need to feel helpful and to know that their contribution is valued. This may include physical care (e.g. bathing, mouth care). Families and friends should not be made to feel like intruders in the care of their loved one. They must be given every opportunity to stay with the patient, and visiting arrangements should be flexible. Reassure family members who find it too difficult to be at the bedside that the patient will not be left alone. Explain that even if comatose, the patient may be aware of the family's presence. They may still be heard by the patient.

The importance of religion and ritual in dying

For those patients who possess a strong religious conviction as part of their spirituality, rituals around death are very important. Professionals should be respectful of this and act with sensitivity to these requirements. Table 21.2 gives a brief outline of some of the traditional practices of the main religious and cultural groups in the

Table 21.2 Overview of rituals around death for main UK religious/cultural groups.

Religion/ culture	Death rituals	Disposal of the body
Christianity	• Traditionally a priest performs the last rites prior to death (prayers of forgiveness and sacrament if possible) • Individuals may wish to pray with the dying patient	• Body can be touched by non-christians • Body is cleaned and covered with a white sheet • Body can be buried or cremated • Funeral directors assist in much of this preparation • The religious component of bereavement occurs at the funeral service
Islam	• Patient should face Mecca if possible (ie south east direction) May keep beard once they have been on pilgrimage to Mecca & wear a Topi (head gear). Not to be removed May prefer to die at home as hospital is seen as for cure only • Mullah (religious leader) may whisper prayers in patient's ear	• Traditionally the body should not be touched by non-muslims • Washing and preparing the body follows precise rules • Burial should occur within 24 hours or as soon as possible • Post-mortems and organ donation are resisted • Burial is the traditional means of disposal of the body
Hinduism	• Brahmin priests may perform rituals that allow forgiveness of sins • A thread may be left around the wrist to show that the patient has received a priest's blessing • Devout Hindus may wish to die on the floor, being close to mother earth	• Correct funeral rites are believed to be important for the salvation of the deceased's soul • Body is washed and put in normal clothes • Only men can perform funeral rites, preferably the eldest son • Cremation is used to dispose of the body • Bereavement involves 10 days of mourning, each day has a particular ceremony

Continued on p. 390

Table 21.2 *Continued*

Religion/ culture	Death rituals	Disposal of the body
Sikhism	• A reader from the temple will recite hymns, if the patient is too weak to do this personally • At death attendants may utter words of praise (Wonderful lord, Wonderful lord)	• The body is washed and placed in a shroud • Religious artefacts worn by patient will be left on the body—'the 5 K's' **Kangha**—wooden comb, **Kara**—iron wrist band, **Kirpan**—short sword, **Kachha**—undershorts, **Kesh**—uncut hair) • Traditionally Sikhs are cremated • Friends and family consider visiting the bereaved as a duty and may provide food
Judaism	• Psalms are recited and the patient should not be left alone • Pillows should not be removed from beneath the head (is believed to hasten death)	• The body should be left for 10 minutes after death • The body may be laid on the floor, with feet pointing to the door • Preparation of the body can be precise and is performed by Jews who specifically deal with the dead • Burial should occur within 24 hours of death • Bereavement is structured with religious ceremony
Buddhism	• The patient will wish to die with a 'clear mind' and may use chanting to achieve this. This influences the nature of the next incarnation • There may be a wish to avoid distractions, e.g. sedating drugs, over-crowding of room, intrusions etc.	• Ideally the body should not be moved or washed before the arrival of a Buddhist monk • Disposal of the body may be by burial, cremation or embalming, depending on the nationality of the deceased

Continued

Table 21.2 *Continued*

Religion/ culture	Death rituals	Disposal of the body
	• Most Buddhists believe that consciousness remains in or near the body for 8–12 hours post death. This may mean that some Buddhists would prefer the body not to be touched during this period	
Rastafarianism	Rastafarians are reluctant to undergo treatments it may contaminate God's temple (their body) Western style medicine may come second to complementary therapies such as herbalism Blood transfusion and organ transplant are not acceptable	Orthodox members show their symbol of faith through a dreadlocks hairstyle, which is not cut at all After death Rastafarians have 10 days of scripture reading and praying. Prayers are said in the name of Ras Tafari, the new Messiah

UK. It is beyond this book to give a detailed account of all beliefs and rituals. It is hoped that this introduces professionals to what they may encounter in their care of dying patients. We all have values, beliefs and rituals that influence the way we experience and cope with life and death. Enquiring about the religious needs of patients can be especially appreciated by both patients and their families. What is of vital importance in culturally safe care is that we ask and explore as we would in any other aspect of care.

It is also important to remember that in a pluralistic society such as the UK, religious law can be interpreted in various ways. Consequently, religious practices may be applied differently and should never be assumed.

Treatment of common symptoms in terminal care

The management of many of the symptoms listed in Box 21.1 is covered elsewhere in this book and will therefore be only briefly mentioned here. This chapter will concentrate on those symptoms that are more specific to the terminal phase.

Analgesia and other drugs which are still of benefit may need to be delivered parenterally (usually subcutaneously: see Chapter 22) or rectally. Planning for this eventuality in the availability of drugs in the home is important. The use of the so-called emergency boxes is one way this has been addressed [14].

The dependency of terminally ill patients demands a multidisciplinary approach, the basis of which is quality nursing care.

General nursing care

It is important to try to involve family and loved ones in the nursing care of the patient. This can be particularly reassuring. Problems should be anticipated and actively prevented. Basic nursing care includes the following:

- careful positioning of the patient;
- pressure area care;
- mouth care;
- bladder and bowel care;
- eye care.

Without the attention to detail that this entails, symptom control will be difficult.

Pain control

Given that pain can change rapidly in the terminal phase, it is important to review patients repeatedly. Indeed, patients may often develop a new pain in the last 48 hours of life [15]. Do not assume that a non-communicative/semiconscious patient will not perceive pain. It is useful to ask repeatedly 'is the patient in pain?' (See also Chapter 8.)

Shortness of breath

Shortness of breath is a common symptom in the terminal phase [16]. It can result from direct involvement of the lungs from the primary disease (malignant or non-malignant) or following a secondary complication (e.g. anxiety, anaemia, infection, asthenia, heart failure). It can be distressing to relatives. Be prepared to use non-drug (fans, open window, relaxation techniques etc.) as well as drug treatments (see also Chapter 10).

Nausea and vomiting

The frailty of terminally ill patients puts them at risk of suffering from nausea and vomiting. Polypharmacy, and anxiety, may compound this. Positioning is important in the avoiding respiratory embarrassment and reducing the anxiety of relatives. A suction machine may be useful in such a situation (see Chapter 9).

Confusion, restlessness and agitation

Confusion is common in patients with advanced illness, particularly in older people and those with chronic cognitive impairment (e.g. dementia, brain tumour). It occurs in up to 75% of patients in the last days of their illness. It is usually fluctuating in severity and characterised by:

- drowsiness;
- poor concentration;
- disorientation;
- poor short term memory;
- inappropriate behaviour.

Misperceptions, delusions and hallucinations may also occur.

Most patients are very frightened. Many retain some insight and fear that they are going mad. It is very distressing to carers [17] and is perhaps the most difficult symptom to manage at home.

Severe agitation, anguish or aggression with risk to self or others is fortunately rare. It generally builds up over days to weeks, although it may be acutely worsened or precipitated by a change of environment (e.g. admission). There are often some warning signs; these include: emotional unease or anguish, fluctuating disorientation and psychotic features, particularly visual hallucinations and paranoid ideas.

MANAGEMENT

The management should be based on certain principles. Firstly, make the patient safe. Secondly, if appropriate, treat reversible causes (see Table 21.3 and Box 21.3). Thirdly, manage the patient in a suitable, quiet environment and fourthly acknowledge the distress and fears of the patient and carers and give clear explanations and reassurances where possible.

In spite of the limitations of assessment, it is important to consider the cause of the confusion, agitation and restlessness. In some instances simple specific measures shown in Box 21.3 can alleviate the cause and result in effective symptom control. It is often challenging, however, to

Table 21.3 Causes of confusion, terminal restlessness and agitation.

Physical causes	Mental/emotional causes (terminal anguish)	Drugs	Biochemical causes
• Uncontrolled pain • Full bladder • Constipation/ full rectum • Immobility • Dyspnoea • Hypoxia • Internal bleeding • Cerebral metastases • Infection • Hypotension • Nausea	• Anxiety • Denial of advancing disease • Fear of dying • Fear of losing control • Unfinished business • Distress at leaving family • Spiritual distress • Frustration with predicament	• Opioids • Psychotropics • Benzodiazepines • Anticholinergics • Anticonvulsants • Steroids • Digoxin • Anticonvulsants • Dopamine agonists • Withdrawal of drugs, e.g. opioids, alcohol	• Liver failure • Renal failure • Hypercalcaemia • Hyponatraemia • Hyper and hypoglycaemia • Thiamine deficiency • Adrenal insufficiency

balance the desire to investigate and discern a cause, with the need to protect patients from intrusive tests which will not, even if abnormal, change clinical management or patient outcome. It is sometimes hard to know a test (e.g. serum calcium) is abnormal and not treat it, but the benefit and risks for patients must be weighed up. For instance, hypercalcaemia is not infrequently part of a terminal deterioration in patients with advanced cancer. Admission to hospital for treatment

Box 21.3 Specific simple management of restlessness: treat the cause

A full bladder: easy to determine, and catheterisation is often an acceptable solution

A loaded rectum: appropriate bowel care can result in calm (e.g. suppository, enema, manual evacuation)

Immobility leads to bed-bound patients suffering from joint stiffness, bed sores and frustration Nursing measures (e.g. pressure-relieving mattress, appropriate bedding, regular turning and careful positioning) and suitable pain relief are all important

Unnecessary drugs: steroids can be stopped abruptly in the terminal phase

Hypoxia: Oxygen may be of benefit to some.

may result in the patient dying away from home or spending some of the last, precious days of their life in a medical environment.

Basic care includes the following measures:

- Reassure the patient and make their environment comfortable (e.g. explanation, spiritual help, music, massage, good lighting).
- Reassure the family and friends.
- Ensure patient safety (e.g. prevent accidents). Most patients are frail and at risk of falling. Sedative drugs may cause hypotension and so increase this risk.
- Provide privacy.
- Assume a confident empathic approach.

In many instances however it is inappropriate or not possible to treat the underlying cause, and drugs are the mainstay of treatment. Confused patients may require antipsychotic medication especially if patients become agitated. Respiridone (500 mcg stat and b.d.) olanzapine (2.5 mg stat and o.d.) have fewer Parkinsonian side effects than haloperidol (2–5 mg stat) but no parenteral preparations are available. Benzodiazepines should generally be avoided in patients with psychotic symptoms as the disinhibition can worsen symptoms.

Table 21.4 indicates the drug options for dying patients with anguish, agitation or restlessness. In an emergency situation a loading dose is often required, followed by regular maintenance, titrated according to response. Although large drug dosages are occasionally

Table 21.4 Suggested therapeutic options for agitation and restlessness.

Sedative drug	Preferred Routes	Loading dose	Usual dose range over 24 hours	Comments
Midazolam	s.c.	2–5 mg	5–30 mg	Drug of choice for anxiety/ anguish
Levomepromazine	s.c., oral	12.5–25 mg	12.5–100 mg	Also antiemetic: may be used o.d.
Haloperidol	s.c., oral	2–5 mg	5–10 mg	Also antiemetic: may be used o.d.
Chlorpromazine	i.m., p.r., oral	25–50 mg	50–200 mg	Alternative
Diazepam	oral, p.r.	2–10 mg	6–20 mg	

required, sedation should be kept to the minimum. In situations where repeated dosages have been necessary to induce calm, patients may sleep for long periods as a result of the cumulative effect of the drugs. Occasionally, a combination of antipsychotic and benzodiazepines is more helpful than increasing doses of either alone.

Myoclonus and epilepsy

Terminally ill patients can occasionally suffer myoclonic jerks (brief, shock-like activity in one or more muscle groups). These can be due to biochemical abnormalities, metabolic disturbance or drugs (particularly opioids) or the disease process itself (e.g. Creutzfeldt Jakob disease). The stopping or reduction in dose of causative drugs (e.g. strong opioids, anticholinergics) should be considered.

In the context of the terminal phase, the control of epilepsy includes first-aid measures and the emergency use of drugs until control is achieved. Subsequent prevention of fits relies on the continued use of previously prescribed drugs whenever possible, supplemented by regular use of sedating drugs (see Table 21.5). When patients can no longer take oral medication a subcutaneous midazolam infusion is a common way to prevent fits.

Noisy or 'bubbly' breathing

Noisy 'bubbly' breathing, often referred to as the 'death rattle', occurs because of the inability of the patient to cough up or swallow secretions from the oropharynx and trachea. Although often not troubling to the patient, it may cause considerable distress to relatives and carers.

NON-DRUG MANAGEMENT

Various techniques can assist in improving noisy breathing.

- Careful patient positioning (e.g. sitting up, recovery position, head down tilt);
- Gentle physiotherapy;
- Gentle oropharyngeal suction;
- Mouth care;
- Nebulised normal (0.9%) saline 5 ml;
- Reassurance to family and friends.

Table 21.5 Drugs to control myoclonus and epilepsy.

Drug	Preferred Route	Myoclonus Emergency	Prevention	Epilepsy Emergency	Prevention
Diazepam Diazemuls	p.r., oral i.v.	5–10 mg repeated every hour	10–20 mg at night	5–10 mg repeated every 5–10 minutes	20 mg at night
Midazolam	s.c., i.v.	2.5–5 mg repeated every hour	10–30 mg over 24 hours	2.5–15 mg repeated every 5 minutes	10–30 mg over 24 hours
Phenobarbitone (alternative in difficult cases)	i.v., s.c.		400–800 mg subcutaneously over 24 hours	100 mg i.v. over 2 minutes, or 200 mg s.c. every 15 minutes	400–800 mg s.c. over 24 hours
Clonazepam (particularly useful in myoclonus)	oral, s.c.		1–8 mg orally (0.5–5 mg s.c.) over 24 hours		

Table 21.6 Drugs to control noisy 'bubbly' breathing.

Drug	Route of administration	Regular dose	Maintenance dose
Hyoscine hydrobromide	s.l., s.c.,	200–400 μg every 2–4 hours	600–2400 μg s.c. over 24 hours.
	transdermal patch		transdermal patch: 1.5 mg every 3rd day
Hyoscine butylbromide	oral, s.c.	10–20 mg every 4–6 hours	60–120 mg over 24 hours
Glycopyrronium	s.c.	200 μg 4 hourly	800 μg over 24 hours

DRUG MANAGEMENT

Anticholinergic drugs (Table 21.6) reduce the production of orolaryngeal secretions they also increase their viscosity. Recent guidelines on their use suggest that there is a difference between drugs in speed of onset, duration of effect, side-effect profile and cost but there is none that is of overall superiority [18].

Urinary incontinence and retention

Urinary incontinence is a common problem in the terminal phase, not least due to patient immobility. If ignored it can result in distress and agitation. Practical solutions are needed to overcome the problem: nursing assistance, pads, provision of commode, penile sheath and catheterisation. The incontinence adviser can be a help in complicated cases.

Retention of urine may occur for various reasons, including: prostatic outflow obstruction, drug therapy or constipation. This can be extremely uncomfortable and warrant catheterisation. Clearing any constipation and stopping aggravating drugs (especially anticholinergics) is advisable.

Constipation

A combination of drugs, immobility, dehydration, and low food intake make constipation a particular problem in the terminal phase. As previously noted, it can distress patients to the point of agitation and restlessness. Although patients may be frail, enema and suppositories may be of great help.

Pressure area care/skin care

Terminally ill patients are particularly vulnerable to pressure sores. The team should anticipate this and prevent problems by using pressure-relieving aids and mattresses (see also Chapter 20).

Mouth care, swallowing difficulties, hydration and feeding

Every assessment of a terminally ill patient should include the mouth. Frequent mouth care prevents problems and in most part thirst can be overcome. Patients too weak to access drinks must be offered sips of fluid or a fluid-dipped sponge on a very regular basis. Involving and teaching the relatives in this role is often helpful for both the carers and the patient (see also Chapter 9).

As patients become weak, they slowly lose their ability to swallow freely. Oral medication becomes harder to cope with and this should be seen as another opportunity to rationalise treatment. It is generally inappropriate to commence artificial feeding or hydration (Box 21.4) and this is the time to consider ceasing these interventions [19].

Box 21.4 Considerations in using artificial hydration at the end of life

Arguments FOR	Arguments AGAINST
May reduce thirst	May stop patients being at home
Appears less like 'just letting the patient die'	Makes death less 'natural' and more medicalised
May help circulation of drugs to relieve symptoms	May stop nurse giving mouth care and thereby reduce frequency of nursing contact
May reduce confusion	May cause pulmonary oedema
	May increase incontinence/ restlessness from full bladder
	Cannulas are painful and infusion sets constraining

Distressing acute terminal events

It is fortunate that distressing acute terminal events are rare. In addition, for many cancer patients they can be anticipated and the patient, the carers and the professionals can plan ahead to minimise distress. Acute terminal events are more common for patients dying from non-malignant chronic illness but the impact of these on them or their relatives is not researched. Table 21.7 shows the frequency of very distressing terminal events in hospice in-patients.

When such terminal events are managed badly, patient and carer distress may be magnified, bereavement may be more difficult and abnormal, and the team may feel failure and dissatisfaction. When managed well, the burden of suffering for patients and their carers may be greatly eased and many bereavement problems will be prevented. Great satisfaction may be gained by the team who work together to achieve this.

The principles of management of massive haemorrhage, respiratory distress or other acute terminal incidents are similar irrespective of the type of event or the cause. Prevention may be possible if warning or herald signs are noted. Anticipation, planning and preparation of carers and patients are essential. Families can often cope better with the event itself, and in bereavement, if they are sure that they can contact a professional at any time who knows the patient. Availability of care 24 hours a day, 7 days a week is invaluable in the support of patients at home.

Such events are frightening and distressing for *everyone*—patients, carers and professionals. Since most such events cause death within minutes, the most important aspect of care is to stay with the patient. The urge to do something or get help should be resisted if this requires leaving the patient alone.

Table 21.7 Frequency of very distressing events in hospice in-patients (data from [15]).

Symptom	Frequency (% of patients)
Haemorrhage/haemoptysis	2
Respiratory distress	2
Restlessness	1.5
Pain	1

Box 21.5 Drugs used in the management of distressing acute terminal events

Benzodiazepine	*Opioid*
Diazepam 10–20 mg p.r.	Diamorphine 2 × equivalent 4-hourly dose
Diazemuls 5–20 mg i.v. Midazolam 5–10 mg i.m./i.v.	10 mg i.m./i.v. if opioid naive

Other possible drugs

Ketamine 20–100 mg i.m./i.v.*

*Caution: See text.

The main aims of drug treatment are:

- to reduce fear;
- to reduce pain;
- to reduce the level of awareness of the patient.

The oral administration of drugs is inappropriate since absorption will be too slow for efficacy. The fastest route is the intravenous one. Box 21.5 lists drugs used in the management of distressing acute terminal events.

Ketamine should be used with great caution. It may be useful since it has a rapid onset of action, is both analgesic and anaesthetic and does not require the preparation time of controlled drugs. It has a short-lived effect, however, and causes very unpleasant emergent effects, particularly if administered without a benzodiazepine. It is available only on a named patient basis in the community and probably will only be used by specialists.

Planning ahead

PATIENTS AT RISK

Patients with cancer who are at greater and predictable risk of distressing terminal events, fall into four groups.

- Patients with fungating tumours involving soft tissue around major blood vessels.
- Patients with pelvic tumour associated with fistulae involving the vagina and/or rectum.
- Patients with trachcostomal recurrent tumour.
- Patients with anterior, superior mediastinal or tracheal tumours.

DISCUSSION WITH CARERS, THE PROFESSIONALS AND THE PATIENT

When there is a serious risk of such a terminal event many carers find it much less distressing to be forewarned despite the difficulty and distress of such a discussion. Occasionally, however, this knowledge and uncertainty is very disturbing to a carer (although they may still be better prepared to cope if such an event does happen). The discussion must be handled therefore with great sensitivity and followed-up with repeated support and review of the situation. Such a discussion should have three principal aims:

- First, to give an opportunity for the carer to voice their own suspicions and fears and discuss them in realistic terms.
- Second, to help the carer plan what they might do so that they can feel less helpless and fearful.
- Third, to ensure that the carer understands the optimum sources of professional support and how to contact them; for example, *not* to call 999, but instead to have the telephone numbers of the GP and emergency hospice/palliative care team beside the telephone.

Discussion of the possibility of a distressing terminal event with the patient is sometimes helpful. If a patient asks or is reported to be (or appears to be) worrying about such an event, facilitating discussion may allow a more realistic scenario to be portrayed with the opportunity to reassure the patient and the carer that suffering would be transitory and unconsciousness would develop quickly, and to develop a plan of care together. It is also an opportunity to reassure many patients that such distressing terminal events are, in fact, very rare.

It is worth noting that many patients and carers worry about such catastrophic events when they are highly unlikely to occur in their particular circumstances. It is often helpful to ask if this is a significant fear in order to reassure the patient and carer that it *will not* happen. For example, the authors have met several patients who thought that their enlarging liver would eventually burst through their abdomen. Explaining that this would not happen brought tremendous relief.

There should also be discussion among the members of the professional team to:

- establish a clear plan of management and delegation of responsibilities;
- ensure all aspects of the plan are carried out;
- allow support and evaluation within the team should a distressing terminal event occur.

AVAILABILITY OF DRUGS IN THE HOME

When there is a possibility of an acute, distressing terminal event it is useful to ensure that the necessary drugs (see Box 21.5) are readily available. A specific 'emergency box' within the home is a helpful way of planning this.

MASSIVE HAEMORRHAGE

In addition to the general measures already outlined, it is useful to have at hand dark-coloured towels or blankets to reduce the visual and psychological impact of massive blood loss. Pressure on the bleeding site with a pillow or large pad may help (but may be very painful because of the tumour).

HAEMOPTYSIS

In patients with cancer massive haemoptysis usually occurs in those with a primary lung cancer or as a consequence of a systemic coagulation dysfunction or in the case of fungal pneumonia in profoundly neutropenic patients. Patients with lung metastases and tracheolaryngeal primary tumours very rarely have massive haemoptysis.

There is often a warning of increasing, fresh haemoptysis.

CAROTID BLOW-OUT

Carotid blow-out is more likely to occur in patients with recurrent tumour in a site previously treated with both surgery and radiotherapy. Death occurs within 2–3 minutes. There is often a herald bleed (see Chapter 12).

PELVIC BLEEDING

Tumours of the cervix, uterus and rectum may erode into major pelvic blood vessels. This is often preceded by the formation of vesico-vaginal, recto-vaginal, or vesico-rectal fistulae, and with increasing loss of fresh blood.

Vaginal packing may be useful in some patients.

Many patients with pelvic tumours will have experienced venous obstruction and some may have been treated with warfarin. This is obviously an extra risk factor for massive haemorrhage.

GASTROINTESTINAL BLEEDING

Massive haematemesis is usually due to peptic ulceration or oesophageal varices rather than tumour erosion into a major vessel. Patients with advanced cancer are often taking non-steroidal anti-inflammatory drugs (NSAIDs) and many are also taking steroids. They are therefore greatly at risk of peptic ulceration and there should be a proactive approach to watch for and treat characteristic warning signs in order to prevent catastrophic bleeding. Patients with, or with high likelihood of, oesophageal varices are generally well identified and appropriate planning can be made well in advance.

Procedures after death

Diagnosing death

It is usually the responsibility of a doctor to diagnose death; however, in some hospices, nursing staff can perform this task. This can be done in various ways, although in terminal care a confirmation of somatic death is made by observing the following:
- fixed dilated pupils;
- no heart sounds;
- no respiratory effort;
- no pulse.

How to prepare bodies after death

Relatives should be allowed the choice to see and spend time with the deceased person, not only during the act of dying but also afterwards. They may need a lot of support in this and preparation of the body may play a part in this support. Some relatives may wish to be involved in the 'laying out' of the body. Institutional policies with regard to laying out should be followed with sensitivity to the wishes of family and friends. In particular, different cultural or religious practices should be respected (see Table 21.2).

Wounds should be covered with waterproof dressings and pads used to absorb body fluid and leakage. Catheters and infusion lines, should be removed (unless the case is being referred to the coroner). Those handling the body should be warned of any risk of infection and some bodies may need to be placed in body bags.

A list of funeral directors can be given to patients; indeed the general practitioner (GP) or district nurse may be in a position to contact a firm for the family. Undertakers are available 24 hours a day and can prepare the body. Although not immediately necessary, the body is often taken from the patient's home to the funeral parlour.

Organ donation

Patients carrying a donor card, or whose family consent, may be able to donate various organs and tissues. Table 21.2 illustrates some potential cultural differences in approach. Generally speaking, organs are retrieved from patients who have died from cerebral trauma, intercranial haemorrhage, anoxic brain damage following cardiopulmonary arrest, or primary brain tumours. Further guidance is available from the British Transplantation Society [20].

Tissue and organ donation is rarely considered and although terminally ill patients may not satisfy the criteria, this does not apply universally and families should be given an opportunity to provide consent, if they wish. For instance corneal donation is a fairly frequent experience for hospices.

Obviously it is important for professionals to be fully conversant with local policy and approach relatives with appropriate sensitivity. Additional advice is provided by local tissue transplant co-ordinators. They are able to speak to relatives and arrange tissue retrieval.

Death certificates (Medical Certificate of Cause of Death)

The death certificate (Figure 21.2) must be issued by a registered medical practitioner. It cannot be issued in the following circumstances:

- Patient not attended in their last illness by a medical practitioner.
- The certifying doctor has not examined the body or seen the patient in the 14 days prior to the death.
- The cause of death is unknown or appears unnatural.
- The cause of death is associated with an anaesthetic, industrial disease, surgery, fracture, violence or suicide.

In these cases the coroner must be informed and a post-mortem may subsequently be performed. If doubt exists, it is always worthwhile discussing the case with the coroner or the coroner's officer (police representative of the coroner).

Details on how to fill out death certificates are outlined at the front of the certificate book. The certificate is then taken to the Registrar of Births, Marriages and Deaths (usually by a relative), whereupon a Certificate for Disposal is issued; this needs to be given to the undertaker.

MED A 20 275821

BIRTHS AND DEATHS REGISTRATION ACT 1953
(Form prescribed by the Registration of Births and Deaths Regulations 1987)

MEDICAL CERTIFICATE OF CAUSE OF DEATH

For use only by a Registered Medical Practitioner WHO HAS BEEN IN ATTENDANCE during the deceased's last illness, and to be delivered by him forthwith to the Registrar of Births and Deaths.

Registrar to enter No. of Death Entry ....

Name of deceased .... JOHN SMITH

Date of death as stated to me .... 23RD day of JANUARY 1998 Age as stated to me 68

Place of death .... 32 ANY STREET, HOME TOWN

Last seen alive by me .... 22ND day of JANUARY 1998

1. The certified cause of death takes account of information obtained from post-mortem.
2. Information from post-mortem may be available later.
3. (3) Post-mortem not being held.
4. I have reported this death to the Coroner for further action.

[See overleaf]

Please ring appropriate digit(s) and letter.

(a) Seen after death by me.
b Seen after death by another medical practitioner but not by me.
c Not seen after death by a medical practitioner.

CAUSE OF DEATH

The condition thought to be the 'Underlying Cause of Death' should appear in the lowest completed line of Part I.

	These particulars not to be entered in death register Approximate interval between onset and death
I(a) Disease or condition directly leading to death† .... LUNG CANCER	18 MONTHS
(b) Other disease or condition, if any, leading to I(a)	
(c) Other disease or condition, if any, leading to I(b)	
II Other significant conditions CONTRIBUTING TO THE DEATH but not related to the disease or condition causing it.	

The death might have been due to or contributed to by the employment followed at some time by the deceased. ☐ Please tick where applicable

†This does not mean the mode of dying, such as heart failure, asphyxia, asthenia, etc: it means the disease, injury, or complication which caused death.

I hereby certify that I was in medical attendance during the above named deceased's last illness, and that the particulars and cause of death above written are true to the best of my knowledge and belief.

Signature .... Qualifications as registered by General Medical Council } MBBS

Residence .... MY PRACTICE, HOME TOWN Date 23RD JANUARY 1998

For deaths in hospital: Please give the name of the consultant responsible for the above-named as a patient. ....

MED A 20 275821

(Form prescribed by the Registration of Births and Deaths Regulations 1987)

NOTICE TO INFORMANT

I hereby give notice that I have this day signed a medical certificate of cause of death of

JOHN SMITH

Signature ....

Date 23/1/98

This notice is to be delivered by the informant to the registrar of births and deaths for the sub-district in which the death occurred.

The certifying medical practitioner must give this notice to the person who is qualified and liable to act as informant for the registration of death (see list overleaf).

DUTIES OF INFORMANT

Failure to deliver this notice to the registrar renders the informant liable to prosecution. The death cannot be registered until the medical certificate has reached the registrar.

When the death is registered the informant must be prepared to give to the registrar the following particulars relating to the deceased:

1. The date and place of death.
2. The full name and surname (and the maiden surname if the deceased was a woman who had married).
3. The date and place of birth.
4. The occupation (and if the deceased was a married woman or a widow the name and occupation of her husband).
5. The usual address.
6. Whether the deceased was in receipt of a pension or allowance from public funds.
7. If the deceased was married, the date of birth of the surviving widow or widower.

THE DECEASED'S MEDICAL CARD SHOULD BE DELIVERED TO THE REGISTRAR

Fig. 21.2 The Medical Certificate of Cause of Death.

If the body is to be cremated, a second form needs to be completed by two independent doctors (usually the certifying doctor and another doctor who is at least 5 years post-registration).

Post-mortem

A post-mortem may be a mandatory requirement (cases referred to the coroner). This is a legal requirement and cannot be refused. Post-mortems can also be requested in order to clarify medical details of the death relatives can refuse these even if the patient had wished it.

Summary

Care for patients who have reached the terminal phase of their illness poses many challenges to professionals. Good quality care at this point often requires increased professional support of patients and their loved ones. The development of care pathways has provided a method to improve the quality of such care in the last days and hours of life. Following a death there are certain practical requirements that need to be dealt with professionally and with sensitivity to the feelings of the bereaved.

References

1 O'Connor S, Schatzberger P, Payne S. A death photographed: one patient's story. *BMJ* 2003; 327: 233.
2 Addington Hall J, McCarthy M. Dying from cancer: results of a national population based investigation. *Palliat Med* 1995; 9: 295–305.
3 Townsend J, Frank AO, Fermont D, et al. Terminal cancer care and patients' preference for place of death. *BMJ* 1990; 301: 415–417.
4 Cartwright A. Changes in life and care in the year before death 1967–1987. *J Public Health Med* 1991; 13: 81–87.
5 MacCabee J. The effect of transfer from a palliative care unit to nursing homesare patients' and relatives' needs met? *Palliat Med* 1994; 8: 211–214.
6 Fukui S, Kawagoe H, Masako S, et al. Determinants of the place of death among terminally ill cancer patients under home hospice care in Japan. *Palliat Med.* 2003; 17: 445–453.
7 Exley C, Field D, McKinley RK, Stokes T. *An evaluation of Primary care based palliative care for cancer and non-malignant disease in two cancer accredited primary care practices in Leicestershire.* University of Leicester, Department of Epidemiology and Public Health, 2003.
8 Hofmann JC, Wenger NS, Davis RB, et al. Patient preferences for communication with physicians about end-of-life decisions. SUPPORT Investigators. Study to Understand Prognoses and Preference for Outcomes and Risks of Treatment. *Ann Intern Med.* 1997; 127: 1–12.

9 National Council for Hospice and Specialist Care Services. *Specialist Palliative Care: A Statement of Definitions*. Occasional Paper, No. 8, London: NCHSCS, 1995.

10 Clinical Guidelines Working Party. *Changing Gear: Guidelines for Managing the Last Days of Life*. London: National Council for Hospice and Specialist Palliative Care Services, 1997.

11 Ellershaw J, Wilkinson S. *Care of the Dying. A Pathway to Excellence*. Oxford: Oxford University Press, 2003.

12 Ellershaw J, Ward C. Care of the dying patients; the last hours or days of life. *BMJ* 2003; 326: 30–34.

13 Commission for Health Improvement. *Investigation into the Portsmouth Healthcare NHS Trust Gosport War Memorial Hospital*. London: Commission for Health Improvement, 2002.

14 Thomas K. *Out of Hours Palliative Care in the Community*. London: Macmillan Cancer Relief, 2001.

15 Lichter I, Hunt E. The last 48 hours of life. *J Palliat Care* 1990; 6: 7–15.

16 Boyd KJ. Short terminal admissions to a hospice. *Palliat Med* 1993; 7: 289–294.

17 Brajtman S. The impact on the family of terminal restlessness and its management. *Palliat Med*. 2003;17: 454–460.

18 Bennett M, Lucas V, Brennan M, et al Association for Palliative Medicine's Science Committee. Using anti-muscarinic drugs in the management of death rattle: evidence-based guidelines for palliative care. *Palliat Med*. 2002; 16: 369–374.

19 British Medical Association. Withholding and withdrawing life sustaining treatments. *Report of the British Medical Association*. London: BMJ Publishing Group, 2001.

20 *Towards standards for organ and tissue transplantation in the United Kingdom*. Surrey, The British Transplantation Society, 1998. or www.bts.org.uk

22: Medicines Management in Palliative Care

CHRISTINE HIRSCH, JEREMY JOHNSON AND CHRISTINA FAULL

Introduction

The complex mix of symptoms that arise in advanced illness may often require the patient to take a large number of medicines, which require frequent review and modification to achieve optimal management. The acquisition and administration of medication is not always straightforward and can lead to the development of practical and pharmacological problems for the patient, carers and the health care team. To achieve high quality care, often crossing boundaries of responsibility, requires close teamwork, efficient organisation and good communication.

This chapter will describe how pharmacists can make a valuable contribution to the care of patients with advanced illness, through the application of their expertise in medicines management. Some of the unusual prescribing issues in advanced illness will be highlighted, particularly problems of access to drugs in the community and the prescribing of controlled drugs. This chapter also includes a section on the use of the syringe driver for the administration of drugs by subcutaneous infusion.

The pharmacist in palliative care: a key team member

By definition, palliative care requires a multiprofessional team approach [1]. Pharmacists, both from community and hospital backgrounds, have become established key members of specialist health care teams [2, 3], helping to optimise drug treatments for individual patients in order to achieve specified therapeutic outcomes, reduce drug-related problems and improve quality of life [4]. Pharmaceutical care plans although traditionally associated with a hospital environment, facilitate many activities essential to reducing drug related problems and improving quality of life, which are of equal importance in

Box 22.1 Outline of a typical hospital pharmaceutical care plan

- Consider patients diagnosis, frequency and severity of symptoms, impact on normal daily activities and ensure optimum choice and use of drugs. Consider prophylaxis for predictable side effects
- Identify and monitor possible drug interactions and adverse drug reactions and ensure reporting of these where appropriate
- Consider the patient's ability to take medicine in prescribed formulation and regimen. Arrange appropriate training for carer/patient, including use of compliance aids if necessary
- Discuss patient and carers understanding of goals of therapy and potential side effects
- Monitor any relevant laboratory tests which may be available

Review all drugs, formulations and doses regularly to ensure that regimen is appropriate for any changes in severity or frequency of symptoms
- Ensure that the drugs prescribed are easily available in the community and if they are not, arrange for their supply
- Anticipation of emergencies, such as haemorrhage or convulsions

the community setting. A typical plan might include the information shown in Box 22.1.

Helping patients understand their medicines

A traditional role of the pharmacist has been to advise patients about their medicines. In one study, 60% of palliative care patients at home were reported to be non-compliant with their medication. [5] The pharmacist can help patients and their carers understand the purpose of each medicine and the instructions of the prescribing doctor. They may also explore the patients' attitude, both social and cultural [6], to their prescribed medication, addressing any anxieties and where necessary provide further information about: the dosage regimen for effective symptom management; specific drugs; requests for over-the-counter remedies and potential interactions; symptoms and other aspects of care.

Use of drugs beyond licence

In palliative care, medications are often used outside their licensed indication or route of administration e.g. antidepressant agents for pain control, many injectable preparations for subcutaneous infusion and administration of medication via feeding tubes. The licensing of drugs by the Medicines Control Agency in the UK regulates the activity of the pharmaceutical companies in relation to the marketing of the drug. It does not restrict prescribing or administration by qualified medical practitioners. In many cases pharmaceutical companies may not have applied for extensions to the terms of the product licence for the product for economic reasons.

A position statement has been prepared on behalf of the Association for Palliative Medicine of Great Britain and Ireland and the Pain Society, which addresses the use of drugs beyond licence in palliative care and pain management. This recommends that:

> *'The use of drugs beyond licence should be seen as a legitimate aspect of clinical practice ... is currently both necessary and common ... Health professionals should inform, change and monitor their practice ... In the light of evidence from audit and published research'* [7].

Patients receive 'package inserts' with their dispensed medicines which can cause anxiety and confusion for the patient or carer if written information regarding the indications and dose regimen is inconsistent with verbal information from their prescriber. The pharmacist can address this at the point of dispensing either verbally or supplement it with specifically designed written information.

Administration of drugs via feeding tubes is an unlicensed activity, but necessary for those palliative care patients unable to swallow. There is little published data about the administration of drugs via feeding tubes and in many areas local policies have been developed. Guidance should be sought from the pharmacist on the suitability of formulations, possibility of interaction with other medication and feed, and maintaining tube patency [8, 9].

Occasionally patients require drugs that are available only as unlicensed 'specials', or on a named patient basis from the pharmaceutical industry. Community pharmacists may have to call on the local hospital pharmacy department, or pharmaceutical manufacturing specialist, to obtain these medicines. Time and advanced warning are particularly important in these situations.

Medication compliance aids

Patients taking a large number of different medicines may have difficulty, for a variety of reasons, in adhering to the correct regimen. This is a complex issue and although compliance aids may be helpful, patients' potential ability to cope at home with a particular device should be assessed and considered [10, 11]. The pharmacist will be able to advise on re-fillable and blister-pack systems or use of large print labels, diaries and charts.

- *Blister packs.* These are prepared by a pharmacist and usually contain at least one week's medications.
- *Daily pill dispensers.* These contain the supply of pills for a single day in up to four dosage times. Each dosage time is labelled with the time, part of the day, and a number and/or 'braille' character. Some pill dispensers, such as Redidose (Fig. 22.1), come in sets of seven so that the system can be recharged weekly but the tablets required for each day can be issued or carried separately.
- *Weekly pill dispensers.* Weekly pill dispensers include the Dosett (see Fig. 22.2). A tray of medicines for the week is accessed through clearly labelled compartments allowing up to four dosage times daily.

At present these devices are not prescribable on FP10 prescription (GP prescriptions). Primary Health Care Trusts may fund the devices following individual patient assessment.

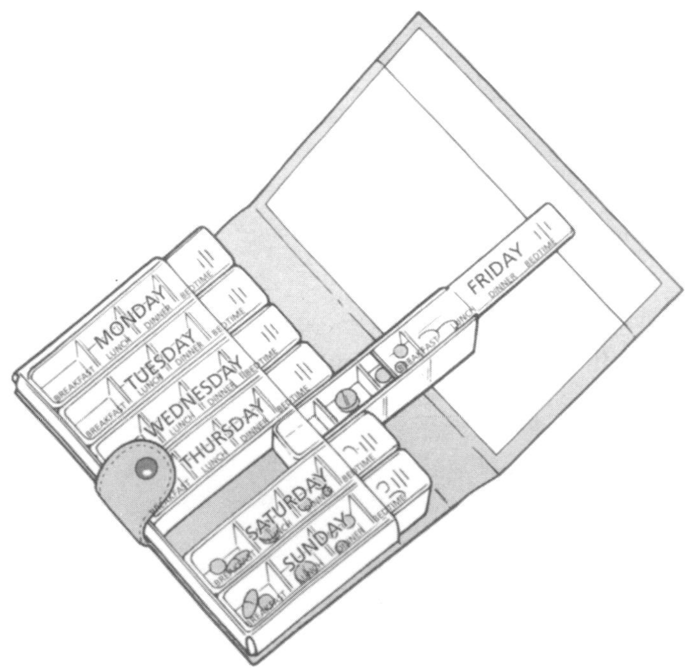

Fig. 22.1 The Redidose seven-day pill dispenser.

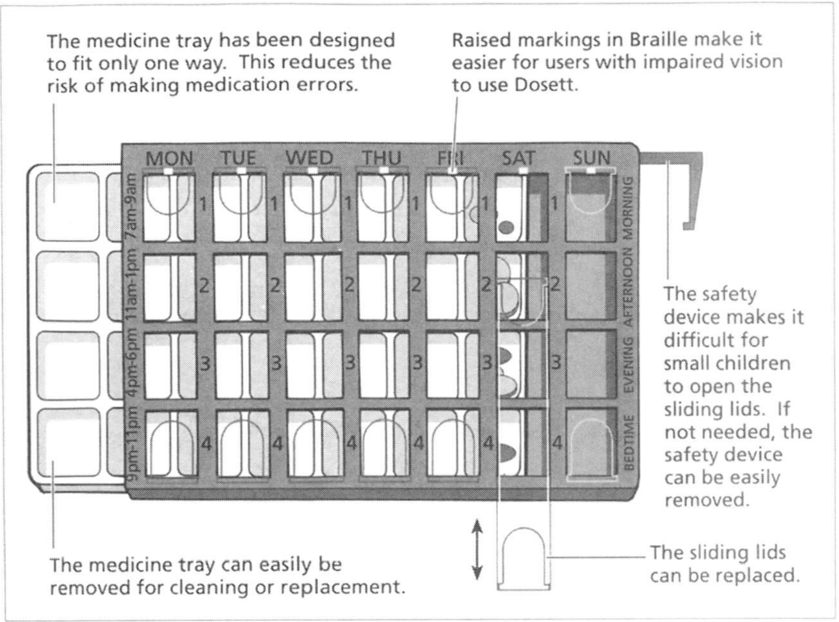

Fig. 22.2 The Dosett weekly pill dispenser.

The use of the syringe driver in palliative care

When patients become unable to take medications via the oral route, drug administration by subcutaneous infusion can be an alternative way to achieve symptom control, particularly if the rectal or transdermal route is not appropriate. In most instances subcutaneous administration is preferable to the intravenous or intramuscular routes.

In palliative care the role of the syringe driver has been firmly established by its ability to administer subcutaneous infusions of analgesics, either as single agents, or in combination with other compounds such as antiemetics, sedatives or anticholinergic drugs [12–18]. The syringe driver provides 'steady-state' plasma concentrations of drugs, avoiding the necessity for repeated injections (this is important in frail, cachectic patients) and allows more than one drug to be combined in the syringe.

However, prescribing involves anticipation of the patient's requirements over the next 24 hours. Any alteration in symptoms may necessitate additional injections to supplement the infusion regimen, therefore medication should also be prescribed for immediate administration in case of breakthrough symptoms. The boost button (available on the Graseby MS26 syringe driver) should not be used as this method is unlikely to give an adequate dose of analgesia. Moreover, frequent boosting will cause the syringe driver to run through early, exposing the patient to the risk of uncontrolled pain and boosting would also infuse all drugs in the driver [19].

Overenthusiastic and indiscriminate use of the syringe driver should be avoided. For those who can take and absorb oral medication, a subcutaneous infusion delivered by a syringe driver is unlikely to improve symptom control. Some drugs with long half lives may be given by bolus s.c. injections. Many drugs can be given effectively by other routes (e.g. sublingual, buccal, rectal, transdermal). Long-term use is rarely indicated, but if required, may be maintained as long as necessary. Once symptoms are controlled, it is often possible to reconvert medications to the oral formulations.

Syringe drivers commonly used in palliative care in the UK are lightweight, portable infusion pumps, usually electrically or mechanically operated, capable of delivering precise doses of medication over a set period of time, most commonly 24 hours (Figure 22.3).

Further information on setting up the syringe driver may be found in the Appendix.

Indications

The syringe driver may be indicated in the following situations:

- persistent nausea or vomiting;
- oral/pharyngeal lesions;
- difficulty in swallowing;
- poor alimentary absorption;
- intestinal obstruction;
- profound weakness/cachexia;
- comatose or moribund patient.

Explanation to the patient and carers

Prior to commencing an infusion, time should be spent with the patient and their carers explaining the nature and intention of the procedure. Some patients find the syringe driver obtrusive and disconcerting; many have reservations and some fear that the institution of a syringe driver equates with impending death. Questions should be invited, anxieties acknowledged and reassurance given where appropriate.

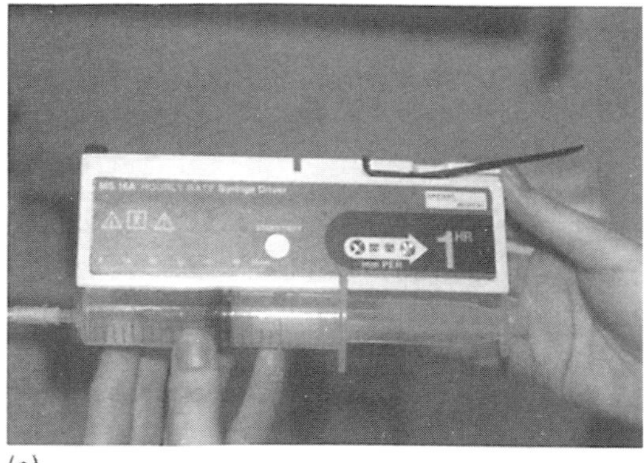

(a)

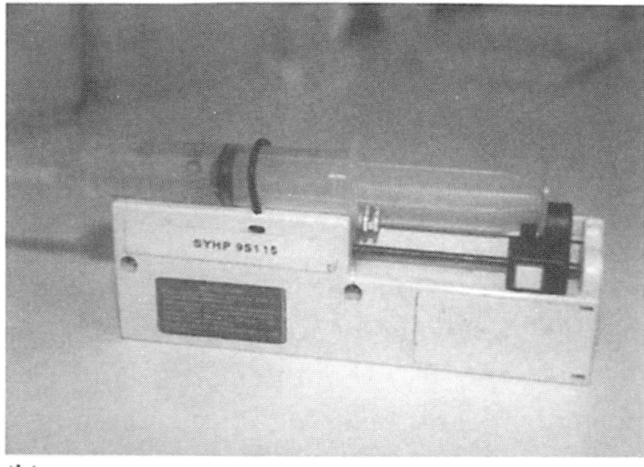

(b)

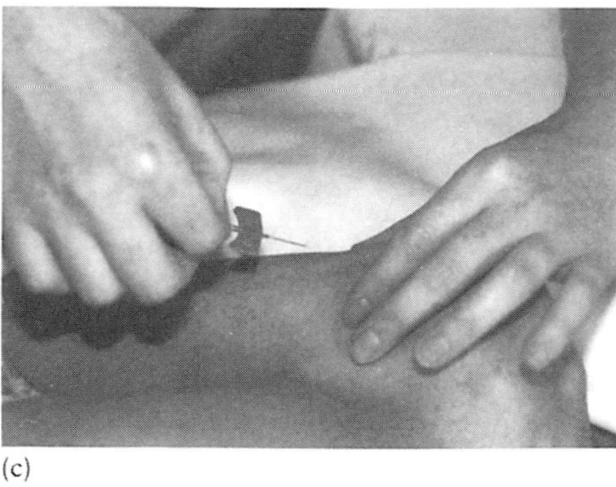

(c)

Fig. 22.3 Setting up a syringe driver. (a) Draw up medication and set rate of delivery. (b) Attach loaded syringe and clamp to driver. (c) and (d) Insert fine-gauge butterfly needle into skin. (e) Loop tubing and secure with transparent dressing. (f) Final set up.

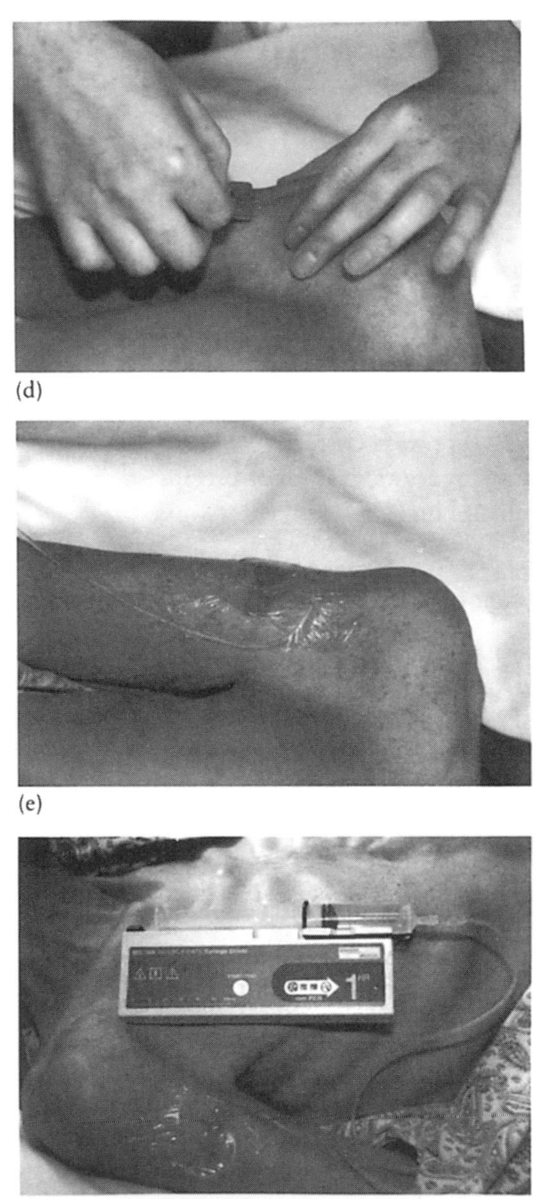

(d)

(e)

(f)

Fig. 22.3 *Continued*

Drugs used in syringe drivers

Mention will be made here of the more commonly used drugs in symptom management (Table 22.1), highlighting some of the important issues to be considered when prescribing drugs for subcutaneous infusion. The choice of drug may be directed by local or national guidelines. Other chapters in this book should be consulted for more detail about the use of drugs in symptom management. Advice should be sought from local palliative care specialists on unusual drugs or combinations and there are several sources of readily available information on drugs, and combinations, which may be successfully used in syringe drivers [9, 20–22]. If drug dosages need to be altered, a new syringe should be set up rather than the infusion rate altered. Alteration of the rate will deliver all of the drugs at an increased or decreased rate. It will also alter the time of next recharge of the syringe, and may lead to times without infusion if district nurses are planning visits at the same time each day.

Changing the infusion rate can potentially lead to an overdosage (or underdosage) if the rate is not checked and reset at each syringe recharge. It also complicates the calculation of the actual dose of each drug the patient is receiving daily.

COMBINING DRUGS IN SYRINGES

Diamorphine has become established as the opioid of choice for use in syringe drivers since it has a high water solubility. The maximum recommended concentration for single-agent diamorphine is 250 mg/ml.

Many different drug and dosage combinations have been used in syringe drivers [23]. An invariable component of this UK hospice survey was diamorphine, usually administered with an antiemetic and/or sedative. However, 18 of the 28 drugs reported had been used infrequently and by fewer than 5% of the hospices. For the majority of these less frequently used drugs there is little evidence confirming efficacy by this route of delivery and no reliable data regarding their compatibility or stability with other drugs.

Drugs should be diluted with water for injection unless there is a specific requirement to use sodium chloride. In particular do not use 0.9% saline to dilute cyclizine as there is a high risk of precipitation. Always keep the number of drugs combined in a single syringe to a minimum (generally two, sometimes three), check compatibility data and seek advice.

Table 22.1 Drugs used in syringe drivers. This list is not exhaustive; it covers many of the drugs used in palliative care. See other chapters for specific indications and usage.

Medication	Trade name and ampoule size	Indication	Dose range per 24 hours	Comments
Analgesics				
Diamorphine hydrochloride [43]	Crystalline powder 5, 10, 30, 100, 500 mg Reconstitute with water	Pain	Start: One-third total daily dose of oral morphine.	• Opioid of choice for s.c. infusion • Highly soluble • Do not exceed 250 mg/ml • Loading dose (equivalent to 4 h) may be required initially s.c.
		Dyspnoea	10–20 mg in opioid naive patients Increase as necessary by 30–50% increments No maximum dose	
Hydromorphone (*symbol for rarely used*)	10 mg/ml, 20 mg/ml, 50 mg/ml	Diamorphine intolerance, on the recommendation of palliative care specialist	Start 1/6 dose of oral Hydromorphone	Unlicensed, available as a special order from Martindale Chemically incompatible with hyaluronidase [44]
Oxycodone [33]	10 mg/ml,1,2 ml	Diamorphine intolerance	7.5 mg in 24 hours in opioid naive patients One half of oral Oxycodone dose	If mixing with cyclizine, do not exceed 3 mg/ml cyclizine

Alfentanil [20] (*symbol for sometimes used*)	1 mg/2 ml, 5 mg/10 ml, 5 mg/ml	Alternative to diamorphine on advice of palliative care specialist, particularly in renal failure.	Opioid-naïve patients start 0.5–1 mg over 24 hours.	
Methadone [45, 46][‡]	10 mg/ml 1, 2, 3.5, 5 ml	On recommendation of palliative care specialist.	Seek advice from palliative care specialist.	• Can have unacceptable adverse reactions at injection site. • Wide variation in individual plasma concentration. • Long half life tendency to accumulate. • Rectal route an alternative
Ketamine [47, 48][†]	Ketalar 10 mg/ml/20 ml amp 50 mg/ml/10 ml amp 100 mg/ml/5 ml	Difficult cancer pain, especially of neuropathic origin on recommendation of palliative care specialist	Start 100 mg/day Titrate against effect Increase to 300–500 mg/day	• Inhibits NMDA receptor • Psychomimetic side-effects (may need midazolam/haloperidol cover) • Contraindicated in raised intracranial pressure and fits • Caution in hypertension/cardiac problems • Available in the community on named patient basis only Irritant, dilute with sodium chloride 0.9% to largest possible volume

Continued on p. 420

Table 22.1 *Continued*

Medication	Trade name and ampoule size	Indication	Dose range per 24 hours	Comments
NSAIDs				
Ketorolac [9] (*symbol for sometimes used*)	Toradol 10 mg/ml 30 mg/ml	Bone pain on recommendation of palliative care specialist	30–60 mg	• Well tolerated • Caution in renal failure • Can be nephrotoxic • Short term use only (few days because of nephrotoxicity) • High incidence of upper GI bleeding, co-prescribe gastroprotective drug • Dilute with 0.9% sodium chloride
Antiemetics				
Metoclopramide*	Maxolon and non-proprietary 5 mg/ml, 2 and 20 ml	Impaired gastric emptying	30–100 mg	• Dopamine receptor antagonist • Non-sedating • Large volume • Possibility of extrapyramidal/dystonic side effects or tardive dyskinesia with prolonged use in younger women
Haloperidol*	Serenace and Haldol 5 mg/ml 10 mg/ml 2 ml	Drug induced nausea Metabolic causes Antipsychotic	2.5–10 mg	• Central dopamine receptor antagonist • Mildly sedating • Settles agitation and psychosis

Cyclizine*	Valoid 50 mg/ml	Intestinal obstruction Movement induced nausea	50–150 mg	• Antihistamine (H_1) and anticholinergic • Drowsiness can be a problem • Compatibility problems. Do dilute with sodium chloride
Ondansetron‡	Zofran 2 mg/ml 2 and 4 ml	Chemotherapy or radiotherapy induced vomiting (not usually s.c. route)	8–24 mg	• $5HT_3$ antagonist If not effective in 3 days discontinue • Expensive
Sedative and antiemetic				
Levomepromazine [9]*	Nozinan 25 mg/ml 1 ml	Nausea Confusion Restlessness Psychosis	6–12.5 mg 12.5–200 mg	• Effective antiemetic • Extremely useful for terminal agitation • Occasional skin reactions • If used as a single agent may be diluted with 0.9% sodium chloride
Sedative				
Midazolam [49]	Hypnovel 2 mg/ml 5 ml 5 mg/ml 2 ml	Anxiety Terminal restlessness Dyspnoea Anticonvulsant Myoclonus	10–90 mg (common range 10–30 mg)	• Water soluble benzodiazepine • Large inter-individual variability in steady-state plasma level

Continued on p. 422

Table 22.1 *Continued*

Medication	Trade name and ampoule size	Indication	Dose range per 24 hours	Comments
Clonazepam†	Rivotril 1 mg/1 ml	Anxiety Terminal restlessness Anticonvulsant Neuropathic pain	0.5–8 mg	• Less water soluble than Midazolam • Irritant • May cause confusion
Anticholinergic				
Hyoscine hydrobromide‡	0.4 mg/ml 1 ml 0.6 mg/ml 1 ml	Terminal bronchial secretions and additional sedation	0.6–2.4 mg	• Dry mouth—extra attention to oral hygiene
Hyoscine butylbromide [9]†	Buscopan 20 mg/ml 1 ml	Severe colic Intestinal obstruction	20–120 mg	May be as effective as the hydrobromide for bronchial secretions—and much cheaper
Glycopyrronium Bromide	Robinu 1 0.2 mg/ml 1.3 ml	Terminal secretions	0.6–1.2 mg	• Less likely to cause confusion than Hyoscine Hydrobromide Slower onset than hysocine hydrobromide

Steroids				
Dexamethasone[†]	Dexamethasone sodium phosphate 5 mg/ml 1, 2ml Dexamethasone sodiumphosphate 4 mg/ml 1.2 ml . 24 mg/ml 5 ml	Spinal cord compression, cauda equina	12–16 mg	• Compatibility difficulties (see Table 22.2) • Use separate syringe driver if necessary
		Raised intracranial pressure	8–16 mg	
		Reduction in peritumour oedema	4–16 mg	
Anticonvulsants				
Clonazepam[†]	See above			
Midazolam[*]	See above			
Miscellaneous				
Octreotide [50][†]	Sandostatin 50 μg 100 μg/ml 1 ml 200 μg/ml 5 ml 500 μg/ml 1 ml	Reduces: GI secretions Volume of vomit in intestinal obstruction Volume of entero-colic fistula	500 μg initially, if ineffective stop after 48 hours, if effective titrate to, lowest effective dose (range 50–600 μg)	Expensive

Frequently used; [†] Sometimes used; [‡] Rarely used; § Solubility of morphine salts: diamorphine HCl = 625 mg/ml, morphine acetate = 400 mg/ml, morphine tartrate = 100 mg/ml, morphine sulphate = 45 mg/ml. Contraindicated: the following are all too irritant to be used subcutaneously; diazepam, prochlorperazine and chlorpromazine.

If the contents of the syringe become cloudy or discoloured before or during infusion, the syringe should be discarded immediately. Should incompatibility problems persist and alternative drugs or routes are not available, then a second syringe driver may be required to infuse drugs separately.

Correct storage temperatures should be observed for all drugs. Where high concentrations of drugs are being infused, change in temperature (particularly cold) can reduce solubility. The syringe driver contents should also be protected from light by placing in an opaque pouch, holster or pocket to prevent photodegradation,

COMPATIBILITY AND STABILITY

Consideration of the compatibility of drugs is vital to ensure efficacy of therapy. Interactions between drugs can be difficult to predict and may produce a number of effects, including a reduction in stability or changes in solubility resulting in precipitation or crystallisation. This may cause the infusion cannula to become blocked, the injection site to become inflamed, and the treatment to be ineffective. Physical examination of the contents (looking for cloudiness or discolouration), although a guide to compatibility, does not guarantee absence of chemical reaction. Ideally, all combinations would be chemically analysed for active ingredients and any toxic breakdown products. This is costly in terms of time and resources and has not been done for the many different combinations of drugs and doses tailored to individual symptoms.

Most drugs used in syringe drivers are water soluble and can be mixed. However, some drugs e.g. phenobarbital (made up in propylene glycol) are immiscible with aqueous solutions and should not be used in the same syringe as other drugs.

The major factor leading to incompatibility is the relative concentration of each drug. Other factors include pH, storage conditions, temperature and ionic strength.

Many salts in aqueous solution undergo degradation: for example diamorphine is hydrolysed to 6-mono-acetylmorphine and morphine. The stability of diamorphine under a variety of conditions has been examined [24–29]. The addition of haloperidol, cyclizine or metoclopramide reduces the stability considerably dependant on relative concentrations, and also leads to loss of the antiemetic from the solution [26, 27, 30, 31]

Table 22.2 indicates the compatibility and stability of two-drug mixtures for at least 24 hours [32, 33]. Higher concentrations may lead to lower efficacy due to instability or precipitation of drugs.

Table 22.2 The compatibility of drugs combined in a syringe for s.c. infusion.

	Diamorphine	Metoclopramide	Haloperidol	Cyclizine	Levomepromazine	Midazolam	Hyoscine hydrobromide	Hyoscine butylbromide	Dexamethasone	Octreotide	Glycopyrronium	Oxycodone
Diamorphine		c[‡]√√	√√	c[*]√√	√√	√√	√√	√√	c	√√	√√	n
Metoclopramide	c[‡]√√		n	n	N	√	n	n	√√	√	n	√√
Haloperidol	√√	N		√	N	√√	√	√	p	√	no data	√√
Cyclizine	c[*]√√	N	√		√	c	c	p	p	NO	no data	p[§]
Levomepromazine	√√	N	n	√		√	√	√	p	NO	no data	√√
Midazolam	√√	√	√√	c	√		√	√	p	no data	√	√√
Hyoscine hydrobromide	√√	N	√	c	√	√		n	no data	no data	n	√√
Hyoscine butylbromide	√√	N	√	p	√	√	n		no data	√	n	√√
Dexamethasone	c	√√	p	p	P	p	no data	no data		p	NO	√√
Octreotide	√√	√	√	NO	NO	no data	no data	√	p		no data	no data
Glycopyrronium	√√	N	no data	no data	no data	√	n	n	No	no data		no data
Oxycodone	n	√√	√√	p[§]	√√	√√	√√	√√	√√	no data	no data	

√√ No problems at usual therapeutic concentrations—published evidence.
√ compatible at usual therapeutic concentrations—common usage but no published evidence.
c = caution at higher concentrations.
p = occasionally precipitates.
NO = definite compatibility problems.
n = generally not a clinically useful combination (same group of drug or counteracting effects).
[*]Stable with diamorphine up to 20 mg/ml + cyclizine up to 20 mg/ml. Higher concentrations of diamorphine are probably only stable with lower concentrations of cyclizine. Diamorphine any concentration + cyclizine up to 6.7 mg/ml . (i.e. maximum 50mg of cyclizine in 8 ml infusion with diamorphine> 160 mg: maximum 100 mg of cyclizine in a 16 ml infusion with diamorphine> 320 mg in 16 ml).
[‡]Stable with diamorphine up to 25 mg/ml + metoclopramide up to 5 mg/ml (i.e. diamorphine 200 mg is stable with up to 40 mg of metoclopramide in a 8 ml infusion).
[§]Cyclizine concentrations should not exceed 3 mg/ml when mixed with oxycodone injection, either diluted or undiluted.

The site of the infusion

An appropriate choice of infusion site as indicated in the Appendix will help to minimise site problems. Change the infusion site only when necessary, i.e. if it is painful, or appears to be inflamed or swollen. The frequency of this will vary between patients and depend on the combination of drugs used. Single-agent diamorphine infusions can last for several days, whereas if cyclizine or levomepromazine is used, daily changes may be necessary. The extension set and needle should generally be changed at each re-siting [34].

Should there be persistent problems with irritation at the injection site, consider the following options:

- reducing the concentration of drugs (i.e. larger volume);
- changing the drug or considering an alternative route;
- mixing drugs with 0.9% saline (if compatible);
- using a plastic (Teflon or Vialon) cannula;
- adding hydrocortisone 50–100 mg or dexamethasone 0.5–1 mg to the infusion(if compatible) [9];
- 1500 units of hyaluronidase can be injected into the site before starting the infusion. (It should not be added to the infusion.) This is an enzyme that breaks down connective tissue locally and increases diffusion.

The Boost Button (MS26 Graseby models)

The 'boost button' must not be used for top-up medication or breakthrough analgesia unless there are exceptional circumstances. Each boost advances the plunger 0.23 mm: this will shorten the total infusion time by about 7–8 minutes. The equivalent of a 4-hourly dose of analgesics would require approximately 30 clicks of the button! Furthermore all other drugs present in the infusion will also be given with each bolus.

Obtaining the drugs for the palliative care patient–hospital/hospice/community—seamless care

Although palliative care patients may spend some periods in a hospital or hospice, the majority of patients receive palliative care in the community. It is vital that drugs required for symptom control are easily accessible within the community and that the necessary communication channels exist for responding to changing requirements.

Domiciliary services

Many community pharmacists offer a home delivery service for patients without carers or those who are too frail or unwell to collect medicines from the pharmacy. Some operate prescription collection services or repeat medication services where a pharmacy receives prescriptions directly from a GP surgery. This service must be requested by the patient or carer [35].

Drugs used frequently in palliative care

The range of drugs required to treat palliative symptoms are not always routinely stocked by pharmacies and it has been recognised that in many areas patients and health care workers have experienced difficulties in obtaining medicines easily, resulting in uncontrolled symptoms for the patient and distress for carers. The patient and their carers may need assistance in organisation of supplies so that essential equipment and medications are always available. For example, they may be advised to obtain their prescriptions well before their current stock of medicines runs out. There are now increasing examples of systems operating across the country where identified pharmacies stock an agreed range of medicines for palliative care [36, 37].

Examples of prescription medicines which may not be routinely stocked by community pharmacists are shown in Box 22.2.

The complexity of medicines used in the care of terminally ill patients in the community serves to highlight the importance of careful planning of the discharge of a patient from secondary to primary care,

Box 22.2 Examples of prescription medicines that may not be routinely stocked by community pharmacists

- Large quantities or high dosages of morphine-containing analgesics
- Alternative strong opioids (diamorphine injection, transdermal fentanyl, oxycodone, hydromorphone)
- Midazolam injection
- Levomepromazine injection
- Haloperidol injection
- Metoclopramide injection
- Dexamethasone tablets in high doses and injection
- Hyoscine hydrobromide, butylbromide or glycopyrronium injection
- Diazepam suppositories or rectal liquid

or from hospice to home. Good communication between health care professionals is the key to the smooth operating of such systems. This applies equally when patients are discharged from hospital or specialist palliative care units. Faxing medication details (where a patient has identified a regular community pharmacist) can ensure that supplies of medication are available when required, as the pharmacist is able to anticipate prescriptions and have all drugs to hand [38].

The problem of availability of medication becomes more acute outside normal working hours. This is being addressed in different ways: by making palliative care drugs available at central 'out-of-hours' medical locations, using pre-filled drug bags ('Bearder bags') available at access points such as a deputising agency, or hospice [39] or by using a network of dedicated on-call palliative care community pharmacists such as these provided by Lothian Primary Care NHS Trust [40].

Unwanted medicines

A patient, or his or her representative, may return unwanted medicines, including controlled drugs, to any pharmacist for destruction.

The prescribing and dispensing of controlled drugs

Controlled drugs are subject to the requirements of the Misuse of Drugs Regulations 2001 as amended. The legislation is split into five Schedules. Schedule 1 lists drugs such as LSD, ecstasy-type substances and cannabis, which have virtually no therapeutic use and have the strictest control imposed on them. Schedule 2 drugs include the principal opioids and major stimulants (e.g. amfetamine), while buprenorphine and most barbiturates fall into Schedule 3. Schedule 4 drugs consist mainly of the benzodiazepines. Schedule 5 covers the low dose and dilute preparations of some of the Schedule 2 drugs and has the lowest level of control. Controlled Drugs are distinguished in the *British National Formulary* by the symbol CD (Controlled Drugs). The status of compounds can be checked in the *Medicines, Ethics and Practice Guide* obtained from the RSPGB [35].

The prescription

It is an offence for a doctor to issue an incomplete prescription and it is illegal for a pharmacist to dispense a controlled drug unless all

Box 22.3 Details required for a controlled drug prescription

- The name and address of the patient
- In the case of preparations, the form (i.e. tablets, capsules, mixture etc.) and where appropriate the strength (if there is more than one available) of the preparation
- The total quantity of the preparation, or the number of dosage units, in both words and figures
- The specified dose: for example, the instruction 'one as directed' constitutes a dose but 'as directed' does not indicate the specific dose.

the information required by law is given on the prescription. Failure to comply with the handwriting regulations (see below) will result in inconvenience to the patient and delay in supplying the necessary medicines.

The Misuse of Drugs Regulations 2001, as amended, requires that prescriptions for Schedule 2 and 3 drugs (all strong opioids, barbiturates and temazepam) must be completed in the following manner:

- Prescriptions ordering controlled drugs must be signed and dated by the prescriber and specify the prescriber's address.
- The prescription must always be written in the prescriber's own handwriting in ink or be otherwise indelible and include the details shown in Box 22.3. Examples of prescriptions are given in Figure 22.4. The use of computer-generated forms for repeat prescriptions of controlled drugs is thus generally inappropriate.

EXEMPTIONS TO PRESCRIPTION REQUIREMENTS

Exemptions to the requirement for the prescriber's own handwriting include prescriptions for Schedule 3 drugs temazepam and phenobarbital and controlled drugs in Schedule 4 (anabolic steroids and benzodiazepines). In addition, temazepam prescriptions do not have to contain all the usual controlled drug requirements, such as 'total quantity in words and figures'. For the purpose of prescription writing temazepam can be written up as for any other prescription-only medicine.

Taking controlled drugs abroad

Patients who wish to holiday abroad and who need to take their own supply of Schedule 2 or 3 controlled drugs, such as morphine, with

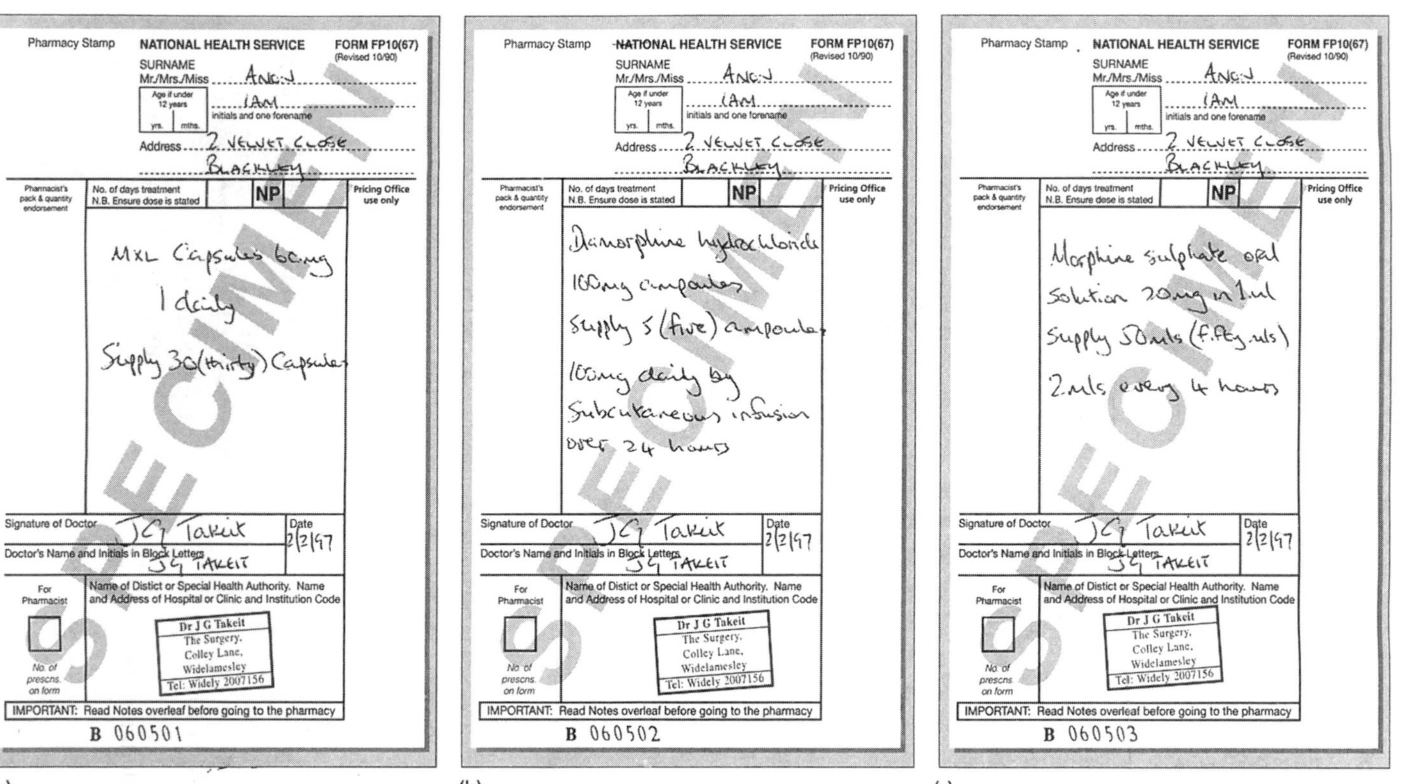

(a)

Pharmacy Stamp NATIONAL HEALTH SERVICE FORM FP10(67) (Revised 10/90)
SURNAME Mr./Mrs./Miss ANON
Age if under 12 years yrs. mths.
IAM initials and one forename
Address 2 VELVET CLOSE BLACKLEY
Pharmacist's pack & quantity endorsement
No. of days treatment N.B. Ensure dose is stated
NP
Pricing Office use only
MXL Capsules 60mg
1 daily
Supply 30(thirty) Capsules
Signature of Doctor JG Takeit
Date 2/2/97
Doctor's Name and Initials in Block Letters JG TAKEIT
For Pharmacist
No. of prescns. on form
Name of Distict or Special Health Authority. Name and Address of Hospital or Clinic and Institution Code
Dr J G Takeit
The Surgery,
Colley Lane,
Widelamesley
Tel: Widely 2007156
IMPORTANT: Read Notes overleaf before going to the pharmacy
B 060501

(b)

Pharmacy Stamp NATIONAL HEALTH SERVICE FORM FP10(67) (Revised 10/90)
SURNAME Mr./Mrs./Miss ANON
Age if under 12 years yrs. mths.
IAM initials and one forename
Address 2 VELVET CLOSE BLACKLEY
Pharmacist's pack & quantity endorsement
No. of days treatment N.B. Ensure dose is stated
NP
Pricing Office use only
Diamorphine hydrochloride
100mg ampoules
Supply 5 (five) ampoules
100mg daily by
Subcutaneous infusion
over 24 hours
Signature of Doctor JG Takeit
Date 2/2/97
Doctor's Name and Initials in Block Letters JG TAKEIT
For Pharmacist
No. of prescns. on form
Name of Distict or Special Health Authority. Name and Address of Hospital or Clinic and Institution Code
Dr J G Takeit
The Surgery,
Colley Lane,
Widelamesley
Tel: Widely 2007156
IMPORTANT: Read Notes overleaf before going to the pharmacy
B 060502

(c)

Pharmacy Stamp NATIONAL HEALTH SERVICE FORM FP10(67) (Revised 10/90)
SURNAME Mr./Mrs./Miss ANON
Age if under 12 years yrs. mths.
IAM initials and one forename
Address 2 VELVET CLOSE BLACKLEY
Pharmacist's pack & quantity endorsement
No. of days treatment N.B. Ensure dose is stated
NP
Pricing Office use only
Morphine sulphate oral
Solution 20mg in 1ml
Supply 50mls (fifty mls)
2mls every 4 hours
Signature of Doctor JG Takeit
Date 2/2/97
Doctor's Name and Initials in Block Letters JG TAKEIT
For Pharmacist
No. of prescns. on form
Name of Distict or Special Health Authority. Name and Address of Hospital or Clinic and Institution Code
Dr J G Takeit
The Surgery,
Colley Lane,
Widelamesley
Tel: Widely 2007156
IMPORTANT: Read Notes overleaf before going to the pharmacy
B 060503

Fig. 22.4 Examples of controlled drug prescriptions.

them may need to seek a licence from the Home Office. Up to 15 days worth of opioids may usually be taken without licence unless the dose of opioids is particularly high (no clear definition of this is available). The patient's prescribing doctor will need to write a letter to the Home Office. The letter will need to include the following information:

- patient's full name and address and date of birth;
- country of destination;
- medication details, including: name, form, strength and total quantity of each controlled drug to be taken out of the UK;
- departure date and return date.

The Home Office will, if the quantity or type of opioid requires it, issue a licence, allowing the patient to take the drug(s) through British customs. They will also issue, if necessary, the telephone number of the destination country's embassy. Ten days should be allowed for processing of the licence. It has no legal status outside the UK and does not ensure safe passage through the customs of the country of destination. The patient will need to contact that country's embassy to clarify the requirements for taking controlled drugs through the customs of the destination country.

Disposal of controlled drugs after a death at home

Controlled drugs can be returned to any pharmacist by a patient's representative for destruction.

Pharmacy and Palliative Care: The future

Technological developments will continue to allow more patient care to be undertaken in the community. For example, the use of ambulatory infusion pumps has led to effective home-based chemotherapy and epidural infusion of analgesia for improved pain control. The RPSGB encourages community pharmacists to become involved with this specialist type of care and recent government directives have identified the importance of the pharmacists' role.Exploratory studies have examined the potential effects of community pharmacists' interventions in palliative care and attempted to benchmark current levels of knowledge in the UK [41, 42].

Clearly there is a need for hospital, community and hospice pharmacists to work together and for all to work closely with the primary health care teams and specialist teams to provide comprehensive care for patients [1].

The pharmaceutical needs of patients with advanced disease demand the development of specialist knowledge amongst pharmacists, particularly community pharmacists. A network of pharmacists with a particular role and expertise in palliative care could improve care for terminally ill patients in the community.

References

1 World Health Organization WHO Expert Committee Report: *Cancer Pain Relief and Palliative Care*. Technical report series 804.Geneva: 1990.
2 Blackshaw CA. An investigation into the current services available for the provisions and use of medicines in the care of terminally ill patients in the community. MSc Thesis, University of Keele, 1995.
3 Gilbar P, Stefanuik K. The role of the pharmacist in palliative care: results of a survey conducted in Australia and Canada. *J Palliat Care*, 2000; 18(4): 287–292.
4 Hepler CD, Strand LM. Opportunities and responsibilities in pharmaceutical care. *Am J Hosp Pharm* 1990; 47: 533–543.
5 Zeppetella G. How do terminally ill patients at home take their medication? *Palliat Med* 1999; 13(6): 469–475.
6 Aslam M. Pharmacists, Medicines and the fast of Ramadan. *Pharm J* 1997; 259: 973–976.
7 The Association for Palliative Medicine and The Pain Society. *The Use of Drugs Beyond Licence in Palliative Care and Pain Management*. 2002.
8 Gilbar PJ. A guide to enteral drug administration in palliative care. *J Pain Symptom Manage* 1999; 17(3): 197–207
9 Twycross R,Wilcock A, Charlesworth S, Dickman A. Palliative Care Formulary 2nd edition. Oxford: Radcliffe Medical Press, 2002.
10 Aronson JK, Hardman M. Patient compliance. *BMJ* 1992; 305: 1009–1011.
11 Mullen D. Compliance becomes concordance. *BMJ* 1997; 314: 691–692.
12 Russell PSB. Analgesia in terminal malignant disease. *BMJ* 1979; 1: 1561.
13 Dickinson RJ, Howard B, Campbell J. The relief of pain by subcutaneous infusion of diamorphine. In: Wilkes E, Lenz J, eds. *Advances in Morphine Therapy*. The 1983 International Symposium on Pain Control. Royal Society of Medicine International Symposium series, no. 64. London: Royal Society of Medicine, 1984: 105–110.
14 Oliver DJ. The use of the syringe driver in terminal care. *Br J Clin Pharmacol* 1985; 20: 515–516.
15 Coyle N, Mauskop A, Maggard J, Foley KM. Continuous subcutaneous infusions of opiates in cancer patients with pain. *Oncol Nurs For* 1986; 13: 53–57.
16 Beswick DT. Use of syringe driver in terminal care. *Pharm J* 1987; 239: 656–658.
17 Burera E, Brenneis C, Michaud M, Chadwick S, MacDonald RN. Continuous subcutaneous infusion of narcotics using a portable disposable device in patients with advanced cancer. *Ca Treat Rep* 1987; 71: 635–637.
18 Bottomley DM, Hanks GW Subcutaneous midazolam infusion in palliative care. *J Pain Symptom Manage* 1990; 5: 2, 59–261.
19 Evans N, Palmer A. Controlling breakthrough pain in palliative care. *Nurs Stand* 1998; 13(7): 53–54.

20 Dickman A, Littlewood C, Varga J. *The Syringe Driver: Continuous Subcutaneous Infusions in Palliative Care*. Oxford: Oxford University Press, 2002.

21 Control of pain in patients with cancer. Edinburgh: Scottish Intercollegiate Guidelines Network, Scottish Cancer Therapy Network; June, 2000.SIGN Guideline 44. www.sign.ac.uk

22 Back I. www.pallmed.net Syringe driver drugmix database, 2001.

23 Johnson I, Patterson S. Drugs used in combination in the syringe driver—a survey of hospice practice. *Palliat Med* 1991; 6: 125–130.

24 Allwood MC. Diamorphine mixed with antiemetic drugs in plastic syringes. *Br J Pharmaceutical Pract* 1984; 6: 88–90.

25 Collins AJ, Abethell JA, Holmes SG, Bain R. Stability of diamorphine hydrochloride with haloperidol in prefilled syringes for subcutaneous infusion. *J Pharm Pharmacol* 1986; 38(Suppl.): 511.

26 Regnard C, Pashley S, Westrope E Anti-emetic/diamorphine compatibility in infusion pumps. *Br J Pharm Pract* 1986; 8: 218–220.

27 Allwood MC. The compatibility of high dose diamorphine with cyclizine or haloperidol in plastic syringes. *Int J Pharm Pract* 1991; 5: 120.

28 Allwood MC. The stability of diamorphine alone and in combination with antiemetics in plastic syringes. *Palliat Med* 1991; 5: 330–333.

29 Allwood MC, Brown PC, Lee M. Stability of injections containing diamorphine and midazolam in plastic syringes. *Int J Pharm Pract* 1994; 3: 57–59.

30 Grassby PF, Hutchings L. Drug combinations in syringe drivers: the compatibility and stability of diamorphine with cyclizine and haloperidol. *Palliat Med* 1997; 11: 217–224.

31 Fawcett JP, Woods DJ, Munasiri B, Becket G. Compatibility of cyclizine lactate and haloperidol lactate. *Am J Hosp Pharm* 1994; 51: 2292.

32 Grassby PF Personal communication 1996.

33 Gardiner PR. Compatibility of an injectable oxycodone formulation with typical diluents, syringes, tubings, infusion bags and drugs for potential co-administration. *Hosp Pharm* 2003; 10: 354–361.

34 Mitten T. Subcutaneous infusions: a review of problems and solutions. *Int J Palliat Nurs* 2001; 7(2): 75–85.

35 The Royal Pharmceutical Society of Great Britain. Medicines, *Ethics & Practice A Guide for Pharmacists*. Oxford: Pharmceutical Press, 2003:27.36. Allen M. What is palliative care? *Pharm J* 1995; 254: 193–194.

36 Chapman M. The community pharmacist's role in terminal care. *Pharm J* 1995; 254: 868–869.

37 Thomas C, Groves K. Two way drug traffic. *Pharm Manage* 2000; 16(4): 50–51.

38 Thomas K. Out-of-hours palliative care in the community. Continuing care for the dying at home.London: Macmillan Cancer Relief, 2001.

39 Pharmaceutical Care Awards 2000. *Pharm J* 2001; 266: 883.

40 Asghar M.N, McManus P. Give terminal care more support. *Pharm Pract* 2000; 10(4): 47–49.

41 Needham DS, Wong IC, Campion PD. Evaluation of the effectiveness of UK community pharmacists' interventions in community palliative care. *Pall Med* 2002; 16: 219–225.

42 Jones VA, Murphy A, Hanks GW. Solubility of diamorphine. *Pharm J* 1985; 235: 426.

43 Walker SE , Lau DWC.Compatibility and stability of hyaluronidase and Hydromorphone. *Can J Hosp Pharm* 1992; 45: 187–192.
44 Bruera E, Fainsinger R, Moore M, et al. Clinical note: local toxicity with subcutaneous methadone. Experience of two centres. *Pain* 1991; 45: 141–143.
45 Fainsinger R, Schoeller T, Bruera E. Methadone in the management of cancer pain: a review. *Pain* 1993; 52: 137–147.
46 Luczak J, Dickenson AH, Kotlinska-Lemieszek A. The role of Ketamine, an NMDA receptor antagonist, in the management of pain. *Prog Palliat Care* 1995; 3: 127–134.
47 Mercadante S. Ketamine in cancer pain: an update. *Palliat Med* 1996; 10: 225–230.
48 Bleasel MD, Peterson GM, Dunne PF. Plasma concentrations of Midazolam during continuous subcutaneous administration in palliative care. *Palliat Med* 1994; 8: 231–236.
49 Fielding H, Kyaterekera N, Skellern G, et al. The compatibility and stability of octreotide acetate in the presence of diamorphine hydrochloride in polypropylene syringes. *Palliat Med* 2000; 14: 205–207.

Further reading

Urie J et al. Pharmaceutical Care (10) Palliative Care. *Pharm J* 2000; 256: 603–614
Bernard SA, Bruera E. Drug interactions in palliative care. *J Clin Oncol* 2000; 18(8): 1780–1799.
British National Formulary. Guidance on prescribing in terminal care (in the first section of the book).
Controlled dosage systems for residential homes. *Pharm J* 1990; 244: 385–386.
David J. A survey of the use of syringe drivers in Marie Curie Centres. *Euro J Cancer Care* 1992; 1: 23–28.
Stewart BJ. *Terminal Care in the Community*. Oxford: Radcliffe Medical Press, 1996.
Trissel LA. *Handbook on Injectable Drugs*, 11th edition. Houston, TX: American Society of Health-System Pharmacists Inc: 2001.

Appendix: Setting up a syringe driver for subcutaneous infusion

The Graseby MS26 syringe driver has been used to illustrate the principles. The manufacturer's leaflet and local Guidelines should always be consulted for any variation.

Equipment

The following equipment should be assembled before setting up a syringe driver: the syringe driver; a battery; a Luer-Lok syringe (usually 10 or 20 ml); an infusion-giving set (choose the smallest volume) with fine-gauge (23 or 25G) butterfly needle or alternative plastic cannula; clear adhesive dressing (Opsite or Tegaderm); medication as prescribed and a suitable diluent, i.e. sterile water for injection; and a syringe driver plus label for attaching to the syringe.

Instructions for the use of Graseby model syringe drivers

Set the rate of delivery. Since the syringe bore varies with different manufacturers what is important is not the volume but the *length* of the infusion fluid.

The rate of delivery is calculated as:

length of infusion volume (e.g. 48 mm)
delivery time (e.g. 1 day)

e.g. with 48 mm of infusion:

The MS 16 model is set at mm/hour (02 mm/hour).
The MS 26 model is set at mm/day (48 mm/day).

- Drugs are drawn up diluted with diluent, usually water, for injection. The syringe is inverted several times to ensure good mixing.
- Opinion is divided regarding whether to prime the line, then measure the length of fluid in the syringe or measure the length of fluid then prime the line in order to set the rate [34]. It is most important that practice is safe and consistent and local policies should be adhered to in order to prevent error. Measuring then priming means that the first infusion will run through slightly earlier, whereas priming then measuring means that slightly less drug will be available for that 24-hour period.
- The loaded syringe is attached and secured to the driver with the neoprene flange and the infusion started by pressing start/boost button. A light will flash every 20–25 seconds.

Note: Driver can only be switched off by removing battery.

- Replace the syringe driver guard. Protect mixture from light by using a holster or carry-case.

Choice of site for the infusion cannula

Suitable sites for placement of the butterfly needle include: the upper chest; outer upper arm; anterior abdomen; and thighs. The exact placement may be influenced by the patient's preference, by the disease process and by common sense. The area over the scapula may be used in confused or disorientated patients.

Take care to avoid the deltoid area in bed-bound patients who require regular turning and sites over bony prominences in cachectic patients. Also avoid broken skin, areas of inflammation, recently irradiated areas, sites of tumour and oedematous/lymphadematous areas.

Care of the Infusion Regular checks

It is essential that the following checks are made regularly throughout the period of use, preferably using a dedicated syringe driver monitoring chart:drug and doses

- for signs of irritation or inflammation at the injection site;
- for evidence of leakage at the various connections;
- that the driver is working (light flashing/intermittent motor noise);
- that the set rate is correct and the corresponding amount of fluid infused
- for signs of crystallization or precipitation (cloudiness);
- that the tubing is not kinked.

23: Complementary Approaches to Palliative Care

ELIZABETH THOMPSON AND
CATHERINE ZOLLMAN

Introduction

The last 25 years have seen a dramatic increase in the use of complementary medicine (CM). Palliative care settings appear to be no exception to this observation. The only published survey of UK hospices in 1992 showed 70% of respondents offering massage and aromatherapy services [1]. Of 55 oncology departments surveyed in England and Wales in 1998, 38 were offering at least one complementary therapy [2]. Of the total number of women with breast cancer in UK in the year 2000, 31.5% had consulted a CM practitioner since their diagnosis [3]. The vast majority of patients and service providers use a combination of complementary approaches and orthodox palliative care, and there are similarities between these two approaches which makes the resulting package of care potentially attractive. This chapter will explore these similarities and show how CM and orthodox palliative medicine might truly 'complement' each other.

Confusion surrounds the term 'complementary medicine' and other terms that are sometimes used interchangeably (Table 23.1). One possible definition of CM is:

> *Areas of medicine that are generally outside current accepted medical thought, scientific knowledge or university teaching* [4].

However it is defined, CM describes a very heterogeneous group of approaches, some of which have features in common, while others have conflicting theories and practice. For the purpose of this chapter, we have not considered psychotherapy, cognitive/behavioural approaches or counselling under our definition of CM.

The appropriateness of CM in holistic palliative care

Palliative care acknowledges that a patient's physical symptoms cannot be fully understood or helped without an appreciation of emotional,

Table 23.1 Assumptions about complementary medicine (CM).

Statement	Comments
Alternative	Implies used instead of orthodox treatment. In fact the majority of CM users appear not to have abandoned orthodox medicine.
Not provided by the NHS	CM is increasingly available on NHS. Of the total number of GP practices in UK, 39% provide access to CM for NHS patients [5].
Unregulated	Osteopaths and chiropractors are now state registered and regulated. Other CM disciplines will probably soon follow.
Natural	Many conventional pharmacological products are derived from natural products e.g. plants and minerals. Conversely CM can involve unnatural practices.
Holistic	As in conventional medicine, there are practitioners who take a holistic approach to their patient and there are those who are more reductionist in outlook.
Unproven	There is a growing body of evidence that supports the claim that certain types of CM are effective in certain clinical conditions.
Irrational—no scientific basis	Basic science research is beginning to give an understanding of the mechanisms of some types of CM (e.g. acupuncture, hypnosis [6, 7])
Harmless	There are reports of rare but serious adverse effects associated with some CM use [8].

psychological and social factors. Likewise, many CM practitioners claim to have a holistic perspective. The central tenets of anthroposophy, a philosophical and therapeutic system developed by Rudolf Steiner, are a good example of this approach (see Box 23.1).

Palliative care and many CM disciplines take an 'individualised' approach, i.e. that what is of greatest importance is not the underlying

Box 23.1 Central tenets of anthroposophy

- Each individual is unique
- Scientific, artistic and spiritual insights may need to be applied together to restore health
- Life has meaning and purpose—the loss of this sense may lead to a deterioration in health
- Illness may provide opportunities for positive change and a new balance in our lives

diagnosis, but how it affects the individual patient and their quality of life. Many CM treatments also contribute to a pleasurable sense of being cared for and thereby improve quality of life.

Existential questions and concerns form a regular feature of work with people with advanced disease. Some CM disciplines include a spiritual dimension and can recognize and address symptoms at this level. Many CM practitioners will explicitly acknowledge potential spiritual concerns. Both palliative and complementary medicine, which are person-centred rather than disease-centred, have strategies that ensure it is never the case that 'there is nothing more to be done'; patients' symptoms can be improved, relationships healed, preparations for death embraced, etc. Realistic hope can sustain people.

As with the best of palliative care nursing, many CM approaches involve practitioners and patients in a degree of physical contact which legitimises touch and human contact.

The benefit of any intervention, particularly in advanced illness must clearly outweigh any harm. Except for some notable exceptions (see later sections) CM approaches have very few harmful effects if used appropriately.

Most palliative care units have a 'low-tech' atmosphere where patients are helped to feel at home. Most CM approaches require a minimum of equipment and can be readily practised by the bedside, at home or in a day care centre. Techniques can even be taught to relatives or patients themselves as well as volunteers and medical and nursing staff.

The above features, common to many CM therapies and to holistic palliative care, have led many cancer patients to seek out CM treatments. They have also led many existing palliative care services to incorporate a range of these approaches. The rest of this chapter will describe some of the CM treatments most commonly used and encountered in these settings, considering the background to each therapy as well as the research evidence, indications and contra-indications for its use. We will then consider some of the problems patients may experience related to their use of CM, and discuss ways in which these can be minimised by appropriate advice and involvement from the palliative care team.

Acupuncture

Acupuncture, the ancient Chinese art of healing using the insertion of fine needles to 'cure' or palliate symptoms, has origins dating back to at least 2500 BC. The *Yellow Emperor's Classic of Internal Medicine* [9] describes, amongst other concepts, an elaborate system of diagnosis based on vital energy, or 'Qi', and meridians, which are a series of invisible lines joining acupuncture points together.

The patient is treated using thin needles inserted in a carefully chosen combination of specific acupuncture points. The needles are left *in situ* or stimulated by hand for up to 20 minutes. In addition, some needles are stimulated using electro-acupuncture equipment, using 'moxibustion' (a technique involving heat and herbs), or given painless stimulation using low-level laser therapy.

Over the last 30 years, solid evidence has accumulated on many of the basic mechanisms of action of acupuncture [6], including stimulation of multiple endogenous opioids, release of serotonin (which can influence mood), autonomic effects, alteration in blood supply and increased production of corticosteroids. However, more basic scientific research is needed.

Many patients feel very relaxed and some feel slightly drowsy after their first acupuncture treatment. Some even feel somewhat euphoric. Patients can be treated lying down or sitting up. They often feel a combination of sensations such as heaviness, numbness, tingling and soreness around the needles, a phenomenon called 'de Qi' (pronounced 'ter chi').

Indications for acupuncture

Acupuncture is used for a wide variety of problems and symptoms, and the WHO has published a list of common conditions helped by acupuncture [10].

PAINFUL CONDITIONS

Painful conditions, such as those affecting muscles and bones, are especially amenable to treatment using acupuncture. Uncontrolled studies in patients with malignancy show that a reduction in consumption and side-effects of conventional analgesics is sometimes possible using acupuncture to treat bone pain, nerve pain and pain due to soft tissue disease [11]. However, pain relief for malignant conditions is generally of shorter duration than for non-malignant conditions and tolerance to the effects of acupuncture may be more of a problem in the former. If disease progression occurs, duration of pain relief can decrease. Acupuncture can also be helpful for syndromes including post-surgical and post-radiotherapy pain syndromes.

BREATHLESSNESS

In a series of 20 patients with disabling, advanced cancer-related breathlessness, use of acupuncture was associated with clinical improvements measured both subjectively and objectively [11].

NAUSEA AND VOMITING

Nausea and vomiting (including chemotherapy-induced symptoms) have been reduced by acupuncture and transcutaneous electrical nerve stimulation (TENS), and these effects appear to be reproducible. A systematic review of acupuncture antiemesis found that 11 out of 12 good-quality, randomised, placebo-controlled trials favoured acupuncture [12].

HOT FLUSHES

Pilot data suggests a benefit using acupuncture for vasomotor symptoms both in prostate cancer and breast cancer [13, 14].

XEROSTOMIA

A recent study evaluated acupuncture-like transcutaneous nerve stimulation in the treatment of radiation-induced xerostomia in head and neck cancer patients treated with radical radiotherapy [15]. Results showed improved whole saliva production and related symptoms that were sustained at 6 months.

Other conditions

Miscellaneous problems such as changes in bowel habit due to radiation, ulcers, bedsores, depression, itch and hiccup may also be helped by acupuncture [11].

SAFETY, ADVERSE EFFECTS AND RECOMMENDED CONTRAINDICATIONS

Generally acupuncture has a low side-effect profile. Acupuncturists should have a thorough knowledge of anatomy and physiology and of the diagnostic process. Deep needling, where needles could cause internal damage, should be avoided. Disposable needles should be used to prevent the risk of infection to patients.

Acupuncture should not be used for patients with significantly impaired clotting. Needles should not be used in a lymphoedematous limb. Patients with an unstable spine should not have treatment over the spine. Patients fitted with pacemakers should not have electro-acupuncture.

DIETARY INTERVENTIONS

Although 'healthy eating' advice is a mainstay of general health promotion and disease prevention strategies, the use of diet as a *treatment* for established disease (other than certain well-defined deficiency or intolerance syndromes) is rare in contemporary Western medicine. Complementary medicine encompasses a wide spectrum of possible dietary interventions (Table 23.2). Cancer patients may use these interventions with a variety of aims in mind (Table 23.3). The link between various dietary factors and development of certain cancers in humans seems well established [16], however the evidence for dietary approaches in the management of established cancer remains less clear. The scope of this chapter precludes a detailed review [17] but the tables below give an idea of the types of intervention, their possible adverse effects and some examples of relevant research findings.

With terminally ill patients, it is particularly important to balance realistic chances of benefit with the likely adverse effects. While most dietary interventions are safe and well-tolerated, complete dietary regimes can be arduous, prolonged and involve an upheaval of daily life. Playing an active part by choosing and maintaining a dietary intervention can be, for some, an important self-help coping strategy.

Healing

Spiritual healing is a process whereby a practitioner focuses intention to produce a change in another living system. Although viewed by many orthodox practitioners as one of the 'fringe' complementary therapies, patients find healing acceptable and helpful with few, if any, side effects. It is not necessary for patients or healers to hold any particular religious or spiritual belief.

Healing is practised under various names (therapeutic touch, non-manual touch therapy, psychic healing, etc.) but can be broadly classified into two differing approaches.

- *Laying on of hands*—Where the healer's hands are placed gently on or near the body of the patient with a 'healing intention'. The process usually takes 15–20 minutes. Patients may experience warmth, tingling or relaxation during or immediately after the procedure. Reiki is a distinct form of healing originating in Japan. It involves the laying

Table 23.2 Types of dietary intervention relevant to palliative care.

Type of intervention	Principles on which intervention is based	Details of intervention	Potential adverse effects of intervention.
Ingestion of nutritional supplements (vitamins, minerals, etc. normally found in the diet): different philosophies.	1 Ingestion at RDA (recommended daily allowances) prevents deficiency due to inadequate dietary consumption, e.g. treatment or disease-related anorexia.	For example, vitamin C, beta carotene, vitamin B complex, CoQ10, selenium, zinc, evening primrose oil and vitamin E.	None
	2 Ingestion at doses higher than RDA used to compensate for increased nutritional need, e.g. during cancer treatment, post-operative.	Supplements often available in liquid or powder preparations.	Evening primrose oil can exacerbate temporal lobe epilepsy.
	3 Ingestion at mega-doses uses supplements as pharmacological agents to treat disease.	Can involve taking more than 18 tablets a day at doses such as 8 mg vitamin C per day.	Tablet fatigue. Megadose vit. C can cause diarrhoea. Hypervitaminosis A occasionally in prolonged use, esp. if liver function deranged. Copper deficiency with prolonged zinc supplementation. High dose folic acid may antagonise methotrexate; very high dose Vitamin C may increase methotrexate toxicity.
Ingestion of nutritional products or extracts	Eating substances are not a normal dietary constituent. (NB much overlap with herbal medicine products).	e.g. laetrile-extract from apricot kernels, shark's cartilage.	Laetrile has considerable toxicity. Most products are expensive and unproven.
Complete dietary regimes	Dietary regimes used as complete treatments for disease, e.g. the metabolic therapy described by Dr Max Gerson in the 1950s; Livingstone-Wheeler regime; macrobiotic diet, etc.	*Gerson*—strict vegetarian diet; salt, alcohol and nicotine excluded; freshly pressed vegetable juices, coffee enemas, potassium supplements and enzymes. *Livingstone-Wheeler*—diet as above plus vaccine prepared from patient's own blood.	Lifestyle disruption: some regimes are time-consuming and arduous. Malnutrition has been described anecdotally in patients with advanced disease on strict anticancer dietary regimes.

Table 23.3 Range of reasons why patients may use dietary interventions and examples of related evidence.

Reasons why patients may try dietary intervention as part of cancer care	Examples of interventions used for this purpose	Examples of relevant research evidence
Improving immune function	IP6	Phytic acid active ingredient of high fibre diet significantly inhibited DMBA- rat mammary cancer in vivo
	MGN 3	Early studies of MGN-3 (rice bran extract) supplementation show enhanced lymphocyte NK cell activity.
Reducing risk of cancer (primary prevention)	Supplementation above RDA	Antioxidantvitamin supplementation shown to reverse pre-cancerous changes, but possibly only in populations where vitamin deficiency is endemic
		Studies showed unexpected increase of lung cancer among men who received beta carotene (20 mg per day) compared with those who did not [18]
Reducing risk of cancer recurrence or spread (secondary prevention).	Change to more healthy eating pattern	Fat intake negatively correlated with disease-free survival in breast cancer
Improved survival	Mega-dose vitamin supplementation	High dose vitamin C trials seem on balance to show no benefit although methodological disputes are ongoing
		Breast cancer-specific survival were not improved for a mega-dose vitamin and mineral supplemented group compared with matched controls [19]
	Nutritional products such as laetrile (apricot kernel extract)	Controlled trials show no benefits
	Complete dietary regimes	Gerson [20]
	Dairy free	Relationship between IGF-1 present in high levels in dairy produce which is known to enhance tumour cell proliferation. Higher circulating levels of IGF-1 have been assoc. with increased risk of prostate cancer [21]

on of hands in a particular routine, which is thought to channelise energy into the patient and increase their own healing energy in a way which is both relaxing and health promoting. There are many accounts of Reiki being beneficial in a palliative care setting [22] but no systematic studies are available.

- *Distance healing*—Where the patient and healer(s) may be physically separated by large distances and where meditation, prayer or other focused intent is used by the healer(s). The patient may not necessarily know that healing is taking place.

Both approaches may involve visualisation techniques such as seeing patients surrounded in light, picturing them fit and well or clearing images of disease from their bodies.

Evidence for the effectiveness of healing

One study in the palliative care setting showed that for 10 patients who had three non-contact Therapeutic Touch sessions the sensation of well-being increased as measured by the Well-Being Scale [23]. Despite the lack of a clear mechanism of action, there is a body of evidence which suggests that healing can have statistically significant effects. Two examples of distance healing are given here. In the first example, 393 patients admitted to a coronary care unit (CCU) were randomly allocated to receive intercessionary prayer (IP) from a group of Christians based outside the hospital, or to receive no distant healing. Patients and assessors were unaware of the treatment allocation. Treatment group patients had significantly fewer complications (cardiac arrest, pneumonia, intubation, requirement for antibiotics or diuretics) during their CCU stay [24].

The second example concerns studies in psychiatric and hospitalised patients. These have demonstrated significant anxiolytic effects of healing when compared to sham or placebo procedures [25].

Adverse effects and safety issues

There are no published reports of adverse reactions to the procedure of healing itself, although there are anecdotal reports of patients stopping necessary medication after seeing faith healers. The Confederation of Healing Organizations (CHO), which represents healers in the UK, has published a Code of Conduct for members which advises them against making diagnoses and giving medical advice.

Provided that practitioners and patients are clear about the limitations of therapy, and there is regular reassessment by medically trained professionals, healing can be considered a very safe therapy. However, sensitivity concerning the religious beliefs and customs of the patient is necessary.

Herbalism

Herbalism, or phytotherapy, is the study and practice of using plant material for medicinal and health promotion purposes. Much of modern pharmacological prescribing has its roots in ancient herbal traditions. However, herbalists hold that isolation and extraction reduces efficacy and increases toxicity. They believe in a wider and more balanced pharmacology of plants, and therefore prefer to use organically grown, whole plant preparations.

For clarity we can divide the topic into its main branches: Chinese herbalism, Western herbalism and specific herbal 'cures'.

Chinese herbalism

Chinese herbalists use a traditional system of diagnosis, observing the pulse and the tongue, to decide on an individual prescription, often containing a number of herbs. They may combine this with acupuncture treatment.

Western herbalism

A Western herbalist takes a case history, exploring physical, psychological and emotional dimensions, that centres on looking for a pattern of disturbance or disease. Individualised prescriptions are determined by key symptoms thought to correspond to dysfunction in certain organs. Herbs are usually administered as tinctures or alcohol-water extracts, but elixirs, pills, ointments, pessaries and suppositories are also used.

Specific herbal 'cures'

Some individual herbal preparations are purported to have anticancer effects or to enhance conventional cancer treatments by reducing toxicity or increasing efficacy. They can be used singly or as part of regimes, such as the Gerson therapy. Some commonly encountered remedies are listed below.

- Iscador, a preparation, of the mistletoe plant, is part of a wider medical approach known as anthroposophy, founded by Rudolf Steiner in 1920.

- 'Juzentaihoto' (JTT), a Chinese herbal preparation is popular in Japan and the USA;
- 'Essiac' (burdock, sheep sorrel, turkey rhubarb and slippery elm bark);
- Astralagus membranaceus or 'huang qi', from the root of the milk vetch plant—claimed to have tonic and immunostimulant properties;
- 'Kombucha'—a mixture of bacteria and yeast grown in birch leaf tea;
- Sutherlandia—a plant from South Africa sold to enhance well being and immune support

Evidence for effectiveness of herbal medicine

Iscador has been shown to have immunostimulatory properties and increase natural killer cell activity [26]. Reduction of radiotherapy induced T-cell suppression has been seen in mice. A retrolective cohort study of women with breast cancer treated post-operatively with mistletoe extract showed that adverse effects of orthodox treatment, quality of life and relapse-free intervals were all improved compared to standard treatment-matched controls [27].

Preliminary research from Japan claims that JTT can improve chemotherapy-associated myelosuppression and quality of life in advanced breast cancer patients [28]. JTT can aid biological recovery from radiation in mice, and has been associated with an increase in natural killer-cell activity in post-operative patients with gastrointestinal cancers [29].

One laboratory-based study of Astralagus membranaceus with interleukin-2 showed a 10-fold potentiation of interleukin activity when the combination was used compared to interleukin used alone [30]. Another study using a distilled fraction of the same herb showed a reversal of cyclophosphamide-induced immunosuppression in rats [31].

A meta-analysis of randomised clinical trials comparing Hypericum (St John's wort) with conventional antidepressants in mild depression showed similar efficacy with considerably lower toxicity for the herbal product [32].

There are no clinical trials that substantiate the claims made for Essiac, Kombucha or Sutherlandia.

Experienced herbalists anecdotally report success in treating nausea in the terminally ill patient when other conventional methods have failed.

Adverse effects

Although an extensive review of herbal safety published in the *Food and Drug Law Journal* in 1992 states that 'there is no substantial evidence that toxic reactions to herbal products are a major source of concern' [33], there have since been a few reports of severe idiosyncratic reactions such as acute hepatitis and irreversible rapidly progressive interstitial renal fibrosis following the ingestion of traditional Chinese herbs [8]. Side-effects of Iscador are similar to those of Interferon, with high fever, headaches and muscle pains; liver pain has been observed in patients with liver metastases.

Given the large number of people using herbal remedies, there are very few reports of serious adverse effects. A recent cross-sectional survey of patients attending the out-patient department at a specialist cancer centre, identified potential risks of herbal products and supplements and issued a health warning in 20 cases (12.2%) [34]. The National Poisons Unit and the University of Exeter are also establishing databases of validated reports of adverse events attributed to herbal products.

Homoeopathy

Homoeopathy from the Geek 'homoeo' similar, plus 'pathos' illness, is based on the 'law of similars'. This is the principle of treating like with like where symptoms of disease are treated with medicines capable of producing similar symptoms when given to healthy individuals. Information about each remedy is built up from proven evidence of the remedy on healthy volunteers or though clinical cases where the outcome has been good.

The homoeopathic method was described in 1790 by the German physician, Samuel Hahnemann who conducted the first proving or trial of a medicine from Chinchona, the Peruvian Bark. During experiments to reduce adverse effects, he discovered that serial dilution made medicines less toxic but paradoxically more active, particularly when dilution was combined with vigorous shaking known as succussion. This process is called 'potentisation' and is considered to increase the therapeutic action of the remedy. The remedies are thought to stimulate a self-healing, self-regulating response within the body.

The homoeopath identifies patterns emerging from a holistic clinical history and matches these with features of known homoeopathic remedies to make an individual prescription. Remedies can be prescribed in tablet or liquid form and are easily administered in the terminal phase without interfering with other medications.

Evidence and indications for homoeopathy

Over 100 controlled clinical trials of homoeopathy have been systematically reviewed [35]. Although many were methodologically poor, over three-quarters of the trials favoured homoeopathy. A meta-analysis of 89 trials in various clinical conditions showed homoeopathy to be consistently superior to placebo [36]. Published work has shown homoeopathy to be useful for a range of symptoms in the diagnosis of cancer in particular fatigue, hot flushes, mood disturbance and chemotherapy-induced stomatitis [37–39]. Case studies suggest that one remedy may not produce any response whereas another, which fits the symptom pattern more closely, may be followed by dramatic improvement in key symptoms as well as non-specific improvements in anxiety and psychological adjustment.

Adverse effects

There are no known toxic effects of homoeopathy. However, patients and homoeopaths describe a number of remedy reactions suggestive of a shift within the self-regulating mechanism thought to orchestrate the body. These include the transient development of new or previous symptoms or a worsening of existing symptoms called a homeopathic aggravation. In a recent audit of 116 patients in routine out-patient practice, a third of the patients described aggravations and new symptoms and 5 patients regarded the aggravation as adverse. These reactions are transient and respond quickly to decreasing the frequency or stopping the remedy.

Pat's story

Pat attended the homoeopathic hospital in September 2000 with recurrent ovarian cancer unresponsive to second-line chemotherapy. She was on a syringe driver containing diamorphine for pain relief, and her kidneys were stented due to obstructed ureteric flow due to the cancer. Over the following few months following treatment with the individualised homoeopathic remedy, Lachesis (Bushmaster snake venom) combined with Iscador,

Continued on p. 450

> *Continued*
>
> Pat was able to come off the syringe driver and a year later the stents were removed and she was well enough for debulking surgery. Three years on, she requires occasional Coproxamol and is still prone to cystitis. These are her words. "Coming to the homeopathic hospital was a turning point for me. The doctor was interested in me as a whole and the way I thought. This was powerful as up till then the doctors only wanted to ask about how the cancer was affecting me. Not only has the homeopathy helped slow the progress of the cancer down but other symptoms such as nightmares and flatulence have been helped. I know the homeopathy has worked combined with excellent conventional care and the support from my health shop."

Massage, aromatherapy and reflexology

The use of touch to relieve discomfort is probably one of the most instinctive and oldest therapies in existence.

Massage, which can be defined as therapeutic soft tissue manipulation, is a component of many traditional systems of medicine. Swedish massage is the form on which most current European techniques are based. Indian Head Massage is a type of head and shoulders massage often given without undressing the client. It is adapted from traditional Indian Ayurvedic practice and may be particularly suited to situations where a full body massage is impractical.

Aromatherapy is massage using essential oils—aromatic plant extracts prepared by distillation—which are said to have different properties (relaxing, invigorating, antiseptic, purifying etc.). A combination of diluted essential oils will be selected to suit the preference and nature of the patient.

Reflexology is a technique whereby the feet are massaged in a way which is claimed to affect the functioning of the organs of the body. Specific areas of the feet (reflex zones) are said to correspond to individual organs, and massaging these areas can either give the therapist diagnostic information or lead to therapeutic change in the corresponding organ.

Massage techniques have been extensively employed in palliative care settings [1] and have been adapted for these circumstances, for example by using gentle massage strokes to avoid overtreating frail patients. Treatments can be given by independent massage therapists but increasingly trained nurses, physiotherapists and occupational therapists are providing massage and aromatherapy. If essential oils are used, they must be diluted with a carrier oil (e.g. sweet almond oil) and can be used singly or in established combinations of 4–5 low-toxicity oils.

Indications and effects of massage therapies

Practitioners using massage in palliative care settings have reported psychological, emotional and physical benefits for patients and staff. The research base is rigorously and extensively reviewed elsewhere [40]. Key points emerging are summarised below.

Psychological effects. A small number of well-conducted randomised controlled trials support the claim that massage is effective in relieving anxiety in institutional settings. Effects on depression are less clear.

Emotional effects. The pampering and pleasure received during a massage can be one of the few positive physical experiences for a patient with advanced disease. In the words of one patient: 'it was done so lovingly and gently. The whole experience has made me feel I was worth caring about' [41]. Practitioners also report an effect of massage in improving the body image of patients who have undergone mutilating surgery.

Massage may lead to emotional release although patients can be nurtured and supported without feeling they have to 'open up' and talk.

Physical effects. Massage is frequently used for pain relief, perhaps alleviating pain through reduction in anxiety and muscle tension, although there are almost no reliable research data on the subject. Lymphoedema is now widely treated by using specialist massage and bandaging techniques.

There are also anecdotal reports describing improvements in sleep patterns, lethargy, fatigue, terminal agitation, and restlessness after massage.

Interpersonal significance. Massage gives staff and relatives a way of spending time and being with the dying patient.

Use among staff. Staff support systems sometimes include massage, and practitioners report that these sessions are used to 'unload' problems. As one member of staff puts it: 'Massage allows me to "take in" so that I can "give out"' [40].

Evidence comparing the different massage therapies

Randomised trials comparing aromatherapy massage with massage using carrier oil alone [41, 42] have provided results which are difficult to interpret owing to a number of methodological flaws. There seems at least to be a suggestion that essential oils may augment the effects of massage in reducing anxiety and some physical symptoms.

Reflexology is one of the most sparsely researched of the complementary disciplines, and claims that it has greater efficacy than a simple foot massage are currently unsubstantiated.

Adverse effects and recommended contraindications

Providing massage is gentle and care is taken in moving and lifting patients; adverse effects are rare. As with other CM disciplines, contraindications reflect established practice rather than documented side-effects. No serious adverse events with aromatherapy have been documented.

Limbs affected by deep-vein thrombosis should not be massaged, and extreme caution should be exercised when massaging close to bone metastases. Skin recovering from radiotherapy should generally be avoided. Patients with abnormal clotting or platelets should be massaged with great care.

The variety and concentration of aromatherapy oils is limited to avoid theoretical risks of overexposure or interaction with concurrent medication. Although vigorous massage close to active tumour sites is generally avoided, there are no known reports of metastatic spread being promoted by massage.

Mind–body techniques: hypnosis, meditation, relaxation and visualisation

Mind–body medicine encompasses a wide range of therapeutic interventions that address psychological and emotional issues with the aim of altering physical symptoms and possibly disease processes.

Techniques encompassed by the term 'mind-body approaches' include counselling, psychotherapy, therapy involving hypnosis, cognitive-behavioural techniques, neurolinguistic programming (NLP), relaxation, yoga, visualization and meditation.

Hypnosis

Hypnotic techniques increase a patient's suggestibility and responsiveness to psychological approaches by using an altered state of consciousness, or 'trance'. Hypnotic techniques can be used to augment any number of psychotherapeutic or psychological techniques, from hypno-analysis to cognitive behavioural techniques. Therapy incorporating hypnosis is only as good as the underlying therapy and therapist. However, a recent meta-analysis of trials comparing identical cognitive-behavioural interventions delivered alone or with hypnosis, showed a substantial enhancement in treatment outcome with adjunctive hypnosis [43]. One hospice reports the use of a retrospective questionnaire to evaluate hypnotherapy in a day care setting. Out of 256 patients who had hypnotherapy 52 surviving patients were set the questionnaire. Forty one patients responded and 61% of these patients reported improved coping.

Meditation

Meditation is a process by which the mind is stilled to facilitate a calm and pleasant experience of the present moment. It may also, but does not necessarily, have a spiritual dimension (Table 23.4).

Visualisation and imagery

Imagined scenes, objects, places or people are used in many mind–body techniques to enable a change in subjective experience. A favourite beach or beautiful garden are popular images.

Most of these techniques can be taught and applied in one-to-one sessions or facilitated groups by therapists or doctors and nurses with appropriate training. Using audio tapes and headphones, patients can practise the technique anywhere, at home or in hospital, and many learn to 'customise' the methods to suit themselves.

Table 23.4 Categories of meditation techniques.

Concentrative meditation
Involves focusing the mind on the breath, an image (real or imagined) or a sound (often repeated). Through this concentration the mind becomes more tranquil and aware.
Mindfulness meditation
Attention is opened to whatever enters the mind without judgement or worries, so that eventually the mind becomes more calm and clear.

Indications and effects of mind–body techniques

Relaxation and visualisation techniques have been used to promote relaxation and a general feeling of well-being whilst undergoing stressful experiences such as chemotherapy or bone marrow aspiration.

Studies have indicated efficacy of mind-body techniques in certain situations. For example, the pain of oral mucositis was much reduced in patients undergoing bone marrow transplantation who had relaxation and imagery training [44]. Pain in patients with advanced cancer was reduced by deep-breathing, progressive muscle relaxation and imagery training [45].

Several studies have demonstrated that anxiety and nausea related to chemotherapy respond well to mind-body approaches, especially in children and adolescents. Anticipatory nausea and vomiting have been helped by hypnosis [46].

Altering the course of the disease

Very few studies have examined the effects of mind–body interventions on the progression of cancer. Results are contradictory and it is too early to draw definite conclusions in this controversial area.

Carl Simonton encouraged cancer patients to use images such as sharks eating cancer cells or armies of soldiers in battle, to enhance immune function and augment the effect of conventional treatment. An uncontrolled study in 225 selected cancer patients reported survival figures 'as much as twice as long' as national averages [47]. However, the study had profound methodological flaws, such as non-representative sample and lack of any staging or prognostic data.

Spiegel and co-workers, while conducting a randomised study of a 12-month psychosocial group intervention to improve quality of life in patients with metastatic breast cancer, found a clinically and statistically significant survival advantage in intervention patients compared with controls [48]. Further work has suggested that it is the application of such psychological interventions that may be the key to improving survival [49].

Adverse effects and contraindications

Providing that any therapist who employs hypnotic techniques has the appropriate training and background experience, mind–body therapies are generally very safe. Therapists need to be aware of the psychological vulnerability of cancer patients and the limited time available for patients with terminal illness to deal with deep trauma or ingrained patterns of behaviour. Realistic goals of therapy need to be agreed and often techniques used symptomatically are more appropriate than an analytic approach.

The World Health Organization (WHO) cautions that hypnosis should not be used in patients with psychosis, organic psychiatric conditions or antisocial personality disorders.

Documented adverse effects of sustained meditation include grand-mal seizures in established epileptics and acute psychosis in individuals with a history of schizophrenia.

Robert was initially diagnosed in March 1996 with adenoid cystic cancer (of the tongue), and in January 1997 scans revealed secondaries on his liver and both lungs. He has recently had a cancer recurrence at the base of his skull, but is pleased that this is currently not growing and the last scan showed no change. He attended the Bristol Cancer Help Centre and describes "a typical day's holistic treatment (mind, body and spirit) included individual sessions with the doctor, counsellor, nutritionist, art therapist and healer and group sessions on guided meditation and relaxation. There was also empowering, informal interaction with other patients . . . I remember saying to my wife that I would always appreciate their complementary therapy for helping me to live with cancer, even if I lived no longer than forecast." With visualisation "my imagination runs riot with a rich mixture of themes including peace, war and humour. The regular hero is my immune system known affectionately as 'Baldrick' because of his indefatigable optimism and cunning plans. I discovered how to graft my wicked sense of humour onto their creative therapies in order to ensure that my cancer cells die laughing. At first the techniques such as meditation and visualisation seemed to be separate, until I quickly discovered how they inter-relate: for example I have powerful visualisations during healing sessions."

Potential problems with CM approaches in palliative care settings

Guilt and responsibility

One of the most important potential adverse effects of CM that has been observed is the generation of guilt. Many CM disciplines support the belief that the way people behave and look after their bodies influences their state of health. They also place great emphasis on the role of self-healing. These two axioms can develop into a two-edged sword. On the one hand they can promote greater independence and self-esteem by reversing the patient's traditional role of sitting back and letting the doctors do the work. On the other hand, they can create a burden of responsibility and guilt in patients who come to believe that they are the cause of their own illness and that the reason they are not getting better is because they are not trying hard enough, eating well enough, or being good enough to people. CM practitioners, particularly those who are unused to working with patients with a terminal disease, must be very aware of these risks.

Increasing denial

CM can be used as a psychological or emotional support in the face of progressing disease or impending death. However, there is a fine line between this and a potential for increasing an unhelpful pattern of denial, which can risk delaying or even preventing appropriate adjustment and acceptance. This is not unique to CM: inappropriate use of conventional oncological treatments may have similar effects.

Masking important symptoms

Use of CM can mask or disguise the development of complications which require urgent conventional medical treatment (e.g. incipient cord compression). It may also mask disease progression for which further conventional symptomatic treatment is superior (e.g. radiotherapy to bony metastases). Regular medical reassessment of all patients with new or persistent symptoms is mandatory.

Antagonism and communication difficulties

There is often an element of faith in some of the principles of CM, and disagreement about the effectiveness of various techniques. It is possible that those who do not share these beliefs (either family members or conventional medical carers) will feel antagonised by a patient's decision to seek CM treatments. This can lead to isolation and fragmentation of care, placing patients in the difficult position of having to choose between conflicting advice.

Financial

The financial implications of CM for both patient and health service purchasers need to be carefully considered. CM treatments are labour intensive but generally cost little in terms of medication or equipment. Cost-effectiveness is not established.

Supervision and responsibility

CM practitioners will often be working outside the conventional management structures of the NHS. Some may be working as volunteers. Job descriptions, limits to practice, review procedures, lines of clinical and management responsibility and codes of conduct all need to be clearly and carefully defined.

Interprofessional issues

Many conventional health care professionals have undergone CM training but other CM practitioners will have trained outside the multiprofessional environment of an NHS hospital. The language they use and the way in which they conduct their practice may therefore be unfamiliar to medical, nursing and other health care professionals. This can lead to misunderstandings and frustration. The presence of CM practitioners at multi-disciplinary team meetings can be problematic initially, but with time, familiarity and mutual respect can develop.

Conclusions

This chapter has begun to explore the similarities between palliative care and complementary approaches, and to examine the relevance of individual complementary therapies to the palliative care setting. As practitioners individualise their patients' care they may be asked about therapies with which they are unfamiliar and inexperienced. Although there is no evidence that any of the complementary approaches can cure cancer, there is much that demonstrates their ability to improve symptoms and quality of life. Discussing the relevance of complementary medicine (CM) in individual cases openly and with an awareness of this evidence can facilitate a profound and therapeutic patient/carer relationship.

By integrating the best of orthodox and complementary care, it may be possible to meet more of the needs of palliative care patients.

However, well designed research is necessary to establish the most appropriate strategy for future developments [50].

Acknowledgements

The authors would like to thank Dr Jacqueline Filshie of the Royal Marsden Hospital, Sutton, for her section on acupuncture, and to acknowledge the contributions and advice of Keith Robertson, Director of Education, Scottish School of Herbal Medicine; they also thank Pat and Robert for consenting to the use of their case histories.

References

1 Wilkes E. *Complementary Therapy in Hospice and Palliative Care*. Sheffield: Trent Palliative Care Centre, 1992.
2 White P. Complementary medicine treatment of cancer a survey of provision. *Complement Ther Med.* 1998; 6: 10–13.
3 Rees R. et al. Prevalence of complementary therapy use by women with breast cancer: a population-based survey. E. *J Cancer* 2000; 36: 1359–1364.
4 Ernst E, Henstschel C. Diagnostic method in complementary medicine. Which craft is witchcraft? *Int J Risk Saf Med* 1995; 7: 55–63.
5 Thomas K, Fall M, Parry G, Nicholl J. *National Survey of Access to Complementary Health Care via General Practice*. Sheffield: Medical Care Research Unit, 1995.
6 Pomeranz B, Stux G, eds. *Scientific Bases of Acupuncture*. Berlin, Heidelberg, New York: Springer Verlag, 1989.
7 Crawford HJ, Gruzelier JH. A midstream view of the neuropsychophysiology of hypnosis: recent research and future directions. In: Fromm E, Nash MR, eds. *Contemporary Hypnosis Research*. New York: Guilford Press, 1992: 227–266.
8 Vanherweghem JL, Depierreux M, Tielemans C et al. Rapidly progressive interstitial renal fibrosis in young women: association with slimming regimen including Chinese herbs. *Lancet* 1993; 341: 387–391.
9 Veith I. *The Yellow Emperor's Classic of Internal Medicine*. Berkeley: University of California Press, 1972.
10 Bannerman R. Acupuncture: the World Health Organisation view. *World Health* 27/28 December 1979: 24–29.
11 Thompson JW, Filshie J. Transcutaneous electrical nerve stimulation (TENS) and acupuncture. In: Doyle D, Hanks G, McDonald N, eds. *The Oxford Textbook of Palliative Medicine*, 2nd edition. Oxford: Oxford University Press, 1997: 421–437.
12 Vickers AJ. Can acupuncture have specific effects on health? A systematic literature review of acupuncture anti-emesis trials. *J Roy Soc Med* 1996; 89: 303–311.
13 Porzio, Giampiero et al. Acupuncture in the treatment of menopause-related symptoms in women taking tamoxifen. Tumori. 2002; 88(2): 128–130.

14 Hammar M et al. Acupuncture treatment of vasomotor symptoms in men with prostatic carcinoma: a pilot study. *J Urol.* 1999; 161(3): 853–856.
15 Blom M. Acupuncture treatment of patients with radiation induced xerostomia. *Eur J Cancer B Oral Oncol* 1996; 32B(3): 182–190.
16 Doll R. *Causes of Cancer.* Oxford: Oxford University Press, 1981.
17 Goodman S. The role of nutrition *Intregrated Cancer Care* Jenny Baraclough edited.
18 Albaneset AL. The effect of Vitamin E and beta-carotene on the incidence of lung cancer and other cancers in male smokers. *New Eng J Med* 1994; 330(15): 1029–1035.
19 Lesperance ML, Olivotto I A, Forde N, et al. Mega-dose vitamins and minerals in the treatment of non-metastatic breast cancer: an historical cohort study. *Breast Cancer Res Treat.* 2002; 76(2): 137–143.
20 Gar Hildenbrand GL, Hildenbrand LC, Bradford K, Cavin SW. Five-year survival rates of melanoma patients treated by diet therapy after the manner of Gerson: a retrospective review. *Alternat Ther Health Med* 1995; 1(4): 29–37.
21 Oliver SE et al. Screen-detected prostate cancer and the insulin-like growth factor axis: results of a population-basedcase-controlstudy. *Int J Cancer.* 2004; 108(6): 887–892.
22 Demmer C, Sauer J. Assessing complementary therapy services in a hospice program. *Am J Hosp Palliat Care.* 2002; 19(5): 306–314.
23 Giasson M, Bouchard L. Effect of therapeutic touch on the well-being of persons with terminal cancer. *J Holist Nurs.* 1998; 16(3): 383–398.
24 Byrd RC. Positive therapeutic effects of intercessory prayer in a coronary care unit population. *South Med J* 1988; 81(7): 826–829.
25 Simington JA, Laing GP. Effects of therapeutic touch on anxiety in the institutionalised elderly. *Clin Nurs Res* 1993; 2(4): 438–450.
26 Hajto T. Immunomodulatory effects of Iscador: A viscum album preparation. *Oncology* 1986; 43 (Suppl. 11): 51–65.
27 Schumacher K et al. Influence of postoperative complementary treatment with lectin-standardized mistletoe extract on breast cancer patients. A controlled epidemiological melticentric retrolective cohort study. *Anticancer Res* 2003; 23: 5081–5088.
28 Adachi I. Role of supporting therapy of Juzentaihoto (JTT) in advanced breast cancer patients. *Jap J Cancer Chemother* 1989; 16(4): 1538–1543.
29 Okamoto T. Clinical effects of Juzendaiho-to on immunologic and fatty metabolic states in post-operative patients with gastrointestinal cancer. *Jap J Cancer Chemother* 1989; 16(4): 1533–1537.
30 Chu DT, Sun Y, Lin JR. A fractionated extract of *Astralagus membranaceus* potentiates lymphokine-activated killer cell cytotoxicity generated by low-dose recombinant interleukin-2. *Chin J Mod Develop Trad Med* 1989; 9(6): 325, 348–349.
31 Chu DT, Sun Y. Lin JR. Immune restoration of local xenogenic graft-vs.-host reaction in cancer patients in vitro and reversal of cyclophosphamide-induced immune suppression in the rat *in vivo* by fractionated membranaceus. *Chin J Mod Develop Trad Med* 1989; (6): 326, 351–354.
32 Linde K, Ramirez G, Mulrow CD, Pauls A, Weidenhammer W Melchart D. St John's wort for depression: an overview and meta-analysis of randomised clinical trials. *BMJ* 1996; 313: 253–258.

33 McCalels RS. Food ingredient safety evaluation. *J Food Drug Law* 1992; 47: 657–665.
34 Werneke U et al Potential health risks of complementary alternative medicines in cancer patients. *Br J Cancer*. 2004; 90(2): 408–413.
35 Kleijnen J, Knipschild P, Ter Riet G. Clinical trials of homoeopathy. *BMJ* 1991; 302: 316–323.
36 Linde K, Clausius N, Ramirez G. Are the clinical effects of homeopathy placebo effects? A meta-analysis of placebo-controlled trials. *Lancet* 1997; 350: 834–343.
37 Thompson E. Reilly D. The homeopathic approach to symptom control in the cancer patient: a prospective observational study. *Palliat Med*. 2002; 16(3): 227–233.
38 Thompson E, Reilly D. The homeopathic approach to the treatment of symptoms of oestrogen withdrawal in breast cancer patients. Aprospective observational study. *Homeopathy*. 2003; 92(3): 131–134.
39 Oberbaum M et al. A randomized, controlled clinical trial of the homeopathic medication TRAUMEEL S in the treatment of chemotherapy-induced stomatitis in children undergoing stem cell transplantation. *Cancer*. 2001 Aug 1; 92(3): 684–690.
40 Vickers A. *Massage and Aromatherapy: A Guide for Health Professionals*. London: Chapman & Hall, 1996.
41 Corner J, Cawley N, Hildebrand S. An evaluation of the use of massage and essential oils on the wellbeing of cancer patients. *Int J Palliat Nurs* 1995; 1(2): 67–73.
42 Wilkinson S. Aromatherapy and massage in palliative care. *Int J Palliat Nurs* 1995; 1 (1): 21–30.
43 Kirsch I, Montgomery G, Saperstein G. Hypnosis as an adjunct to cognitive behavioural psychotherapy: a meta-analysis. *J Consult Clin Psycholol* 1995; 63: 214–220.
44 Syrjala KL, Donaldson GW, Davis MW, Kippes ME, Carr JE. Relaxation and imagery and cognitive-behavioural training reduce pain during cancer treatement: a controlled clinical trial. *Pain* 1995; 63(2): 189–198.
45 Sloman R, Brown P, Aldana E, Chee E. The use of relaxation for the promotion of comfort and pain relief in persons with advanced cancer. *Contemp Nurse* 1994; 3(1): 6–12.
46 Redd WH, Andresen GV, Minagawa RY. Hypnotic control of anticipatory emesis in patients receiving cancer chemotherapy. *J Consult Clin Psychol* 1982; 50: 14–19.
47 Simonton OC, Matthews-Simonton S, Sparkes TE Psychological intervention in the treatment of cancer. *Psychosomatics* 1980; 21(3): 226–233.
48 Spiegel D, Bloom JR, Kraemer HC. Effects of psychosocial treatment on survival in patients with metastatic breast cancer. *Lancet* 1989; 2, 98: 291–293.
49 Cunningham AJ Edmonds CVI Phillips C. A prospective, longitudinal study of the relationship of psychological work to duration of survival in patients with metastatic cancer. *Psychooncology*. 2000; 9(4): 323–339.
50 Ernst E, Filshie J, Hardy J. Evidence-based complementary medicine for palliative cancer care: does it make sense? *Palliat Med*. 2003 Dec; 17(8): 704–707.

Further reading

Lerner M. *Choices in Healing*. Cambridge, MA: MIT Press, 1996.

Vickers A. *Massage and Aromatherapy: A Guide for Health Professionals*. London: Chapman & Hall, 1996.

Defining the Question: Research Issues in Complementary Medicine, Parts I & II. London: Research Council for Complementary Medicine, 1997.

Directory of Complementary Therapy Services in UK Cancer Care Macmillan cancer relief.

Tavares M. National Guidelines for the Use of Complementary Therapies in Supportive and Palliative Care. Foundation of Integrated Health and National Council for Hospice and Specialist Palliative Care.

Resources/Useful Addresses

Palliative care services information

Association for Palliative Medicine of Great Britain and Ireland
11 Westwood Road, Southampton, SO17 1DL
Tel. 02380672888 www.palliative-medicine.org

British Lymphology Society
1, Webbs Court, Buckhurst Ave, SevenOaks, Kent, TN3 1LZ
Tel. 01732 740850 www.lymphoedema.org/bls

Help the Hospices
Hospice House, 34–44 Britannia Street, London WC1X 9JG
Tel. 02075208200 www.helpthehospices.org.uk

Hospice Information Service
St Christopher's Hospice, 51–59 Lawrie Park Road, Sydenham, London SE26 6D2
Tel. 0181 7789252 www.hospiceinformation.info

Hospice Pharmacists' Association
Membership Secretary: Tel. 01727858657 ext. 217
Professional Relations Officer (Mary Allen): Tel. 01442252314

Macmillan Cancer Relief
89 Albert Embankment, London SE1 7UQ.
Helpline 0808 8082020 www.macmillan.org.uk

Marie Curie Cancer Care
89 Albert Embankment, London SE1 7UQ.
Tel. 020 7599 7777 www.mariecurie.org.uk

Mildmay Mission Hospital (AIDS Hospice)
Hackney Road, London E2 7NA
Tel. 0171 7392331 www.mildmay.org.uk

National Council for Hospice and Specialist Palliative Care Services
7th Floor, 1 Great Cumberland Place,
London, W1H 7AL
Tel. 0171 7231639 www.hospice-spc-council.org.uk

Research Council for Complementary Medicine
60 Great Ormond Street, London, WCIN 3JF
Tel. 0171 8338897 www.rccm.org.uk

Scottish Partnership for Palliative Care
1A Cambridge Street, Edinburgh, EH1 2DY
Tel. 0131 229 0538 www.palliativecarescotland.org.uk

Sue Ryder
2nd Floor, 114–118 Southampton Row, London, WC1B 5AA
Tel. 020 7400 0440 www.sueryder.care.org

Patient/carer support groups

Alzheimer's Disease Society
Gordon House, 10 Greencoat Place, London SWIP IPH
Tel. 0171 3060606 www.alzheimers.org.uk

British Liver Trust
Portman House, 44 High Street, Ringwood BH24 1AG
Tel. 01425 463080 www.info@britishlivertrust.org.uk

Cancer Care Society
21 Zetland Road, Redland, Bristol BS6 7AH
Tel. 0117 9427419

Cancer Link (directory of cancer support and self-help)
17 Britannia Street, London WCIX 9JN
Tel. 0171 8332451 www.cancerlink.org

Carers' National Association
20–25 Glasshouse Yard, London ECIA 4JS
Tel. 0171 4908818

'Changing Faces' (support for people with head and neck cancers)
1 & 2 Junction Mews, London W2 IPN
Tel. 0171 7064232 www.changingfaces.co.uk

Cruise Bereavement Care
Mon-Fri 3pm–9pm. Also local branches
0845 7585565

Disabled Living Centre Information Service
Disabled Living Foundation (DLF), 380–384 Harrow Road, London W9 2HU
Tel. 0171 2896111 www.dlc.org.uk www.dlf.org.uk

Haemophilia Society
Chesterfield House, 385 Euston Rd, London NW1 3AU
Free Helpline: 08000186068 www.haemophilia.org.uk

Huntington's Disease Association
108 Battersea High Street, London SW11 3HP
Tel. 0171 2237000 www.hda.org.uk

Lets' Face It (support for people with head and neck cancers)
14 Fallowfield, Yateley, Surrey GU17 7LW
Tel. 0181 9312827 (London office) www.letsfaceit.org

Lymphoedema Support Network
St. Luke's Crypt, Sydney Street, London SW3 6NH
Tel. 02073514480 www.lymphoedema.org/bls

MacFarlane Trust (haemophilia)
PO Box 627, London SW1H 0QH
Tel. 0171 2330342

Motor Neurone Disease Association
David Niven House, 10–15 Notre Dame Mews,
Northampton NN1 2PR
Tel. 01604 250505
MNDA Helpline: Tel. 0345 626262 www.mndassociation.org

Multiple Sclerosis Society
25 Effie Road, Fulham, London SW6 1EE
Tel. 0171 6107171 www.mssociety.org.uk

The Multiple Sclerosis Resource Centre
7 Peartree Business Centre, Peartree Rd Stanway, Colchester, Essex CO3 5JN
Helpline 0800783 0518
Tel. 01206 505444 www.msrc.co.uk

National Association of Citizen's Advice Bureaux
115–123 Pentonville Road, London N1 9LZ
Tel. 0171 8332181 and in local directories www.nacab.org.uk

Parkinson's Disease Society
215 Vauxhall Bridge Road, London SW1V 1EJ
Tel. 0171 9318080 www.parkinsons.org.uk

Groups for AIDS/HIV:

AIDS Ahead (for the deaf)
Unit 17, Macon Court, Herald Drive, Crewe, Cheshire CW1 1EA
Voice: 01270 250736 *or*
Text: 01270 250743

Blackliners (HIV/AIDs ethnic minorities)
Eurolink Centre, 49 Effra Road, London SW2 1BZ
Tel. 0171 7387468

Body Positive (HIV Support)
51B Philbeach Gardens, London SW5 9EB
Tel. 0171 3735237 www.bodypositive.org

HIV-Aids Carers and Family Support Group
Suite 226, Baltic Chambers, 50 Wellington Street, Glasgow G2 6HJ
Tel. 0141 221 8100 www.hiv-aids-carers.org.uk

London Lighthouse (AIDS hospice: information and support)
111–117 Lancaster Road, London W11 1QT
Tel. 0171 7921200

Mainliners (HIV/Drugs/Hepatitis C)
38–40 Kennington Park Road, London SE11 4RS
Tel. 0171 5825434 www.mainliners.org.uk

National AIDS Trust
New City Cloisters, 196 Old Street, London EC1V 9FR
Tel. 020 7814 6767

Naz Project (Asian HIV/AIDS)
Palingswick House, 241 King Street, London W6 9LP
Tel. 0181 7411879 www.naz.org.uk

Positive Partners and Positively Children
The Annexe, Jan Rebane Centre, 12–14 Thornston Street, London SW9 0BL
Tel. 0171 7387333

Terrence Higgins Trust
52–54 Grays Inn Road, London WC1X 8JU
Tel. 0171 8310330 www.tht.org.uk

Children's Palliative Care Services

Association for Children with life threatening or Terminal conditions and their families (ACT)
Orchard House, Orchard Lane, Bristol BS1 5DT
Tel. 0117 922 1556 www.act.org.uk

Association of Children's Hospices
Kings House, 14 Orchard Street, Bristol BS1 5EH
Tel. 0117 905 5082 www.childhospice.org.uk

Cancer and Leukaemia in Childhood
Abbey Wood Business Park, Filton, Bristol BS4 7JU
Tel. 0845 301 0031 www.clic.org.uk

Child Death Helpline (A freephone helpline for anyone affected by the death of a child, operating from Alder Hey and Gt Ormond Street Hospitals)
Tel. 08002829 86 www.childdeathhelpline.org.uk

Children with AIDS Charity
Lion House, 3 Plough Yard, London EC2A 3LP
Tel. 020 7247 91155 www.info@cwac.org

Compassionate Friends (For parents who have had a child die of any age)
53 North Street, Bristol BS3 1EN
Tel. 0117 953 9639 www.compassionatefriends.org

Contact A Family (Provides information and access to specific support groups for families with children with a very wide range of serious conditions)
209–211 City Rd, London EC1V 1JN
Tel. 020 7608 8700
0808 808 3555 www.cafamily.org.uk

Make A Wish Foundation (Aims to grant the favourite wish of children suffering from life-threatening illnesses)
329/331 London Rd, Camberley, Surrey GU15 3HQ
Tel. 01276 24127 www.make-a-wish.org.uk

Sargent Cancer Care for Children (Support, counselling, respite, via work of Sargent Social Workers)
Griffin House, 161 Hammersmith Rd, London W6 8SG
Tel. 020 8752 2800 www.sargent.org

Winston's Wish (Helps bereaved children and young adults rebuild their life after a family death; includes books, guidance, practical support)
Clara Burgess Centre, Bayshill Rd, Cheltenham GL50 3AW
Tel. 01242 515157
0845 2030405 www.winstonswish.org.uk

Childhood Bereavement Network (A national resource for bereaved children, young people and their families)
8 Wakley Street, London EC1V 7QE
Tel. 0117 953 9639 www.ncb.org.uk

Useful Websites

(see also useful addresses for other websites)

UK Organisations

www.doh.gov.uk/cancer/: Department of Health website for cancer

www.doh.gov.uk/pricare/gp-specialinterests/palliativecare.pdf: guidelines for GP's on developing palliative care services as a special interest

www.nof.org.uk: Details New Opportunities Funding in the field of cancer and palliative care within the UK

www.palliative-medicine.org: Association of Palliative Medicine

www.palliativecareglasgow.info: information on palliative care services

www.hospiceathome.org.uk: national forum for hospice @ home

International organisations

www.who.int/cancer/palliative/definition/en/: World Health Organisation Directory

www.eolc-observatory.net/global_analysis/index.htm: International Observatory on End of Life resources

www.hospicecare.com: International Association for Hospice and Palliative Care

www.isncc.org: International Society of Nurses in Cancer Care

Clinical issues

www.pain.com

www.partnersagainstpain.com

www.painconnection.org

www.aromacaring.co.uk/palliative_care.htm: aromatherapy in palliative care

www.breastcancercare.org.uk

www.coloncancer.org.uk

www.nlcfn.org.uk:UK lung cancer forum

www.prostate-cancer.org.uk

www.msif.org: Multiple Sclerosis International Federation

www.hand-in-hand.org.uk: Information on multiple sclerosis for professionals

HIV/AIDS

www.bhiva.org/guidelines.pdf: British HIV Association (BHIVA) www.bhiva.org/chiva/index: children's HIV association for the UK and Ireland

www.doh.gov.uk/eaga: Expert Advisory Group on AIDS (EAGA)

www.doh.gov.uk/chcguid1.htm: Guidance for clinical health care workers: Protection against infection with blood-borne viruses guidance

www.hiv-druginteractions.org/: Liverpool University HIV Pharmacology Group

www.medfash.org.uk: The Medical Foundation for AIDS & Sexual Health

www.unaids.org: United Nations' fight against HIV infection and AIDS

www.hivinsite.com: Information on HIV/AIDS treatment, prevention and policy

Education and Research

www.growthhouse.org: Net guides for cancer and palliative care

www.cancerindex.org: Guide to internet resources for cancer

www.eperc.mcw.edu: End of life/Palliative Education Resource Centre

www.edc.org/lastacts: Innovations in End-of-Life Care

www.mailbase.org.uk/lists/palliative-medicine: Palliative medicine discussion site

www.pallcare.info: Palliative Care Matters- information website for professionals

www.cancerresearchuk.org

www.nelc.org.uk: national electronic library for health

www.palliativedrugs.com: drug information for professionals

www.bereavementarena.com: information on grief and bereavement for professionals

www.jr2.ox.ac.uk/cochrane: cochrane review group on pain, palliative care and supportive care www.pcrs.sghms.ac.uk: palliative care research society

www.isoqol.org: International society for quality of life research

Websites: Patient/carer support

www.hospicenet.org: resource for non-professional carer

www.lastchapters.org: support for patients with life-limited illness

www.roycastle.org: Lung cancer patient support and information network

www.livingwithit: information on lung and breast cancer

www.carersonline.org.uk: carer support

www.carers.org: The Princess Royal Trust for Carers

www.cancerbacup.org.uk: information resource

www.cancerhelp.org.uk: information on specific cancers

www.bereavmentuk.co.uk: online support group for bereaved individuals

www.the-bereavement-register.org.uk: a free service which removes names/addresses of deceased people from mailing lists to reduce distress to bereaved families

www.bbc.co.uk/health/bereavement: information regarding coping

Index